European Respiratory Monograph

# Surgery for Non-Neoplastic Disorders of the Chest: a Clinical Update

Edited by

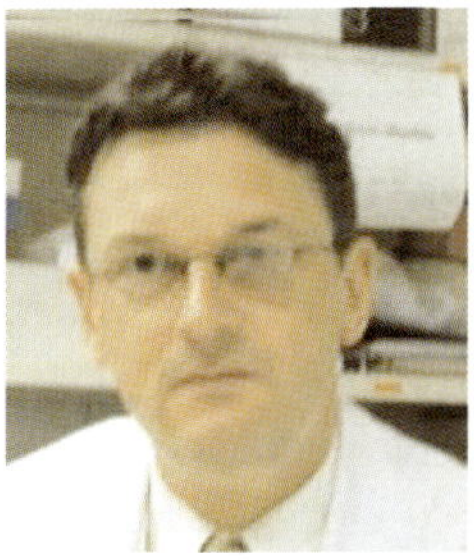

G.M. Verleden

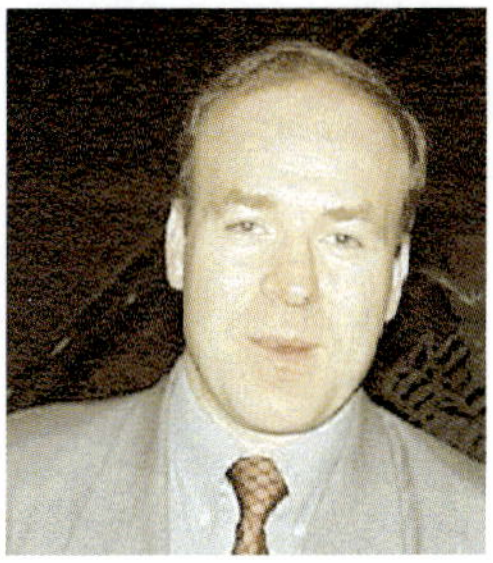

D. Van Raemdonck

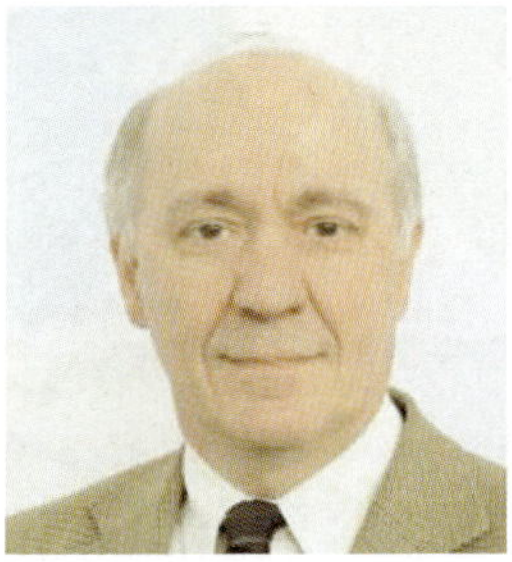

T. Lerut

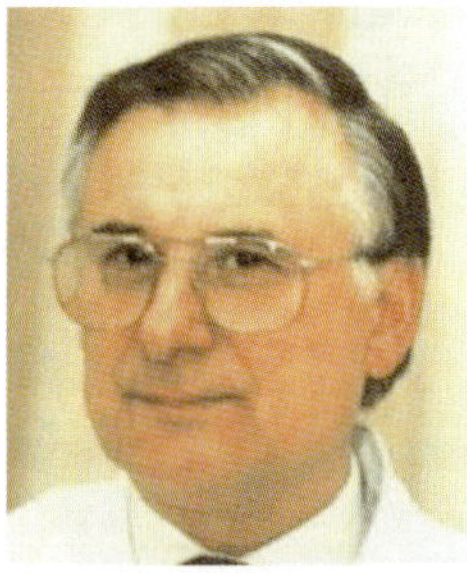

M. Demedts

G.M. Verleden is currently Associate Professor of Pulmonary Medicine at the Catholic University of Leuven and at the University Hospital Gasthuisberg, Leuven, Belgium. He is responsible for the care of asthmatics and is the medical director of the Leuven Lung Transplant programme. His research interests are primarily in the area of inflammation of the airways with particular interest in the role of the airway smooth muscle in asthma and chronic rejection after lung transplantation. The mechanisms underlying symptom perception in asthmatics are also explored in his different experimental set-ups. G.M. Verleden is a member of several international societies, dedicated to respiratory and transplant medicine.

D. Van Raemdonck is Professor of Surgery and Director of the Thoracic Surgery Research Unit in the Center for Experimental Surgery and Anaesthesiology at the Catholic University of Leuven, Belgium. He is Head of Clinic and Surgical Director of the lung transplant programme at the University Hospitals Leuven, Belgium. His research group has published several experimental papers on transplantation of lungs from non-heart-beating donors and clinical papers on lung preservation and *ex vivo* lung reperfusion.

T. Lerut is currently Professor at the Catholic University of Leuven, Belgium and Chief of Thoracic Surgery since 1994. His areas of interests are oesophageal surgery, paediatric thoracic surgery and he started the programme of lung transplantation in 1991. He is member of the Royal Academy of Medicine of Belgium. He is the Chairman of the UEMS European Board of Thoracic and Cardiovascular Surgery. He is author/co-author of over 200 scientific papers in national and international journals.

M. Demedts is currently Professor of Pulmonary Medicine at the Catholic University of Leuven, Belgium, and Chief of Pneumology since 1990. His research interests are primarily in the area of interstitial lung diseases and of respiratory pathophysiology and lung function. He is a member of the Royal Academy of Medicine of Belgium, president of the National Certification Board of Pneumology, and was chairman of the "Colloquium and Forum Vlaamse Longartsen" from 1986–1998. M. Demedts is author/co-author of over 20 books and 400 scientific papers in national and international journals.

**Supported by an unrestricted educational grant from GlaxoSmithKline, Belgium**

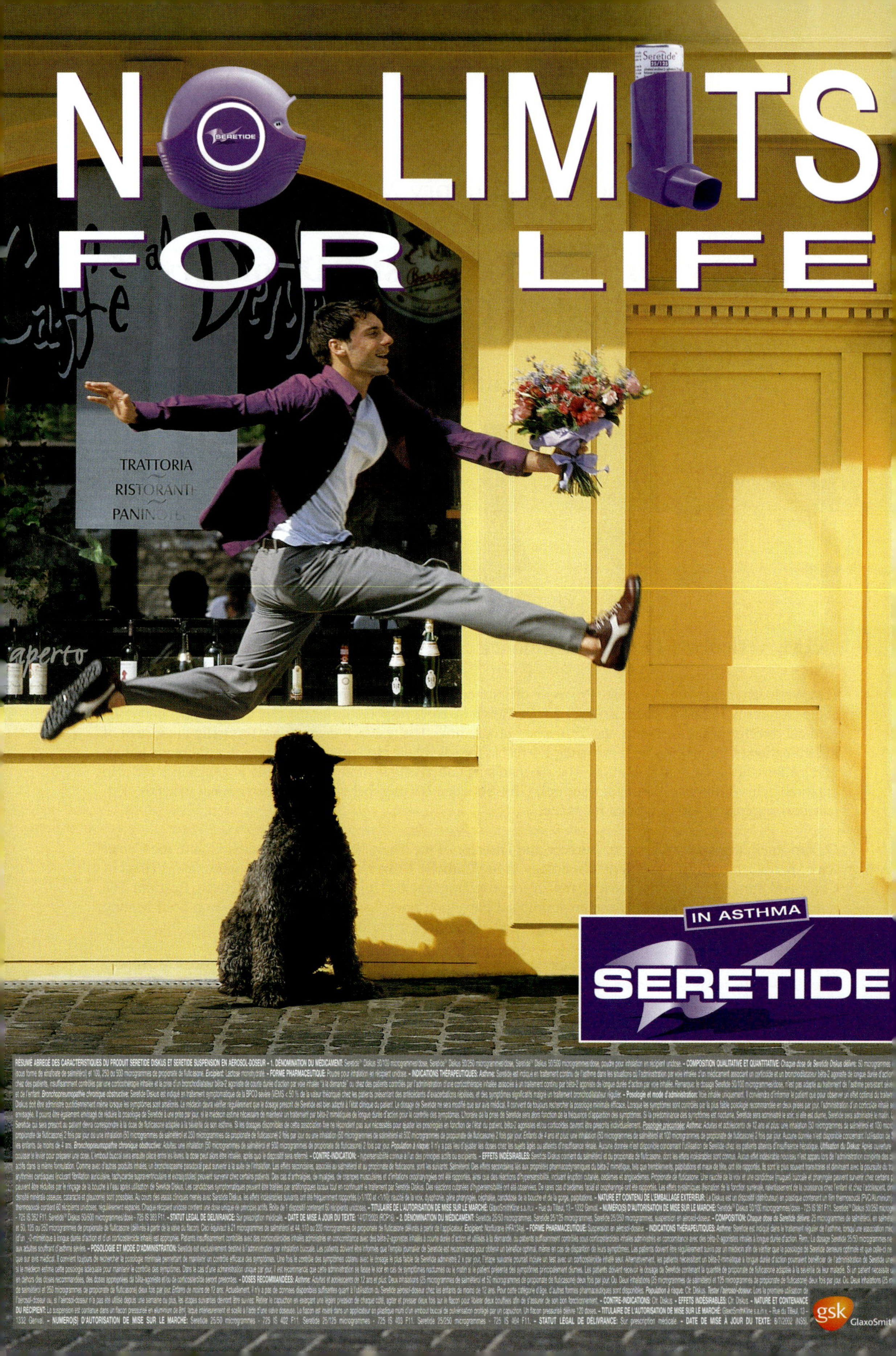
NO LIMITS
FOR LIFE
TRATTORIA
RISTORANTE
IN ASTHMA
SERETIDE
RÉSUMÉ ABRÉGÉ DES CARACTÉRISTIQUES DU PRODUIT SERETIDE DISKUS ET SERETIDE SUSPENSION EN AÉROSOL-DOSEUR
gsk GlaxoSmithKline

The European Respiratory Monograph

Number 29 September 2004

## CONTENTS

# The European Respiratory Monograph

**REVIEWS**

# Preface

Diseases of the chest are numerous and a multidisciplinary approach by the chest physician and thoracic surgeon is often required, not only in the management of chest malignancies, but also in the treatment of non-neoplastic disorders of the chest. Furthermore, many advances and improvements are put forward in the overall management of patients with advanced lung disease; besides lung transplantation, volume reduction surgery is reported as an alternative surgical option for emphysema patients which may delay, or even preclude the need for transplant.

Management of suppurative lung and pleural infections is a challenging problem in clinical practice; classical surgery stands besides thoracoscopic treatment. The frequency of thoracic injuries in trauma victims forms another challenge for the chest physician and thoracic surgeon considering that trauma ranks, at present, only behind cardiovascular disease and cancer. Although disorders of the trachea are relatively uncommon problems that rarely present in routine practice, successful outcomes require judgment in selecting suitable patients and correct timing of surgery, as well as careful determination of the extent of surgery required.

The role of surgery in many of these non-neoplastic disorders is extensively discussed in this issue of the *European Respiratory Monograph*, largely based on discussions and overview reports presented during an international symposium in 2003 organised by the Guest Editors. I, therefore, would like to thank the Guest Editors and the contributors, an international and multidisciplinary group of experienced clinicians, for their generous contributions to this issue of the *European Respiratory Monograph*.

**E.F.M. Wouters**
Editor in Chief

Eur Respir Mon, 2004, 29, a. Printed in UK - all rights reserved. Copyright ERS Journals Ltd 2004; European Respiratory Monograph; ISSN 1025-448x. ISBN 1-904097-33-2.

# *INTRODUCTION*

*G. Verleden, D. Van Raemdonck, T. Lerut, M. Demedts*

The aim of this *European Respiratory Monograph* is to provide a synthesis and update of the indications and results of thoracic surgery for nonmalignant disorders.

Over the last few years, there have indeed been tremendous innovations regarding aspects of thoracic surgery for non-neoplastic disorders of the chest. Especially the field of surgery for emphysema has provided us with a lot of new treatment options, not only lung transplantation, but also lung volume reduction surgery (LVRS) and great efforts have been put into the development of new endoscopic modalities for LVRS. Also the management of suppurative lung and pleural infections has evolved, where classical surgery stands besides the pulmonologist's thoracoscopic treatment. Surgery for congenital bronchopulmonary disorders, extrapulmonary function-improving surgery and the treatment of tracheal and bronchial rupture all deserve renewed attention, because of new insights into their surgical or conservative management.

An international symposium and meeting on "Surgery for non-neoplastic disorders of the chest" was organised by the Dept of Pulmonary Diseases of the University Hospital Gasthuisberg at the Katholieke Universiteit Leuven, Belgium, on 20–22 March, 2003. The purpose was to provide a balanced update of the above mentioned issues, with particular focus on two aspects of lung transplantation: chronic rejection and bronchiolitis obliterans on the one hand, and strategies to prevent and treat reperfusion ischaemia of the donor lung and to decrease organ shortage on the other hand. Some 35 clinical experts and basic researchers in these two fields from all over Europe were gathered for 3 days in Leuven to prepare the present publication. They participated in one of the two working groups (the first on chronic rejection and bronchiolitis obliterans, the second on prevention and treatment of reperfusion and the modalities to decrease the donor organ shortage). Each working group was assigned the task to produce overview reports on these topics. In addition, selected reviews were commissioned on the above mentioned issues.

This symposium was accredited as a "European School of Respiratory Medicine" seminar, and was generously sponsored by GlaxoSmithKline, Belgium, in the framework of the "GSK Chair of Respiratory Pharmacology" attributed to G.M. Verleden.

We are very grateful to E.F.M. Wouters, editor of the *European Respiratory Monograph*, for granting us the privilege of publishing this symposium as a *European Respiratory Monograph*.

*CHAPTER 1*

# Chronic lung allograft rejection: prevalence, pathology, risk factors and pathophysiology

*G.M. Verleden*, J. Egan#, D. Israel-Biet¶, T. Lerut+, J. Lordan§, M. Reynaud-Gaubert[f], G.C. Riise**, L. Sharples##,¶¶, S. Stewart¶¶, B. Vanaudenaerde*, W. van der Bij++, W. Wuyts* and other co-authors of Working Group 1*

**University Hospital Gasthuisberg, Dept of Respiratory Medicine, Lung Transplantation Unit, and +University Hospital Gasthuisberg, Dept Thoracic Surgery, Leuven, Belgium. #The Mater Misericordiae and St Vincents University Hospitals, Advanced Lung Disease and Lung Transplant Program Dublin, Ireland. ¶European Hospital Georges Pompidou, Dept Respir Dis, Paris, and [f] UPRES 3287, University of Medicine, Dept of Respiratory Diseases, Lung Transplant Unit, Marseille, France. §Freeman Hospital, Lung Transplantation Unit, Newcastle upon Tyne, ##MRC Biostatistics Unit, Institute of Public Health and ¶¶Papworth Hospital, Dept of Pathology, Cambridge, UK. **Sahlgrenska University Hospital, Dept Respir Med, Göteborg, Sweden. ¶¶University Hospital Groningen, Lung Transplantation Unit, Groningen, the Netherlands.*

*Correspondence: G.M. Verleden, University Hospital Gasthuisberg, Dept Respir Med, 49 Herestraat, B-3000 Leuven, Belgium.*

Lung and heart-lung transplantation are now an acceptable operative therapy for well selected patients with end-stage heart-lung or lung disease. Although it remains a palliation therapy, these days most of the patients are doing well with, nowadays, a mean actuarial 5-yr survival of 40–50% [1], even increasing to >60–70% for selected indications *e.g.* cystic fibrosis and emphysema in some high volume centres [2, 3]. Although the surgical techniques and the immunosuppressive drug regimen have improved, and new techniques for early detection of chronic rejection have emerged, long-term survival is still hampered by the development of chronic rejection. Indeed bronchiolitis obliterans (BO) or bronchiolitis obliterans syndrome (BOS), the clinical correlate of BO, is now regarded as a manifestation of chronic rejection [4], leading to obliteration and scarring of the terminal bronchioles, and remains the leading cause of morbidity and of late mortality after heart-lung or lung transplant [1].

## The problem of bronchiolitis obliterans or bronchiolitis obliterans syndrome

In a recent review from the University of Stanford by REICHENSPURNER *et al.* [5], the overall prevalence of BO in patients surviving >3 months after transplantation was 64% after heart-lung transplantation and 68% after lung transplantation. The actuarial 1, 3 and 5 yr freedom from BO was 82, 42 and 25% respectively in adults [6] and 76 and 37% after 1 and 3 yrs in children [7]. In the Groningen (the Netherlands) and Leuven (adults only), experience the actuarial freedom from BOS was 55 and 40% respectively after 5 yrs [8, 9]. The incidence is estimated at 12% at 1 yr and >50% at 5 yrs [10].

Chronic rejection after lung transplantation is the single most important factor responsible for late mortality with 40–50% of deaths >3–5 yrs after transplantation occurring due to chronic rejection [1].

Clinically, BO was first described in 1984 in a patient who developed a progressive

Eur Respir Mon, 2004, 29, 1–18. Printed in UK - all rights reserved. Copyright ERS Journals Ltd 2004; European Respiratory Monograph; ISSN 1025-448x. ISBN 1-904097-33-2.

decline in forced expiratory volume in one second (FEV1) after a heart-lung transplantation [11]. Chronic allograft rejection is indeed consistently characterised by a reduction in pulmonary function parameters, most specifically in FEV1, attributed to the airways obstruction. There is no significant reversibility after inhalation of short acting $\beta_2$-agonists. The onset of symptoms is mostly insidious, with progressive exertional dyspnoea, often accompanied by a cough. Sometimes an airways infection seems to have triggered the onset of BO, with quite acute dyspnoea, wheezing and the development of airways obstruction. In the later course of the disease, airways super infections are frequently seen and colonisation with *Pseudomonas aeruginosa* and *Aspergillus fumigatus* is common. At that time, high resolution computed axial tomography scan of the thorax often reveals bronchiectasis and other signs of chronic infection. Auscultation of the lungs is often normal, however, occasional rhales and in later stages, squeaks may be heard. Once established, BO may develop progressively and lead to severe airway obstruction with respiratory insufficiency and death, resulting from an infectious exacerbation. In other patients, the progression may be arrested, either spontaneously or in response to treatment [12, 13]. Sometimes, episodes of progressive loss of lung function are dispersed with stable intervals.

BO or BOS not only represents the most important cause of late mortality, it also causes a significant morbidity, loss of health-related quality of life (HRQOL) and constitutes a tremendous cost, as shown by two recent studies from the Netherlands.

In one study by Van den Berg *et al.* [14] the relationship between HRQOL and BOS was specifically assessed. HRQOL was measured both cross-sectionally and longitudinally by standardised patient self-administered questionnaires, including the Nottingham Health Profile (NHP), the State-trait Anxiety Inventory (STAI), the Zung Self-Rating Depression Scale, and the Index of Well-Being (IWB). Data were collected at 4 and 7 months, and every 6 months afterwards for up to 49 months post lung transplantation. The number of patients who completed the questionnaires varied from 72 at 4 months, to 27 at 49 months after lung transplantation. Cross-sectionally, the patients with BOS reported persistently and significantly more restrictions on the dimensions energy and physical mobility of the NHP compared with patients without BOS. Other domains, *i.e.* pain, sleep, social interaction, and emotional reactions, were not affected. Additionally, patients with BOS reported significantly more depressive symptoms and anxiety 1 and 2 yrs after lung transplantation. Results from the longitudinal analysis support these findings, although no change in depressive symptoms could be found after onset of BOS. While this and previous studies indicate that all lung transplant recipients improve in HRQOL, the development of BOS is associated with a significantly reduced HRQOL [14].

In a parallel follow-up study by Van den Berg *et al.* [15], costs were prospectively investigated in relation to the development of BOS. First, average follow-up costs per week and per patient were compared with patients who did or did not develop BOS. Secondly, in the BOS group, these costs were compared before and after the onset of BOS.

Data on 53 patients (37 patients without and 16 with BOS) were available. The average follow-up time of these 53 patients was 1.5 yrs. The follow-up costs amounted to an average of €806 per week for non-BOS patients, compared with €1,396 per week for BOS patients (+73%; p=0.002). This difference in costs was largely accounted for by an increase in used health-care resources, in particular hospitalisation and medication. For the BOS patients, the average costs per week before and after the onset of BOS were €1,288 and €1,502, respectively [15].

Such studies clearly demonstrate that BOS is not only associated with a significant loss of HRQOL but also with substantial extra costs, which further emphasises the need to focus efforts on prevention of BOS to enhance the cost-effectiveness of lung transplantation.

## Pathology of chronic rejection

BOS is a term used to describe the graft deterioration secondary to persistent airflow obstruction in lung transplant recipients [4]. The current consensus is that chronic rejection causes, or at least significantly contributes, to this functional deterioration and that the associated pathological lesion is that of BO [16]. BOS is defined clinically and functionally and does not necessarily require histological confirmation [17]. Indeed, the patchy nature of BO particularly in its early stages, means that transbronchial biopsy often has a poor yield in this diagnosis. This yield is increased by the use of serial sections and connective tissue stains together with the experience of the reading histopathologist in identifying subtle early changes and some helpful surrogate markers. Transbronchial biopsies and less frequently thoracoscopic or open lung biopsies can also be useful in the clinical setting of BOS in confirming or excluding alternative or concomitant diagnoses, particularly where these are amenable to treatment [18].

Bronchiolitis obliterans is essentially a scarring process affecting the small noncartilage containing airways of the lung graft [16]. The 2001 BOS recommendations state that the pathological term BO should only be used when histology demonstrated dense fibrous scar tissue affecting the small airways [19]. The presence of a lymphocytic submucosal infiltrate or intraluminal granulation tissue is insufficient for a diagnosis of BO. Furthermore, the obliterative lesion can be defined as active when it is associated with the mononuclear cell infiltrate and inactive when inflammatory cells are absent [16]. Histologically, the small airway fibrosis involves both membranous and respiratory bronchioles and can be eccentric or concentric in distribution, thereby reducing the bronchiolar lumen [20]. The initial pathological process appears to be lymphocytic infiltration of the submucosa of the airways and epithelium which is known as lymphocytic bronchiolitis [16, 21]. This can be graded according to severity in an exactly analogous form to the grading of perivascular infiltrates in acute lung rejection.

Lymphocytic bronchiolitis by definition does not show fibrotic changes in the airway, a feature required for the diagnosis of BO. However, refractory airflow obstruction has been described in association with isolated lymphocytic bronchiolitis/bronchitis in lung allografts and it is likely that it can represent the progenitor lesion [22]. Epithelial damage is common in both lymphocytic bronchiolitis and BO with epithelial cell necrosis leading to denudation and umistakable ulceration of the mucosa. The ensuing inflammatory reaction involving fibroblasts and myofibroblast migration into the lumen leads to the formation of intraluminal granulation tissue, often polypoid which can result in subtotal or total obliteration of the small airway. This granulation tissue may organise further with the formation of an eccentric or concentric fibrous plaques in the wall of the airway with varying degrees of occlusion. It is possible that some intraluminal granulation tissue resolves, rather than heals, and that subsequent obliteration of inflamed airways is not necessarily inevitable. Within a given biopsy, or even airway, a spectrum of activity of BO can be seen ranging from intraluminal granulation tissue polyps to occlusive granulation tissue, and eccentric or concentric acellular hyaline plaques.

It has been assumed by some pathologists that active inflammatory and fibroblastic phase of BO precedes the acellular hyaline plaques of inactive disease [23]. However, diffuse or focal plaque-like thickening beneath an intact epithelial surface can be seen in BO which in its earliest form overlaps with the well described basement membrane thickening seen in bronchial asthma. This subepithelial acellular plaque-like pattern of disease can also be associated with squamous metaplasia and attenuation of the overlying epithelium or indeed acute and chronic inflammation of the epithelium and related mucosa. Both the acellular plaque-like and cellular granulation tissue lesions of BO can involve the muscle and adventitial layers of the bronchiolar walls resulting in total destruction. This scarring can extend into the interstitium but is usually easily distinguished from intra-alveolar granulation tissue of organising pneumonia which is a common accompaniment due to associated infections or aspiration. The earliest plaque-like subepithelial fibrosis can be easily overlooked in biopsy material and can equally be easily over interpreted in tangential cuts. The assessment of adequate numbers of bronchioles in serial sections with connective tissue stains is essential to ensure accurate diagnosis. In some patients, most easily seen in open lung biopsy or autopsy material, the acellular plaque-like concentric fibrosis can have superimposed occlusive granulation tissue within the lumen. This may imply a "two hit" process. Certainly more work needs to be done on the relationship between the intraluminal fibromyxoid and fibrotic scarring and submucosal hyaline plaque cicatrisation which may have differing risk factors and time courses.

The obliteration of small airways leads to distal mucostasis with easily identified foamy intra-alveolar macrophages [24]. The presence of such macrophages in biopsy material should raise the possibility of BO in the appropriate clinical BOS setting and as such is a useful surrogate feature. These characteristic macrophages may be more difficult to identify if there is concomitant infection with abundant polymorphs or eosinophils. Other features that may also be seen in association with BO of any stage include: acute rejection with perivascular infiltration; lymphocytic bronchiolitis/bronchitis; infection by common or opportunistic organisms; and organising pneumonia. The distinction between the intraluminal granulation tissue of organising pneumonia involving bronchioles from the intrabronchiolar process of BO can be particularly difficult on biopsy material and may prove impossible [25–27]. Good clinicopathological correlation with radiological input will generally be helpful in this situation but it should also be noted that patients with organising pneumonia on biopsy, particularly if recurrent or persistent, have a higher incidence of BO [28]. Organising pneumonia with or without BO can be seen in cases of aspiration which is a recognised cause of both these pathologies [29]. Although giant cells can occasionally be seen incorporated in the lesions of BO, aspirated foreign material is rarely seen.

The histopathology of BO is now well described in both the immunosuppressed and nonimmunosuppressed settings [30]. Interest in the morphology of the airway has been rekindled by studies of the bronchiolar microvasculature in asthma and other chronic inflammatory lung diseases and indeed vessels have been seen as possible targets for treatment [31–33]. As noted later, in the nonimmunological risk factors section of this paper, it had been suggested that bronchial artery revascularisation could reduce the incidence or postpone the development of BO [34, 35]. This has not been confirmed and it would appear that even in patients free from BO the microvascular density of the small airways is reduced compared with the controls [36]. This reduction includes blood vessels in excess of 0.2 mm in circumference. Partially obliterated airways show similar features to controls, indicating that during the lifespan of the lung allograft there is damage to the microcirculation of the small airways which may modify the response of the airway to immunological and infectious insults. An angiogenic response to this ischaemia is seen with increased numbers of small vessels present in the totally obliterated bronchioles compared with the patent and partially obstructed ones. Interpretation of these findings is confounded by the similarity of pathological changes seen in large airways in BOS at autopsy. These can include the same obliterative features *i.e.* BO with submucosal and intraluminal fibrosis, both cellular and acellular [37, 38]. Whether or not these changes are due to the same risk factors as those of small airways is unclear. Again repeated acute rejection is a probable cause with lymphocytic bronchitis and its accompanying vascular damage to the airway small vessels leading to local ischaemia. It is therefore important to extend these morphological studies of a hitherto rather overlooked aspect of small airway pathology and correlate these with functional and immunological studies.

# Staging of bronchiolitis obliterans syndrome

BO is the histological manifestation of graft failure following lung transplantation and, as previously mentioned, it is difficult to diagnose with transbronchial biopsies As a consequence, in 1993 a clinical classification for graft failure was introduced and the term BOS was introduced [4] (table 1). The application of the term "syndrome" to the clinical disease characterised histologically as BO was an important step forward, because it emphasised the heterogeneous presentation and variable natural history of graft failure. The aim of the clinical classification was to standardise nomenclature, facilitate the description of the natural history of graft failure, to enhance accurate recording of outcome following transplantation and to measure the impact of therapeutic interventions. Importantly, for the first time, it specifically emphasised that a histological diagnosis was not required to make a diagnosis of graft failure. This classification was very successful, but as expected with increasing utilisation, potential areas for improvement emerged. In particular, when the classification was applied, the diagnosis of BOS was commonly made retrospectively. This was believed to be the result of changes in $FEV_1$ being insensitive, relative to early changes in small airways function [39]. An additional problem is that $FEV_1$ is nonspecific for the diagnosis of BO/BOS and the diagnosis is made retrospectively because of the necessity to wait at least one month to see whether there is a return to baseline.

As a consequence, the European Respiratory Society, in partnership with the International Society for Heart and Lung Transplantation (ISHLT) proposed a revision of the classification [19]. The aim was firstly to increase the sensitivity of physiological change for the diagnosis of BOS; and secondly to highlight emerging surrogates for the diagnosis of BO including high resolution computed tomography scan, exhaled nitric oxide (NO) and bronchoalveolar lavage (BAL). The key change was the introduction of a new subcategory referred to as potential BOS stage (BOS 0-p; table 2).

This updated classification builds upon the existing classification of BOS. However, a significant number of factors can confound the diagnosis of BOS especially in single-lung transplant recipients [40]. Therefore it remains to be seen, whether BOS 0-p achieves sufficiently high positive and negative predictive values for the diagnosis of BOS 1 [41]. If this subclassification does not allow pre-emptive therapy for BO it may at least facilitate the introduction of nonphysiological based major and minor criteria for the diagnosis of BOS.

# Risk factors for chronic rejection

BO affects all lung transplant recipients irrespective of age, sex, race, type of lung transplantation procedure and underlying diagnosis. Several risk factors for the development

**Table 1. – Bronchiolitis obliterans syndrome (BOS) stages, based on the percentage of the best postoperative forced expiratory volume in once second ($FEV_1$)**

| BOS stage | $FEV_1$ % of baseline |
|---|---|
| 0 | $\geq 80$ |
| 1 | 66–79 |
| 2 | 51–65 |
| 3 | <50 |

The best postoperative $FEV_1$ is defined as the average of two postoperative best $FEV_1$ measurements, 3–6 weeks apart; Table adapted from [4].

**Table 2. – The new bronchiolitis obliterans syndrome (BOS) classification**

| BOS stage | $FEV_1$ % of baseline# | $FEF_{25-75\%}$ % of baseline# |
|---|---|---|
| 0 | >90 | ≥75 |
| Potential BOS | 81–90 | <75 |
| 1 | 66–80 | |
| 2 | 51–65 | |
| 3 | <50 | |

$FEV_1$: forced expiratory volume in once second; $FEF_{25-75\%}$: forced expiratory flow rate between 25% and 75% of expired volume; #: based on the best postoperative $FEV_1$/ $FEF_{25-75\%}$ which is defined as the average of two postoperative best $FEV_1$/$FEF_{25-75\%}$ measurements, 3–6 weeks apart. Table adapted from [19].

of BO/BOS have been identified, of which late or recurrent/refractory acute rejection and lymphocytic bronchitis/bronchiolitis were the most convincing [42]. Noncompliance with the immunosuppressive medication, human leukocyte antigen (HLA) mismatches at the A locus, total human leukocyte antigen mismatches, cytomegalovirus (CMV) pneumonitis [43] and ischaemia-reperfusion [44] were commonly proposed factors, although evidence for these factors was inconsistent. Other possible factors included: early nonspecific bronchial hyperresponsiveness [45], donor and recipient age; graft ischaemic time, transplantation for primary pulmonary hypertension [46], gastroesophageal reflux [29], and bacterial/fungal/non-CMV viral infection (see chapter three by WARD *et al.* [47] in this Monograph).

Risk factors are generally divided into immunological and nonimmunological factors as follows.

## *Immunological risk factor*

***Acute rejection and lymphocytic bronchitis/bronchiolitis.*** The single most important clinical risk factor for BO is acute rejection, defined as a perivascular infiltration of activated lymphocytes into the graft, but in lung transplant patients was often diagnosed clinically. Acute rejection has been demonstrated in animal models [48]. In addition, from 14 transplant centres that investigated this relationship, 12 reported a significant association with acute rejection. For two of these studies, the effect was only evident for later episodes [43, 44]. Further evidence of the role of acute rejection was provided by an association between BO/BOS and decreased immunosuppression [49]. Nonetheless, there are some patients who develop BO/BOS without having experienced any (documented or treated) acute rejection episodes, which may indicate that it may not be the only factor involved. Conversely, severe or unresponsive acute rejection may directly lead to chronic rejection without a long time interval between them.

Nonfibrosing lymphocytic inflammation of the airways (lymphocytic bronchitis/bronchiolitis) is frequently seen in bronchial biopsies of lung transplant recipients and is now thought to be a manifestation of acute rejection [49], although there are difficulties in attributing histological appearances of lymphocytic bronchitis/bronchiolitis to acute rejection due to the frequent coexistence of infection and the variable presence of bronchioles, if any, in transbronchial biopsy samples [50].

***Human leukocyte antigen mismatches.*** The association between mismatches at specific loci of the major histocompatibility complex (MHC) is not clear. In the largest published series up to date, comprising of some 3,549 lung transplants, no significant association could be found between HLA mismatching and the development of BO. There was, however, an association between mismatching at the HLA-A locus and acute rejection episodes [51].

In studies from individual centres in Pittsburgh (USA) an association between BO was reported and fewer mismatches, which was marginally significant [44]; other centres found an association between BOS onset and mismatches at the A locus [43, 52], or with two DR mismatches [53], or with total mismatches at the A-, B- and DR- loci [43, 50, 54]. In general, studies that have demonstrated the detrimental effects of HLA mismatches have been based on large registries. Single centre studies have limited power due to both the small absolute effect of mismatching and to the lack of prospective tissue matching, resulting in few beneficial transplants.

### *Nonimmunological risk factors*

***Cytomegalovirus infection and other infections.*** Infections are increasingly recognised as a potential risk factor for the development of BO/BOS. CMV infection, pneumonitis and serology mismatching have all been implicated in earlier onset BOS and some studies have shown the introduction of Gancyclovir prophylaxis to be protective. In addition, a small number of centres have implicated bacterial, fungal or community respiratory virus infections and a relationship between the presence of organising pneumonia on transbronchial biopsy and BO. The effect of CMV and other infections on the occurrence of chronic rejection or allograft dysfunction is extensively discussed in the paper by WARD *et al.* [47].

### *Airway ischaemia*

In earlier reports it was suggested that bronchial arterial revascularisation might reduce the incidence [34, 35] or postpone the development of BO [55]. However, this has recently not been substantiated. Indeed, from 11 patients who underwent successful bronchial artery revascularisation, four patients developed BOS. Therefore, the actuarial freedom from BOS was 65 and 50% at 1 and 2 yrs after transplantation respectively [56].

***Other risk factors.*** Younger age at transplantation [57], transplantation for primary pulmonary hypertension [46] and single-lung transplantation [54] have all been associated with BOS or BO.

Donor age, ischaemic time and their interaction was significantly related to BO/BOS in an ISHLT registry report of >5,000 transplants [58]. One study of 500 lung transplant recipients showed increased incidence of BOS in patients with organs from donors with traumatic brain injury death [59] but this needs confirmation. However, despite extensive studies, recipient and donor characteristics such as age, sex, blood group matching, procurement time and ischaemic time were not associated with BO/BOS in any study.

It has been suggested that gastro-oesophageal reflux, as well as reperfusion injury, may pre-dispose to allograft dysfunction [29, 60]. Other studies did not find an association with ischaemia reperfusion injury [61, 62].

## Pathophysiology of bronchiolitis obliterans

In recent years, much effort has been undertaken to unravel the pathophysiological events that initiate and perpetuate the inflammation and scarring of the airways, leading to BO. Several cells (inflammatory as well as structural airway cells), growth factors and cytokines have been implicated in this process.

## *Inflammatory cells*

***Polymorphonuclear neutrophils.*** In the last years, several studies have reported an association between high percentages of polymorphonuclear neutrophils (PMN) in BAL and diagnosis of BO/BOS after lung transplantation [63–66]. DiGiovine *et al.* [63] found BAL neutrophilia to be correlated to increased BAL levels of interleukin (IL)-8, and immunostaining of transbronchial biopsies (TBB) located the IL-8 positivity to the peribronchial region. Chemotactic experiments showed the molecule to be bioactive and capable of attracting neutrophils.

In a cross-sectional study, Riise *et al.* [64] found increased levels of both IL-8 and myeloperoxidase (MPO) in BAL from patients with BOS. Immunohistochemical positivity for MPO was present in the bronchial walls of TBB from BOS patients, but not in matching lung transplanted controls. MPO is an oxidative enzyme released from the azurophilic granules of activated PMN and involved in the production of hypochloric acid, a potent oxidant. Together with low levels of antioxidant markers (vitamins C and E, urate and glutathione: GSH) in BAL fluid in patients with BOS the results made the authors speculate that excess amounts of neutrophil derived proteases could lead to increased oxidative stress and thus contribute to BOS.

More recently, Zheng *et al.* [66] found a positive immunostaining for neutrophil elastase to be largely confined to the airway walls, and not the lung parenchyma, and in the patients with BOS the airway wall neutrophilia correlated with BAL IL-8 levels. Interestingly, BAL neutrophilia and increased levels of IL-8 were also found to be a feature of stable lung transplant recipients without any sign of BOS. Others have confirmed that within the first postoperative month, significantly increased levels of PMN and IL-8 in BAL could be found in patients who later develop BOS [67].

Riise *et al.* [65] investigated the longitudinal pattern of these markers prospectively over a 2-yr period, and found that persistent BAL neutrophilia and signs of neutrophil activation were, indeed, a feature of BOS. BAL fluid levels of both MPO, IL-8 and PMN became significantly elevated over time, and especially for MPO this increase preceded the clinical diagnosis of BOS by several months.

In this context it is interesting to also include recent results from Fisher *et al.* [68] who reported that high concentrations of IL-8 in the donor airways were associated with early graft dysfunction and bad prognosis after lung transplantation. They hypothesised that severe brain injury in the potential donor could set off cytokine activation in the allograft, and hence export a subclinical airway inflammation to the recipient. Early secretion of IL-8 in the allograft would then predispose for later development of BOS.

***Lymphocytes.*** Since a lymphocytic bronchitis/bronchiolitis may be considered as an early manifestation of BO [22], it is apparent that lymphocytes may play a role in the development of BO. Even in stable lung transplant recipients, a significantly increased number of CD8+ cells were found in endobronchial biopsies compared to nontransplanted control subjects [69].

In a mouse model of BO, an increased expression of T-helper cell type I (Th1) and Th2 cytokines was detected in allografts compared with isografts, suggesting that Th1 and Th2 cytotoxic T-cells contribute to the development of BO [70]. It is indeed postulated that macrophage and T-cell activation plays a critical role in the initiation of the delayed-type hypersensitivity reaction leading to cytokine and growth factor production, culminating in epithelial damage, smooth muscle cell proliferation and gradual occlusion of the lumen, characteristic of BO [71]. It has recently also been published that blocking the CD28/B7-2 stimulatory pathway and consequently inhibiting T-cell activation, inhibits the development of BO in rats [71], which again points to the important role of lymphocytes.

***Macrophages/dendritic cells.*** Antigen presentation by lung macrophages/dentric cells (DC) is thought to be important in BO. YOUSEM *et al.* [72] were the first to acknowledge their potential role in chronic rejection, when they showed increased DC in chronically rejecting lung allografts [72]. This was later confirmed in a study by LEONARD *et al.* [73] showing increased numbers of DCs in endobronchial and transbronchial biopsies using specific monoclonal markers such as Class II MHC expression, and DC morphology. Furthermore, a proportion of these DCs expressed co-stimulatory proteins (CD86 and CD80), and were thus capable of activating T-cells [73].

In a mouse airway model of BO, there was an abundant increase in macrophages within 2 weeks after tracheal allograft transplantation, with macrophages predominating after 6–10 weeks [74].

### *Structural airway cells*

***Airway epithelium.*** The airway epithelium seems to play a pivotal role in the initial inflammatory events that lead to BO. It has indeed been demonstrated that the bronchial epithelium is capable of eliciting an allergenic immune response and expresses a number of growth factors, known to stimulate smooth muscle cell migration and proliferation [75]. In epithelial cells, cyclosporine A is also able to induce the production of pro-inflammatory cytokines (IL-6 and IL-8), the latter of which is known to specifically attract neutrophils. Mycophenolate mofetil and tacrolimus also upregulated the expression and production of IL-8, although to a lesser extent, than cyclosporine A [76].

NO has already been implicated in the pathophysiology of graft rejection [77], which may correlate with a strong expression of inducible nitric oxide synthase (iNOS) that has been found in the airway epithelium of patients with chronic rejection [78, 79].

IL-17, which has also been implicated in acute allograft rejection [80], is able to induce IL-8 release from human airway epithelial cells [81], suggesting a role for bronchial epithelium as a bridge between acute and chronic rejection. Recently, it has also been demonstrated that bronchial epithelial cells derived from patients with chronic allograft rejection, are able to upregulate B7-1 and -2, which are known as co-stimulatory molecules for the activation of T-lymphocytes in transplant rejection [82].

***Fibroblasts.*** In a mouse model of BO, it was demonstrated that allografts had myofibroblast predominance, compared with isografts [74]. In 1992, HERTZ *et al.* [83] showed that BAL fluid from BO patients significantly stimulated fibroblast migration, whereas fluid from control patients did not. Furthermore, JONOSONO *et al.* [84] demonstrated a correlation between the fibroblast-proliferative activity in BAL fluid and the decline in forced expiratory flow rate between 25% and 75% of expired volume ($FEF_{25-75\%}$). In a rat transplantation model, onset and progression of BO was associated with changes in morphology of fibroblasts that was accompanied by alterations in their iNOS expression [85].

### *Airway smooth muscle cells*

The airway smooth muscle cell (ASMC) is no longer regarded as an innocent contractile bystander and its potential role in airway inflammation in general, and in BO in particular, is probably being underestimated. As in other inflammatory diseases, like asthma and COPD, it has been proven that ASMC do not only have a contractile but also an active immunomodulating function. ASMC have been shown to be able to respond to an inflammatory stimulus by producing cytokines and chemokines [86, 87]. As a consequence, it became clear that ASMCs have the potential to actively take part in inflammatory processes.

As already mentioned, IL-17 is an important cytokine in acute rejection, whereas IL-8 is especially upregulated in patients with chronic lung rejection. Recently it has been demonstrated that IL-17 is able to induce IL-8 from human ASMC [88], a process that cannot be inhibited by steroids, but is clearly prevented by the addition of N-acetyl cysteine [89]. Since the smooth muscle cell seems to be the largest producer of IL-8 in the airways [63], this may point to a very important role of the ASMC in the transition from acute to chronic rejection. Moreover, it has been described that ASMC, in response to cytokines (granulocyte-macrophage colony-stimulating factor: GM-CSF) secreted by the epithelium, augment their collagen production and expression of tumour growth factor (TGF)-β receptor, leading to fibrosis, the hallmark of BO [90].

## *Role of oxidative stress*

Oxidative stress describes the condition that exists when the level of reactive oxygen species (ROS) produced, exceeds the capacity of antioxidant systems to remove those ROS such that excess oxidants exist in a cell or tissue.

There is indeed some evidence that oxidative stress has a role to play in the pathogenesis of BOS. Riise *et al.* [64] demonstrated that concentrations of ascorbate, urate and GSH, all antioxidant agents, were generally lower whereas the concentration of glutathione persulphide (GSSH) was higher in BAL fluid of patients with BOS, compared with patients without BOS. The reduction in GSH and the increase in GSSH, has meanwhile, been confirmed by Behr *et al.* [91]. It has also been described that all lung transplant recipients had a significant increase of oxidative stress as shown by an elevated Met (O) content, values in patients with BO/BOS being even higher [92].

Generally neutrophils are considered as the most important source of ROS in BO/BOS. It is known that neutrophil MPO catalyses the formation of ROS. Therefore it has been stated that MPO activity is an indicator of oxidative stress due to neutrophil activation [93]. MPO induces the formation of hydrogen peroxide and chloride to hypochloric acid, which leads to the production of chloramines. Due to the fact that it also induces reactive nitrogen species, BAL $NO_2^-$ is strongly correlated with BAL neutrophil percentage in BO/BOS patients [94].

It is thought that an excess of chemically available iron may promote the catalysis of toxic hydroxyl radicals, a major contributor in the pathogenesis of cell injury and airway inflammation following lung transplantation [94]. A potential source of iron within the allograft is ferritin. In BOS patients BAL ferritin was related to BAL albumin, which may indicate that ferritin could contribute to the induction of a microvascular leak syndrome [95]. An increase in lung iron may be part of a final common pathway that ultimately leads to growth factor generation, promotion of collagen gene transcription and airway fibrosis and remodelling [96].

It has also been demonstrated that structural cells, such as ASMCs, are able to produce ROS. Indeed, when ASMCs are stimulated with IL-17, there is an increase in the production of 8-isoprostane, which is a marker of oxidative stress [89]. ROS can provoke an oxidation of GSH, quantitatively the most important antioxidant of the lung leading to a significant reduction of GSH and an increase in oxidised GSH (GSSG), which correlates with $FEV_1$ [91]. This supports the hypothesis that oxidative stress and the effect on GSH/GSSG ratio may be associated with the development of BO/BOS.

### *Cytokines and growth factors*

The mechanisms underlying the development of BO/BOS are not fully understood, but may be hypothesised as follows: an initially immune-mediated response (possibly mediated by anti-HLA antibodies [95]) damages the epithelium, generating different cytokines and chemokines (Th1 and Th2 cytokines; IL-2; interferon-gamma; IL-4; IL-10; and IL-8), that attract lymphocytes and neutrophils to the injured airway [74]. These cytokines not only attract inflammatory cells but it is known that IL-8 also activates neutrophils to release neutrophil elastase, the proteolytic activity of which is physiologically counterbalanced by several antiproteases. The major one, the secretory leukoprotease inhibitor, is especially inhibited by TGF-β, which is present in increased amounts in the BAL of BO/BOS patients [97, 98]. Other proteases, *e.g.* matrix metalloproteinase (MMP)-9 are increased in the sputum of patients with chronic lung rejection and may degrade the extracellular matrix, paving the way for an excessive repair mechanisms and a fibroproliferative phase.

Other chemokines such as RANTES and monocyte chemotactic protein-1 play a crucial role in post-transplant airway obliteration by the recruitment of CD4+ T-cells and mononuclear phagocytes. Indeed, high levels of these chemokines are present in the BAL fluid of lung transplant patients long before BO/BOS is present [67]. The same holds true for a naturally occurring antagonist of the pro-inflammatory cytokine IL-1, its receptor antagonist (IL-1Ra), which attenuates IL-1 bioactivity during the pathogenesis of BO/BOS, creates a local environment that favours fibroproliferation [99].

T-lymphocytes and alveolar macrophages also produce a wide range of inflammatory mediators, profibrotic cytokines and chemokines. Experimental models have demonstrated the deleterious effectors of Th1 cytokines in this context. In rat tracheal allografts for instance, IL-2 and interferon (IFN)-γ are strongly and persistently expressed throughout the development of BO [100]. Furthermore, recent studies have highlighted the strong association between IL-6 and IFN-γ high-expression polymorphism and BOS [101]. Although Th2 cytokines have been associated with tolerance in other solid organ transplantations, an increased expression of IL-4 seems to contribute to the development of BOS in transplanted mice [70]. Conversely, IL-10 has clearly been demonstrated to exert a protective effect, using either IL-10 gene transfer, recombinant IL-10 or anti-IL-10 antibodies in allografted animals [102, 103].

After this early phase of inflammation, there gradually appears a fibroproliferative phase, mediated by several profibrotic mediators, such as platelet-derived growth factor (PDGF) [104], basic fibroblast growth factor [105], transforming growth factor (GF)-β [97, 98, 106] and insulin like GF-1 [107] and endothelin-1 [108], secreted by the epithelium, fibroblasts, inflammatory cells and even smooth muscle cells. These factors attract and activate fibroblasts, leading to extracellular matrix deposition, but also participate in other features of airway remodelling, *i.e.* smooth muscle migration and hyperplasia and neo-angiogenesis. Different antagonists of these mediators have shown their capacity to prevent or to consistently attenuate BO in animal models. Among these, PDGF receptor inhibitors [104], tumour necrosis factor-α soluble receptors [109] or the strong expression of TGF-βIII receptors obtained during gene transfer [110] proved particularly effective.

## Conclusion

Chronic rejection remains the most important and challenging problem after heart-lung and lung transplantation, since it can lead to: obstruction of the airways; loss of quality of life; increased morbidity; increased costs; and a high mortality. In recent years, a lot of new insights into the pathophysiological events of the disease have emerged, although there is no clear evidence, up to now, showing that this has increased the survival of this condition, as effective treatment of this disease is still lacking. Hopefully the near future will bring about better immunosuppressive therapy, leading to a reduction of the acute rejection episodes, which are still considered as the most important risk factor for the development of BO/BOS.

## Summary

Lung and heart-lung transplantations are now considered as effective treatment for highly selected patients with end-stage lung or heart-lung disease. Although the survival rates have improved dramatically in recent years, the development of chronic rejection is still the major cause of late death after transplantation. Histologically chronic rejection is manifested by bronchiolitis obliterans (BO), with a gradual decline in pulmonary function tests and quality of life, eventually leading to respiratory insufficiency and recurrent infections with Gram-negative bacteria and fungi. A lot of research efforts have been put into the detection of possible risk factors for BO and unravelling the pathophysiology of BO. Several key cytokines and growth factors have now been identified. Since the histological diagnosis of chronic rejection remains difficult, a clinical grading system has been proposed, determined as bronchiolitis obliterans syndrome, divided into four, and more recently, five categories, depending on the severity of airflow obstruction. This chapter aims to review the current knowledge on the pathology, the aetiology (*e.g.* risk factors) and the pathophysiology of chronic rejection after heart-lung and lung transplantation.

**Keywords:** Bronchiolitis obliterans, bronchiolitis obliterans syndrome, chronic infection, inflammatory cells, lung transplantation, lymphocytic bronchiolitis.

***Acknowledgements.*** Other co-authors of Working Group 1 include: A. Bankier, A. Boehler, P. Corris, L. Dupont, M. Estenne, S. Fischer, H. Reichenspurner, C. Ward.

## References

1. Trulock EP, Edwards LB, Taylor DO, *et al.* The registry of the International Society for Heart and Lung Transplantation: twentieth official adult heart-lung report – 2003. *J Heart Lung Transplant* 2003; 22: 625–635.
2. Vricella LA, Karamichalis JM, Ahmad S, Robbins RC, Whyte RI, Reitz BA. Lung and heart-lung transplantation in patients with end-stage cystic fibrosis: the Stanfgord experience. *Ann Thorac Surg* 2002; 74: 13–18.
3. Cassivi SD, Meyers BF, Battafarano RJ, *et al.* Thirteen-year experience in lung transplantation for emphysema. *Ann Thorac Surg* 2002; 74: 1663–1670.
4. Cooper JD, Billingham M, Egan T, *et al.* A working formulation for the standardization of nomenclature for clinical staging of chronic dysfunction in lung allografts. *J Heart Lung Transplant* 1993; 12: 713–716.
5. Reichenspurner H, Girgis RE, Robbins BC, *et al.* Stanford experience with obliterative bronchiolitis after lung and heart-lung transplantation. *Ann Thorac Surg* 1996; 62: 1547–1473.

6. Meyers BF, Lynch J, Trulock EP, Guthrie TJ, Cooper JD, Patterson GA. Lung transplantation: a decade of experience. *Ann Surg* 1999; 230: 362–370.
7. Whitehead B, Rees P, Sorensen K, *et al.* Incidence of obliterative bronchiolitis after heart-lung transplantation in children. *J Heart Lung Transplant* 1993; 12: 903–908.
8. Ouwens JP, van der Mark TW, Koëter GH, de Boer WJ, Grevink RG, van der Bij W. Bronchiolar airflow impairment after lung transplantation: an early and common manifestation. *J Heart Lung Transplant* 2002; 21: 1056–1061.
9. Van Raemdonck D, Verleden G, Vanhaecke J, *et al.* The current status of lung transplantation. *Acta Chir Austriaca* 1999; 31: 292–301
10. Tamm M, Sharples L, Higenbottam T, Steward S, Wallwork J. Bronchiolitis obliterans syndrome (BOS) following heart-lung transplantation. *Transpl Int* 1996; 9: Suppl. 1, S299–S302.
11. Burke CM, Theodore J, Dawkins KD, *et al.* Post-transplant obliterative bronchiolitis and other late lung sequelae in human heart-lung transplantation. *Chest* 1984; 86: 824–829.
12. Glanville AR, Baldwin JC, Burke CM, Theodore J, Robin ED. Obliterative bronchiolitis after heart-lung transplantation: apparent arrest by augmented immunosuppression. *Ann Int Med* 1987; 107: 300–304.
13. Verleden GM. Bronchiolitis obliterans syndrome after lung transplantation: medical treatment. *Monaldi Arch Chest Dis* 2000; 55: 140–145.
14. Van den Berg JW, Geertsma A, van der Bij W, *et al.* Bronchiolitis obliterans syndrome after lung transplantation and health-related quality of life. *Am J Respir Crit Care Med* 2000; 161: 1937–1941.
15. Van den Berg JWK, van Enckevort PJ, TenVergert EM, Postma DS, van der Bij W, Koeter GH. Bronchiolitis obliterans syndrome and additional costs of lung transplantation. *Chest* 2000; 118: 1648–1652.
16. Yousem SA, Berry GH, Cagle PT, *et al.* Revision of the 1990 working formulation for the classification of pulmonary allograft rejection: lung rejection study group. *J Heart Lung Transplant* 1996; 15: 1–15.
17. Yousem SA, Paradis I, Griffith BP. Can transbronchial biopsy aid in the diagnosis of bronchiolitis obliterans in lung transplant recipients? *Transplantation* 1994; 57: 151–152.
18. Sibley RK, Berry GJ, Tazelaar HD, *et al.* The role of transbronchial biopsies in the management of lung transplant recipients. *J Heart Lung Transplant* 1993; 12: 308–324.
19. Estenne M, Maurer J, Boehler A, *et al.* Bronchiolitis obliterans syndrome 2001: an update of the diagnostic criteria. *J Heart Lung Transplant* 2002; 21: 297–310.
20. Stewart S. The pathology of lung transplantation. *Sem Diagnostic Pathol* 1992; 9: 210–219.
21. Yousem SA. Lymphocytic bronchitis/bronchiolitis in lung allograft recipients. *Am J Surg Pathol* 1993; 17: 491–496.
22. Ross DJ, Marchevsky A, Kramer M, Kass RM. "Refractoriness" of airflow obstruction associated with isolated lymphocytic bronchiolitis/bronchitis in pulmonary allografts. *J Heart Lung Transplant* 1997; 16: 832–838.
23. Cagle PT, Brown RW, Frost A, Kellar C, Yousem SA. Diagnosis of chronic lung transplant rejection by transbronchial biopsy. *Modern Pathology* 1995; 8: 137–142.
24. Yousem SA. Small airway injury in heart-lung transplant recipients. *Semi in Respir Med* 1992; 13: 85–95.
25. Abernathy EC, Hruban RH, Baumgartner WA, Reitz BA, Hutchins GM. The two forms of bronchiolitis obliterans in heart-lung transplant recipients. *Hum Pathol* 1991; 22: 1102–1110.
26. Yousem SA, Duncan SR, Griffith BP. Interstitial and airspace granulation tissue reactions in lung transplant recipients. *Am J Surg Pathol* 1992; 16: 877–884.
27. Chaparro C, Chamberlain D, Maurer J, Winton T, Dehoyos A, Kesten S. Bronchiolitis obliterans organizing pneumonia (BOOP) in lung transplant recipients. *Chest* 1996; 110: 1150–1154.
28. Milne DS, Gascoigne AD, Ashcroft T, Sviland L, Malcolm AJ, Corris PA. Organizing pneumonia following pulmonary transplantation and the development of obliterative bronchiolitis. *Transplantation* 1994; 57: 1757–1762.

29. Palmer SM, Miralles AP, Howell DN, Brazer SR, Tapson VF, Davis RD. Gastroesophageal reflux as a reversible cause of allograft dysfunction after lung transplantation. *Chest* 2000; 118: 1214–1217.
30. Stewart S, Cary N, Goddard M, Billingham M. An Atlas of the Biopsy Histopathology of Heart and Lung Transplantation. London, Edward Arnold, 2000.
31. Salvato G. Quantitative and morphological analysis of the vascular bed in bronchial biopsy specimens from asthmatic and non-asthmatic subjects. *Thorax* 2001; 56: 902–906.
32. McDonald D. Angiogenesis and remodelling of airway vasculature in chronic inflammation. *Am J Respir Crit Care Med* 2001; 164: 39–45.
33. Wilson JW, Li X. Vessels: new targets for asthma treatment. *Thorax* 2001; 56: 899–900.
34. Baudet EM, Dromer C, Dubrez J, *et al.* Intermediate term results after en-bloc double-lung transplantation with bronchial arterial revasularization. *J Thorac Cardiovasc Surg* 1996; 112: 1292–1299.
35. Yacoub M, Al-Kttan KM, Tadjkarimi S, Eren T, Khaghani A. Medium term results of direct bronchial arterial revascularization using IMA for single lung transplantation (SLT) wth direct revascularization. *Eur J Cardiothor Surg* 1997; 11: 1030–1036.
36. Luckraz H, Goddard M, McNeil K, Atkinson C, Stewart S, Wallwork J. Micro vascular changes in small airways predispose to obliterative bronchiolitis after lung transplantation. *J Heart Lung Transplant* 2002; 21: 154–155.
37. Yousem SA, Suncan SR, Ohori P, Somnmez-Alpan E. Architectural remodeling of lung allografts in acute and chronic rejection. *Arch Pathol Lab Med* 1992; 116: 1175–1180.
38. Yousem SA, Paradis IL, Dauber JA, *et al.* Large airway inflammation in heart-lung transplant recipients--its significance and prognostic implications. *Transplantation* 1990; 49: 654–656.
39. Patterson GM, Wilson S, Whang JL, *et al.* Physiological definitions of obliterative bronchiolitis in heart lung and double lung transplantation: a comparison of the forced expiratory flow between 25% and 75% of the forced vital capacity and forced expiratory volume in one second. *J Heart Lung Transplant* 1996; 15: 175–181.
40. Haider Y, Mogulkoc N, Carroll KB, Yonan N, Egan JJ. The survival of patients with emphysema following the development of BOS. *J Heart Lung Transplant* 2002; 21: 327–333.
41. Hachem RR, Patterson GA, Trulock EP. The predictive value of bronchiolitis obliterans syndrome stage 0-p. *J Heart Lung Transplant* 2003; 22: S78.
42. Sharples LD, Mc Neil K, Stewart S, Wallwork J. Risk factors for bronchiolitis obliterans: a systematic review of recent publications. *J Heart Lung Transplant* 2002; 21: 271–281.
43. Kroshus TJ, Kshettry VR, Savik K, Ranjit J, Hertz MI, Bolman RM. Risk factors for the development of bronchiolitis obliterans syndrome after lung transplantation. *J Thorac Cardiovasc surg* 1997; 114: 195–202.
44. Bando K, Paradis IL, Similo S, *et al.* Obliterative bronchiolitis after lung and heart-lung transplantation. An analysis of risk factors and management. *J Thorac Cardiovasc Surg* 1995; 110: 4–13.
45. Stanbrook MB, Kesten S. Bronchial hyperreactivity after lung transplantation predicts early bronchiolitis obliterans. *Am J Respir Crit Care Med* 1999; 160: 2034–2039.
46. Kshettry VR, Kroshus TJ, Savik K, Hertz MI, Bolman RM. Primary pulmonary hypertension as a risk factor for the development of obliterative bronchiolitis in lung allograft recipients. *Chest* 1996; 110: 704–709.
47. Ward CW, DeSouza T, Keating DT, Lordan J, Egan JJ. Infection and bronchiolitis obliterans syndrome in lung transplant recipients. *Eur Resp Mon* 2004; 29: 44–54.
48. Hirt SW, You XM, Moller F, *et al.* Development of obliterative bronchiolitis after allogeneic lung transplantation: implication of acute rejection and the time point of treatment. *J Heart Lung Transplant* 1999; 18: 542–548.
49. Husain AN, Siddique MT, Holmes EW, *et al.* Analysis of risk factors for the development of bronchiolitis obliterans syndrome. *Am J Respir Crit Care Med* 1999; 159: 829–833.

50. Heng D, Sharples L, McNeil K, Stewart S, Wregitt T, Wallwork J. Bronchiolitis obliterans syndrome: incidence, natural history, prognosis, and risk factors. *J Heart Lung Transplant* 1998; 17: 1255–1263.
51. Quantz MA, Bennett LE, Meyer DM, Novick RJ. Does human leukocyte antigen matching influence the outcome of lung transplantation? An analysis of 3,549 lung transplantations. *J Heart Lung Transplant* 2000; 19: 473–479.
52. Schulman LL, Weinberg AD, McGregor C, Galantowicz ME, Suciu-Foca NM, Itescu S. Mismatches at the HLA-DR and HLA-B loci are risk factors for acute rejection after lung transplantation. *Am J Respir Crit Care Med* 1998; 157: 1833–1837.
53. van den Berg JW, Hepkema BG, Geertsma A, *et al.* Long-term outcome of lung transplantation is predicted by the number of HLA-DR mismatches. *Transplantation* 2001; 71: 368–373.
54. Hadjiliadis D, Davis RD, Palmer SM. Is transplant operation important in determining posttransplant risk of bronchiolitis obliterans syndrome in lung transplant recipients? *Chest* 2002; 122: 1168–1175.
55. Norgaard MA, Andersen CB, Pettersson G. Does bronchial artery revascularization influence results concerning bronchiolitis obliterans syndrome and/or obliterative bronchiolitis after lung transplantation? *Eur J Cardiothor Surg* 1998; 14: 311–317.
56. Daly RC, McGregor CGA, McDougall JC, Midthun DE, Peters SG, Scott JP. Bronchial artery revascularization does not prevent bronchiolitis obliterans syndrome after lung transplantation. Paris, 3rd International Congress on Lung Transplantation, 1998; pp. 22.
57. Girgis RE, Tu I, Berry GJ, *et al.* Risk factors for the development of obliterative bronchiolitis after lung transplantation. *J Heart Lung Transplant* 1996; 15: 1200–1208.
58. Hosenpud JD, Bennett LE, Keck BM, Boucek MM, Novick RJ. The registry of the international society of heart and lung transplantation: seventeenth official report-2000. *J Heart Lung Transplant* 2000; 19: 909–931.
59. Ciccone AM, Stewart KC, Meyers BF, *et al.* Does donor cause of death affect the outcome of lung transplantation? *J Thorac Cardiovasc Surg* 2002; 123: 429–434.
60. Fiser SM, Tribble CG, Long SM, *et al.* Ischemia-reperfusion injury after lung transplantation increases risk of late bronchiolitis obliterans syndrome. *Ann Thorac Surg* 2002; 73: 1041–1047.
61. Fisher AJ, Wardle J, Dark JH, Corris PA. Non-immune acute graft injury after lung transplantation and the risk of subsequent bronchiolitis obliterans syndrome (BOS). *J Heart Lung Transplant* 2002; 21: 1206–1212.
62. Schulman LL, Weinberg AD, McGregor CC, Suciu-Foca NM, Itescu S. Influence of donor and recipient HLA locus mismatching on development of obliterative bronchiolitis after lung transplantation. *Am J Respir Crit Care Med.* 2001; 163: 437–442.
63. DiGiovine B, Lynch JPr, Martinez FJ, *et al.* Bronchoalveolar lavage neutrophilia is associated with obliterative bronchiolitis after lung transplantation: role of IL-8. *J Immunol* 1996; 157: 4194–4202.
64. Riise GC, Williams A, Kjellstrom C, Schersten H, Andersson BA, Kelly FJ. Bronchiolitis obliterans syndrome in lung transplant recipients is associated with increased neutrophil activity and decreased antioxidant status in the lung. *Eur Respir J* 1998; 12: 82–88.
65. Riise GC, Andersson BA, Kjellstrom C, *et al.* Persistent high BAL fluid granulocyte activation marker levels as early indicators of bronchiolitis obliterans after lung transplant. *Eur Respir J* 1999; 14: 1123–1130.
66. Zheng L, Walters EH, Ward C, *et al.* Airway neutrophilia in stable and bronchiolitis obliterans syndrome patients following lung transplantation. *Thorax* 2000; 55: 53–59.
67. Reynaud-Gaubert M, Marin V, Thirion X, *et al.* Upregulation of chemokines in bronchoalveolar lavage fluid as a predictive marker of post-transplant airway obliteration. *J Heart Lung Transplant* 2002; 21: 721–728.
68. Fisher AJ, Donnelly SC, Hirani N, *et al.* Elevated levels of interleukin-8 in donor lungs is associated with early graft failure after lung transplantation. *Am J Respir Crit Care Med* 2001; 163: 259–265.

69. Ward C, Snell GI, Zheng L, *et al.* Endobronchial biopsy and bronchoalveolar lavage in stable lung transplant recipients and chronic rejection. *Am J Respir Crit Care Med* 1998; 158: 84–91.
70. Neuringer IP, Walsh SP, Mannon RB, Gabriel S, Aris RM. Enhanced T cell cytokine gene expression in mouse airway obliterative bronchiolitis. *Transplantation* 2000; 69: 399–405.
71. Tikkanen JM, Lemström KB, Koskinen PK. Blockade of CD28/B7-2 costimulation inhibits experimental obliterative bronchiolitis in rat tracheal allografts. *Am J Respir Crit Care Med* 2002; 165: 724–729.
72. Yousem SA, Ray AL, Paradis IL, Dauber JA, Griffith BP. Potential role of dendritic cells in bronchiolitis obliterans in heart-lung transplantation. *Ann Thorac Surg* 1990; 49: 424–428.
73. Leonard CT, Soccal PM, Singer L, *et al.* Dendritic cells and macrophages in lung allografts. A role in cxg-hronic rejection? *Am J Respir Crit Care Med* 2000; 161: 1349–1354.
74. Neuringer IP, Mannon RB, Coffman TM, *et al.* Immune cells in a mouse airway model of obliterative bronchiolitis. *Am J Respir Cell Mol Biol* 1998; 19: 379–386.
75. Mauck KA, Hosenpud JD. The bronchial epithelium: a potential allogeneic target for chronic rejection after lung transplantation. *J Heart Lung Transplant* 1996; 15: 709–714.
76. Borger P, Kauffman HF, Timmerman JA, Scholma J, van den Berg JW, Koeter GH. Cyclosporine, FK506, mycophenolate mofetil, and prednisolone differentially modulate cytokine gene expression in human airway-derived epithelial cells. *Transplantation* 2000; 69: 1408–1413.
77. Minamoto K, Pinsky DJ. Recipient iNOS but not eNOS deficiency reduces luminal narrowing in tracheal allografts. *J Exp Med* 2002; 197: 1321–1333.
78. McDermott CD, Gavita SM, Shennib H, Giaid A. Immunohistochemical localization of nitric oxide synthase and the oxidant peroxynitrite in lung transplant recipients with obliterative bronchiolitis. *Transplantation* 1997; 64: 270–274.
79. Mason NA, Springall DR, Pomerance A, Evans TJ, Yacoub MH, Polak JM. Expression of inducible nitric oxide synthase and formation of peroxynitrite in posttransplant obliterative bronchiolitis. *J Heart Lung Transplant* 1998; 17: 710–714.
80. Loong CC, Hsich HG, Lui WY, Chen A, Lin CY. Evidence for the early involvement of interleukin 17 in human and experimental renal allograft rejection. *J Pathol* 2002; 197: 322–332.
81. Jones CD, Chan K. Interleukin-17 stimulates the expression of interleukin-8, growth-related oncogene-alpha, and granulocyte-colony-stimulating factor by human airtway epithelial cells. *Am J Respir Cell Mol Biol* 2002; 26: 748–753.
82. Elssner A, Jaumann F, Wolf WP, *et al.* Bronchial epithelial cell B7-1 and B7-2 mRNA expression after lung transplantation: a role in allograft rejection? *Eur Respir J* 2002; 20: 165–169.
83. Hertz MI, Henke CA, Nakhleh RE, *et al.* Obliterative bronchiolitis after lung transplantation: a fibroproliferative disorder associated with platelet-derived growth factor. *Proc Natl Acd Sci USA* 1992; 89: 10385–10389.
84. Jonosono M, Fang KC, Keith FM, *et al.* Measurement of fibroblast proliferative activity in bronchoalveolar lavage fluid in the analysis of obliterative bronchiolitis among lung transplant recipients. *J Heart Lung Transplant* 1999; 18: 972–985.
85. Romanska HM, Ikonen TS, Bishop AE, Morris RE, Polak JM. Up-regulation of inducible nitric oxide synthase in fibroblasts parallels the onset and progression of fibrosis in an experimental model of post-transplant obliterative airway disease. *J Pathol* 2000; 191: 71–77.
86. Pype JL, Dupont LJ, Menten P, *et al.* Expression of monocyte chemotactic protein (MCP)-1, MCP-2, MCP-3 by human airway smooth muscle cells. Modulation by corticosteroids and T-helper 2-cytokines. *Am J Respir Cell Mol Biol* 1999; 21: 528–536.
87. Wuyts WA, Vanaudenaerde BM, Dupont LJ, Demedts MG, Verleden GM. Involvement of p38 MAPK, JNK, p42/p44 ERK and NF-kB in IL-1beta induced chemokine release in human airway smooth muscle cells. *Respir Med* 2003; 97: 811–817.
88. Vanaudenaerde BM, Wuyts WA, Dupont LJ, Van Raemdonck DE, Verleden GM. Interleukin-17 stimulates the release of interleukin-8 by human airway smooth muscle cells in vitro: a potential role for interleukin-17 and human airway smooth muscle cells in bronchiolitis obliterans syndrome? *J Heart Lung Transplant* 2003; 22: 1280–1283.

89. Wuyts WA, Vanaudenaerde BM, Dupont LJ, Van Raemdonck DE, Demedts MG, Verleden GM. N-acetylcysteine inhibits IL-17-induced IL-8 production from human airway smooth muscle cells – a possible role for anti-oxidative treatment in chronic lung rejection? *J Heart Lung Transplant* 2004; 23: 122–127.
90. Chen G, Grotendorst G, Eichholtz T, Khalil N. GM-CSF increases airway smooth muscle cell connective tissue expression by inducing TGF-beta receptors. *Am J Physiol Lung Cell Mol Physiol* 2003; 284: L548–L556.
91. Behr J, Maier K, Braun B, Schwaiblmaier M, Vogelmeier C. Evidence for oxidative stress in bronchiolitis obliterans syndrome after lung and heart-lung transplantation. *Transplantation* 2000; 15: 1856–1860.
92. Hirsch J, Elssner A, Mazyr, *et al.* Bronchiolitis obliterans syndrome after (heart)-lung transplantation. Impaired antiprotease defense and increased oxidant activity. *Am J Respir Crit Care Med* 1999; 160: 1640–1646.
93. Elssner A, Vogelmeier C. The role of neutrophils in the pathogenesis of obliterative bronchiolitis after lung transplantation. *Transpl Infect Dis* 2001; 3: 168–176.
94. Reid D, Snell G, Ward C, *et al.* Iron overload and nitric-oxide-derived oxidative stress following lung transplantation. *J Heart Lung Transplant* 2001; 20: 840–849.
95. Mateos F, Brock JH, Perez-Arellano JL. Iron metabolism in the lower respiratory tract. *Thorax* 1998; 53: 594–600.
96. Sundaresan S, Mohanakumar T, Smith MA, *et al.* HLA-A locus mismatches and development of antibodies to HLA after lung transplantation correlate with the development of bronchiolitis obliterans syndrome. *Transplantation* 1998; 65: 648–653.
97. Elssner A, Jaumann F, Dobmann S, *et al.* Elevated levels of interleukin-8 and transforming growth factor-beta in bronchoalveolar lavage fluid from patients with bronchiolitis obliterans syndrome: proinflammatory role of bronchial epithelial cells. *Transplantation* 2000; 70: 362–367.
98. El Gamel A, Sim E, Hasleton P, *et al.* Transforming growth factor beta (TGF-beta) and obliterative bronchiolitis following pulmonary transplantation. *J Heart Lung Transplant* 1999; 18: 828–837.
99. Belperio J, DiGiovine B, Keane M, *et al.* Interleukin-1 receptor antagonist as a biomarker for bronchiolitis obliterans in lung transplant recipents. *Transplantation* 2002; 73: 591–599.
100. Boehler A, Hui Bai X, Liu M, *et al.* Upregulation of T-helper 1 cytokines and chemokine expression in post-transplant airway obliteration. *Am J Respir Crit Care Med* 1999; 159: 1910–1917.
101. Lu KC, Jaramillo A, Lecha RL, *et al.* Interleukin-6 and interferon-gamma gene polymorphisms in the development of bronchiolitis obliterans syndrome after lung tranbsplantation. *Transplantation* 2002; 74: 1297–1302.
102. Boehler A, Chamberlain D, Zing Z, *et al.* Adenovirus-mediated interleukin-10 gene transfer inhibits post-transplant fibrous airway obliteration in an animal model of bronchiolitis obliterans. *Human gene therapy* 1998; 9: 541–551.
103. Naidu B, Krishnadasan B, Whyte RI, Warner RL, Ward PA, Mulligan MS. Regulatory role of IL-10 in experimental obliterative bronchilitis in rats. *Exp Mol Pathol* 2002; 73: 164–170.
104. Kallio E, Koskinen P, Aavik E, Buchdunger E, Lemstrom K. Role of platelet-derived growth factor in obliterative bronchiolitis (chronic rejection) in te rat. *Am J Respir Crit Care Med* 1999; 160: 1324–1332.
105. Lee AG, Wagner FM, Giaid A, *et al.* Immunohistochemical characterization of inflammatory and proliferative events during chronic rejection in rat lung allografts. *Transplantation* 1997; 64: 465–471.
106. Charpin JM, Valcke J, Kettaneh L, Epardeau B, Stern M, Israel-Biet D. Peaks of transforming growth factor-β mRNA in alveolar cells of lung transplant recipients as an early marker of chronic rejection. *Transplantation* 1998; 65: 752–755.
107. Charpin JM, Stern M, Grenet D, Israel-Biet D. Insulinlike growth factor-1 in lung transplants with obliterative bronchiolitis. *Am J Respir Crit Care Med* 2000; 161: 1991–1998.

108. Charpin JM, Stern M, Lebrun G, Aubin P, Grenet D, Israël-Biet D. Increased endothelin-1 is associated with bacterial infection in lung ransplant recipients. *Transplantation* 2001; 71: 1840–1847.
109. Aris R, Walsh S, Chalermskulrat W, Hathwar V, Neuringer I. Growth factor upregulation during obliterative bronchiolitis in the mouse model. *Am J Respir Crit Care Med* 2002; 166: 417–422.
110. Liu M, Suga M, Maclean A, *et al.* Soluble transforming growth factor-β type III receptor gene transfection inhibits fibrous airway obliteration in a rat model of bronchiolitis obliterans. *Am J Respir Crit Care Med* 2002; 165: 419–423.

CHAPTER 2

# Bronchiolitis obliterans syndrome after lung transplantation: diagnosis and treatment

G.M. Verleden*, A. Bankier#, A. Boehler¶, P. Corris+, L. Dupont*, M. Estenne§, S. Fischerf, T. Lerut**, H. Reichenspurner##, and other co-authors of Working Group 1

*Dept of Respiratory Medicine, Lung Transplantation Unit, **Dept Thoracic Surgery, University Hospital Gasthuisberg, Leuven, §Dept Respiratory Medicine, Hôpital Erasme, Brussels, Belgium, #Dept of Radiology, University of Vienna, Vienna, Austria, ¶Division of Pulmonary Medicine and Lung Transplant Program, University Hospital, Zurich, Switzerland, +Cardiopulmonary Transplantation, Freeman Hospital and University of Newcastle upon Tyne, UK, f Cardiothoracic Surgery, University Hospital, Hannover, and ##Dept Cardiothoracic Surgery, University Hospital, Hamburg, Germany.

Correspondence: G.M. Verleden, University Hospital Gasthuisberg, Dept Respiratory Medicine, 49, Herestraat, B-3000, Leuven, Belgium.

The quality of life of patients with chronic rejection after lung transplantation is severely impaired [1], and mortality is significantly increased. Indeed, in the recent International Society for Heart and Lung Transplantation (ISHLT) registry report, the mortality due to bronchiolitis obliterans syndrome (BOS) increased steadily after transplantation, to become the first cause of death within 3 yrs [2]. Early diagnosis and improved management of BOS has lead to a better survival, although the survival rate is still significantly lower in comparison with lung transplant recipients without BOS. Patients with bronchiolitis obliterans (BO)/BOS have an actuarial 1-, 5- and 10-yr survival of 90, 49 and 29% *versus* 90, 74 and 66% respectively, in patients without chronic rejection [3]. The impact of an early diagnosis of BOS seems important since the survival rate in BOS stages 0 and 1 is better than in stage 3 [4]. Therefore, careful clinical and functional monitoring is essential. This chapter is intended to review the diagnostic criteria of chronic rejection, the possible role of newer surrogate markers, which may be helpful in early diagnosis, and the medical and/or surgical treatment.

## Diagnosis of bronchiolitis obliterans

Although BO diagnosis has to be made by the pathologist, it is often impossible to obtain adequate material or a positive transbronchial biopsy (TBB), demonstrating collagen tissue growing into the bronchioles. In fact, it was demonstrated that the sensitivity of TBB for BO was only 28%, whereas the specificity was 75% [5]. In another study only 15% of TBB showed signs of BO, whereas all investigated patients had clinical BO [6]. This is why in 1993, a committee sponsored by the ISHLT proposed a clinical definition, called BOS [7]. Based on pulmonary function criteria, rather than histology, BOS has been divided into four stages, which is outlined in chapter 1 by VERLEDEN *et al.* [8]. Within each BOS category there are subtypes a and b, which are based upon the following: no pathological evidence of BO, or no pathological material for evaluation (a); or pathological evidence of BO (b). Of course it is evident that other reasons for a decline in the forced expiratory volume in one second ($FEV_1$) *e.g.* acute rejection, infection or suture problems, must be excluded. In a recent revision of these BOS criteria [9], in

Eur Respir Mon, 2004, 29, 19–43. Printed in UK - all rights reserved. Copyright ERS Journals Ltd 2004; European Respiratory Monograph; ISSN 1025-448x. ISBN 1-904097-33-2.

addition to $FEV_1$, the forced expiratory flow rate between 25 and 75% of expired volume ($FEF_{25-75\%}$) was included in the staging parameters. This was included as it had become clear that the latter parameter declined earlier than the $FEV_1$ [10–12]. Alternatively, increased discussions arose regarding whether a 20% drop in $FEV_1$ was not too late to establish a diagnosis of BOS. Therefore, in the revised criteria, a new stage was incorporated, namely potential BOS [9].

## Clinical findings

BO is consistently characterised by a reduction in pulmonary function parameters, most specifically in $FEV_1$, but also in $FEF_{25-75\%}$, which has been attributed to (small) airways obstruction. There is no significant reversibility after inhalation of short-acting $\beta_2$-agonists. The onset of symptoms is mostly insidious, with progressive exertional dyspnoea, often accompanied by cough. Sometimes an airways infection seems to have triggered the onset of BO, with quite acute dyspnoea, wheezing and the development of airways obstruction. In the later course of the disease, airways super infections are frequently seen and colonisation with *Pseudomonas* sp. and *Aspergillus fumigatus* is common. At that time, high resolution computed axial tomography scan of the thorax often reveals bronchiectasis and other signs of chronic infection. Auscultation of the lungs is often normal; however, occasional rhales and in later stages squeaks may be heard. Once established, BO may develop progressively to severe airways obstruction with respiratory insufficiency and death, resulting from an infectious exacerbation. In other patients, the progression may be arrested, either spontaneously or in response to treatment. Sometimes, episodes of progressive loss of lung function are dispersed with stable intervals. Since the loss of lung function in BO is associated with a significant reduction in the quality of life [1] and a high mortality [2], every effort should be directed at early detection of BO prior to severe loss of pulmonary function [13]. The emerging role of surrogate markers, in that respect, may be very important.

## Diagnosis of chronic allograft rejection

As already described previously, the diagnosis of BO/BOS is made either: by transbronchial biopsy, in which typical pathological findings may be seen [7]; and/or by using the BOS criteria, in instances where there is a decline in $FEV_1$ and/or $FEF_{25-75\%}$ without other demonstrable causes. In recent years, it became evident that using these criteria, the diagnosis is often made quite late during the progression, therefore, several surrogate markers for early diagnosis of BO/BOS have been investigated and are summarised below.

### *High resolution computed tomography scan*

Since the introduction of computed tomography (CT) into clinical chest imaging, the application to lung transplant recipients has elicited scientific interest. High-resolution CT demonstrated early signs of chronic rejection such as diminution of peripheral vascular markings, thickening of septal lines and volume reduction. Hyperlucency, air trapping and mosaic phenomenon appeared during more advanced BOS [14]. Early studies were, however, compromised by small patient groups, the lack of follow-up examinations, the lack of expiratory CT examinations, or CT techniques were inadequate to solve the morphological and functional issues raised in this predefined group of patients.

The findings of two substantial studies by WORTHY *et al.* [15] and LEUNG *et al.* [16] later provided evidence that air trapping on expiratory CT scans is an accurate indicator of the bronchiolar obliterations that underlie BOS. This evidence, however, was based on a small numbers of patients. In addition, a control group was not used and air trapping was not compared with the decline of $FEV_1$. Moreover, no information about the evolution of air trapping over time was obtained. Thus, both the potential of air trapping in the diagnosis of BOS and the role of expiratory CT in the follow-up of lung transplant recipients remained unclear.

Focussed on these issues, BANKIER *et al.* [17] reviewed 111 CT examinations performed in 38 patients over a period of 7 yrs. They also determined air trapping scores in eight healthy volunteers. Functional impairment was assessed with the BOS classification. Receiver operating characteristic analysis was performed to determine the optimal threshold of air trapping to distinguish between patients with and those without BOS, and to compute sensitivity and specificity for diagnosing BOS. The group found that the extent of air trapping increased with BOS severity (p=0.001). A threshold of 32% of air trapping was optimal for distinguishing between patients with and without BOS, and provided a sensitivity of 83%, a specificity of 89%, and an accuracy of 88%. The prevalence of BOS and positive predictive value of air trapping increased with postoperative time; however, the negative predictive value of air trapping remained high throughout the study. Patients without BOS who had air trapping exceeding 32% of the parenchyma were at significantly increased risk of developing BOS (p=0.004). It was concluded that at the threshold of 32%, air trapping was sensitive, specific, and accurate for diagnosing BOS [17].

Using spirometrically gated CT, it was shown in another study that the accuracy for diagnosing BO/BOS was 84% [18]. Others, however, demonstrated that none of the typical high resolution CT characteristics of BO/BOS (mosaic perfusion, air trapping, bronchiectasis and tree in bud) could accurately predict the development of BO/BOS [19, 20].

To test whether air trapping is reproducible as a diagnostic sign, BANKIER *et al.* [21] prospectively studied 19 heart-lung transplant recipients. All individuals underwent three expiratory thin section CT examinations within 60 min. Both the anatomical distribution and the extent of air trapping were analysed. The reproducibility of the anatomical distribution of air trapping ranged from 84.2–94.7%. The reproducibility of the extent of air trapping ranged from 97.1–97.7%. No substantial differences in reproducibility were seen between patients with and without BOS. They concluded that in functionally stable heart-lung transplant recipients, both with and without BOS, air trapping is an anatomically and dimensionally stable CT finding [21].

## *Indexes of ventilation*

More than 20 yrs ago, BUIST and ROSS [22] and COSIO *et al.* [23] showed that the single-breath nitrogen washout, which tests the evenness of ventilation, allows early detection of obstruction of peripheral airways in smokers without functional signs of chronic airflow obstruction. Since these studies, considerable theoretical and experimental work has been carried out using single- and multiple-breath washouts of one or more inert gases [24, 25]. This work has produced concepts which support the use of single-breath washouts for the detection of diseases affecting the bronchioles such as BO.

Unlike the conventional single-breath test, single-breath washouts using mixtures containing two inert gases with different diffusivities, *e.g.* sulphur hexafluoride ($SF_6$) and helium (He), may provide information about the sites where ventilation in homogeneities arise. Indeed, whereas the slope of a single gas is determined by both interregional and intra-acinar inequalities, the slope difference ($S_{SF_6}$-$S_{He}$) primarily reflects diffusion-dependent peripheral inhomogeneity. In addition, because theoretical models suggest that the diffusion front for He is located more proximally in the acinus than the diffusion front for $SF_6$, $S_{He}$ is expected to be more sensitive (*i.e.* to increase more) than $S_{SF_6}$ when inhomogeneities arise at the level of terminal and respiratory bronchioles; as a result, $S_{SF_6}$-$S_{He}$ is expected to decrease in disease processes affecting these bronchioles.

In a prospective study by ESTENNE *et al.* [26], a total of 1,929 single-breath tests (median, 30 tests per patient) were performed in 57 heart-lung and bilateral lung transplant recipients who were followed for a median of 1,215 (range=164–2,829) days. A total of 18 of these patients were in stage BOS 1 or greater at the end of the study period. In stable patients, the distribution of ventilation was normal. Conversely, in most patients who developed BOS, slope nitrogen ($S_{N_2}$) and $S_{He}$ increased above the confidence interval, and FEF25–75% decreased below the confidence interval (which corresponded to a 24% decrease), before the criterion for the diagnosis of BOS 1 was reached. The median time interval between the change in the slope of the alveolar plateau and the 20% drop in FEV1 was 356 days for He and 178 days for $N_2$, the corresponding value for FEF25–75% was 102 days.

REYNAUD-GAUBERT *et al.* [27] also conducted a prospective trial aimed at assessing the role of $N_2$ single-breath tests for the detection of BOS. They studied 45 patients who underwent 47 bilateral lung or heart-lung procedures, 22 of whom developed BOS, a total of 765 pulmonary function tests were analysed. On average, $S_{N_2}$ had increased significantly at 151 days and FEF25–75% decreased significantly (*i.e.* >30%) 173 days before the spirometric criteria for BOS 1 was reached. These results are very consistent with those reported by ESTENNE *et al.* [26].

In a study of 15 bilateral lung transplant recipients, ARENS *et al.* [28] reported that nine of the 11 stable patients without BOS and four patients with BOS, had a significant increase in $S_{N_2}$. In the study by ESTENNE *et al.* [26], only seven of 39 patients without BOS (at the end of the study period) demonstrated a significant alteration in ventilation distribution. The corresponding value found by REYNAUD-GAUBERT *et al.* [27], was eight out of 25 patients. It is possible, though speculative at this stage, that alterations in ventilation distribution seen in patients without BOS reflect early lesions which will later produce a gradual decline in FEV1. Data on ventilation distribution, reported so far, seems to be very promising in there is an indication that the $N_2$ or He single-breath test detects post-transplant BO much earlier than conventional pulmonary function tests, in particular the FEV1. The single-breath test appears particularly well suited as a screening test for the following reasons: it takes only a few minutes to be performed; it does not necessitate special operator expertise or patient aptitude; it only requires simple equipment; and it is totally noninvasive. Future studies are needed to examine the relative performance of the single-breath test and the BOS 0-p stage in the early detection of BOS and also its potential use in recipients of single-lung grafts.

## *Exhaled nitric oxide*

Recently it has been demonstrated that patients with BOS have an increased exhaled nitric oxide (eNO) compared with stable lung transplant recipients and also compared with healthy volunteers [29–31]. Furthermore the eNO level was not influenced by the transplantation procedure (single, sequential-single or heart-lung procedure), nor by the diseased native lung in single-lung transplant recipients, which makes it a useful test in all lung transplant recipients [32]. Moreover, in a prospective study it has been shown that an increase of eNO occurs at a mean of 8.6 months before BOS 1 is diagnosed (based on an irreversible decline in $FEV_1$ of $\geq 20\%$) [33]. Decreasing levels of eNO may also accompany the stabilisation of the $FEV_1$ after switching the immunosuppressive therapy from cyclosporin A to tacrolimus in an attempt to treat chronic rejection, indicating that there is a reduction in airways inflammation in the patients who responded to the treatment shift [34]. In a recent study, two consecutive eNO measurements 3–6 weeks apart, using a cut-off value of eNO of $\geq 15$ parts per billion (ppb) had a sensitivity, specificity, positive and negative predictive values of 92, 80, 73 and 94% respectively for the prediction of the development of BO/BOS [35]. Therefore, eNO measurements may be a reliable tool in the early detection of BOS, especially since it is a noninvasive and highly reproducible test, which can be used in all lung transplant recipients. Further studies are definitely needed to establish its exact role in the detection and management of BOS.

### *Other pulmonary function tests*

Since the staging system of BO/BOS is based on spirometry, it is evident that this will have to be repeated at high frequencies, which is therefore often impossible in the hospital setting. Consequently home spirometry is a very interesting tool to detect early changes in spirometric values, albeit without complaints. This was first published in 1990 by OTULANA *et al.* [36]. In their series of 15 heart-lung transplant patients, acute rejection was accompanied by a 10.4±6.9% fall in $FEV_1$ in 20 rejection episodes. In a further study this was also demonstrated in single-lung transplant patients who had been transplanted for emphysema [37]. Recently, home spirometry was also found to be useful in the early detection of chronic rejection. In fact BOS stage 1 was detected an average of 276–341 days earlier with home spirometry than with clinical pulmonary function testing in 17 subjects, depending on the persistence of the decline (1 day or 3 days) [38]. In recent years, the use of home telemetric monitoring of graft function has proved to be of value in the detection of rejection and infection [39]. This method provides very reproducible data; however, it only has mild sensitivity (63%) for the detection of acute allograft dysfunction, using transbronchial biopsies and lavage as a golden standard [40].

The presence of nonspecific hyper-responsiveness has also been correlated with the early detection of BO/BOS. In fact, in a longitudinal study including 111 patients who underwent bilateral lung transplantation, it was demonstrated that a positive methacholine challenge at 3 months after the procedure was associated with the development of BO/BOS, with a positive predictive value of 72% [41]. This may also strengthen the value of eNO measurements since a correlation between eNO and airways hyper-reactivity has been shown, at least in asthmatic patients [42].

### *Bronchoalveolar lavage and induced sputum*

The risk factors and pathogenesis of BO/BOS is discussed in detail by VERLEDEN *et al.* [8] who already discussed that bronchoalveolar lavage (BAL) neutrophilia and increased levels of different chemo/cytokines may precede the diagnosis of BO/BOS. Most of these studies, however, had a cross-sectional design. Recently, REYNAUD-GAUBERT *et al.* [43] published a prospective study using BAL cellular differentiation and the BAL concentration of interleukin (IL)-8, RANTES, monocyte chemotactic protein-1 (MCP-1), soluble intracellular adhesion molecule-1 (sICAM-1) and vascular cellular adhesion molecule-1 (VCAM-1). A total of 13 stable lung transplant patients and eight patients who developed BO/BOS were prospectively followed for analysis of the above parameters. Significantly elevated levels of BAL neutrophilia and IL-8 were found, on average, 151±164 and 307±266 days, respectively, before the clinical diagnosis of chronic rejection. There was also early upregulation of MCP-1 and RANTES, with a mean of 253±323 and 152±80 days respectively before BOS could be diagnosed. These results demonstrate the potential use of these cyto/chemokines as early markers of the onset of BO/BOS [43]. In addition the sustained increase in fibroblast proliferation index of BAL fluid may precede the development of BO/BOS [44]. BAL neutrophilia has also been used as an early marker of BO/BOS, and indeed seems to be very important, as it has been demonstrated that persistent BAL neutrophilia may be a predictor of mortality after lung transplantation [45].

The potential role of induced sputum has not received much attention up until now. BEEH *et al.* [46] demonstrated that it is a safe procedure in lung transplant patients. The group also found an increased total cell count in transplant recipients compared with healthy volunteers, and an increased sputum neutrophilia in lung transplant patients with chronic rejection compared with stable patients, which correlated with the $FEV_1$. The group also demonstrated an increased level of matrix metalloproteinase-9 (MMP-9), tissue inhibitor of metalloproteinase-1 (TIMP-1) and tumour necrosis factor (TNF)-$\alpha$ in induced sputum from lung transplant recipients compared with control subjects and also a higher level of these markers in lung transplant patients with chronic rejection, suggesting that also these matrix-metalloproteinases can be measured in induced sputum and might be involved in the development of BO/BOS and [47].

## Medical treatment of bronchiolitis obliterans and bronchiolitis obliterans syndrome

There are, as yet, no double-blind, randomised studies available that have looked at the effect of a certain intervention (mostly addition of a new immunosuppressive drug or replacement of an immunosuppressive drug) on the further evolution of BO/BOS. Therefore, it remains very difficult to define whether any intervention really constitutes a true effect on the $FEV_1$ evolution or rather is a reflection of the natural history of BO/BOS. The typical evolution of the $FEV_1$ of a heart-lung transplant patient with biopsy-proven BO is depicted in figure 1. This evolution illustrates the natural history of BO/BOS, which implies a gradual decline in $FEV_1$ with a slowing down of the decline once the $FEV_1$ had reached low values. The apparent arrest in the decline in $FEV_1$ could be considered as a hopeful event. However, this patient did not receive any new treatment, except for chronic immunosuppressive medication consisting of cyclosporin A (CsA) and corticosteroids. In fact the only intervention that has been done was a temporary increase in steroid dose, which did not result in any $FEV_1$ improvement. Keeping this in mind, it remains difficult to interpret all the literature data that are available concerning the medical treatment of BO/BOS, as all available studies have looked at an apparent arrest in decline in $FEV_1$, which is, unfortunately difficult to interpret due to the lack of a control group.

Despite these prerogatives, it still remains interesting to give an overview of the possible interventions that may be helpful in the prevention or the treatment of BO/BOS.

### *Prevention of the known risk factors*

Since the acceptable cold-ischaemic-time of a lung remains rather short (varying between 4–7 h) and because of the increasing donor organ shortage (especially lungs and heart-lungs) worldwide, presently it is not possible to routinely perform a prospective

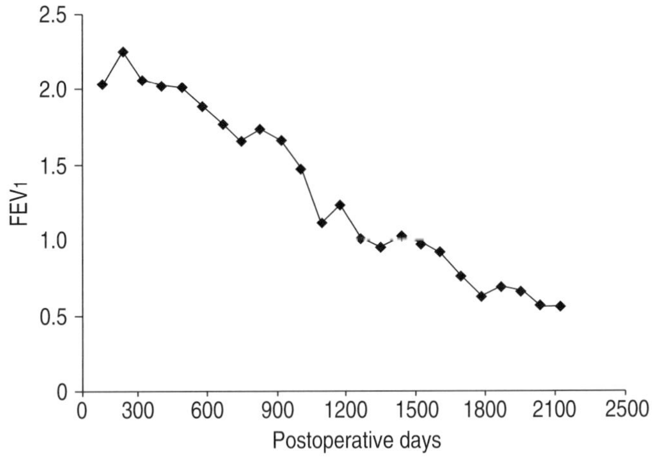


Fig. 1. – Natural evolution of the forced expiratory volume in one second (FEV1) in a heart-lung transplant patient with biopsy-proven bronchiolitis obliterans. The patient received no specific treatment for their chronic rejection, except temporary augmentation of the corticosteroids without significant effect. After an initial rapid decline in the FEV1, there was a spontaneous slowing down of the decline with an apparent arrest during 1.5 yrs.

human leukocyte antigen (HLA) cross match, to overcome the problem of severe HLA mismatch after lung transplantation. Therefore, this will not be discussed further.

Since acute rejection during the first months after transplantation and especially refractory and recurrent acute rejection, is one of the major risk factors to developing BO/BOS [7], several studies have looked at the effect of treating refractory acute rejection and recurrent acute rejections (RAR), hoping to reduce the prevalence of BO/BOS. There is indeed some evidence now which shows that initial therapy with either mycophenolate mofetil (MMF) or tacrolimus, instead of azathioprin, and cyclosporin respectively, or induction therapy with cytolytic agents (rabbit antithymocyte globulin: rATG or a monoclonal antibody against T-cells OKT3) and IL-2 receptor blockers, might reduce the incidence of acute rejections.

### *Role of mycophenolate mofetil*

Nowadays more and more transplant centres are using MMF in *de novo* therapy or intend to switch to MMF in cases of RAR. Data published by the ISHLT registry clearly show an increasing use of MMF in lung transplanted patients over time [2]. Reichenspurner *et al.* [48] showed that combining MMF with CsA reduced the incidence of acute rejections after lung transplantation, an effect that was even more evident when MMF was combined with tacrolimus. The safety profile of this combination was excellent and infection rates were not different from historical controls including azathioprin.

O'Hair *et al.* [49] treated 13 lung transplant patients with an MMF based immunosuppression and compared the linearised rate of acute rejection rate per 100 patient-days during the first 3 months after transplantation with two historical control groups. Only a trend towards a lower rejection rate in the MMF group (0.85 acute rejection episodes per 100 patients-days in the MMF group, *versus* 1.49 and 1.38 in the historical controls) was observed. Ross *et al.* [50] performed a two-centre, nonrandomised, concurrent cohort study and compared an MMF based immunosuppressive regimen *versus* an azathioprin based therapy, as initial treatment after lung transplantation. The MMF group experienced significantly fewer biopsy-proven acute cellular rejection episodes per 100 patient-days, compared with the azathioprin group (0.26±0.34 *versus* 0.72±0.43; p<0.01). Moreover, there was a trend in the MMF group towards a lower prevalence of BOS after 1 yr. ZUCKERMANN *et al.* [51] compared an MMF based immunosuppression, as initial therapy, with an historical control group, who had been treated with azathioprin. The incidence of acute rejections in the MMF treated patients was much lower compared with the historical azathioprin treated control group, although no exact figures are given. Furthermore the group found no increase in infectious episodes occurring in the MMF group.

In another randomised, prospective, multicentre, open study, initial therapy with MMF was compared with azathioprine in 81 consecutive lung transplant recipients. Using biopsy-proven acute rejection and overall survival at 6 months as end-points, no difference was found between the two immunosuppressive regimens in combination with cyclosporin [52].

By contrast, in another small study, lung transplant patients who started with MMF and tacrolimus had fewer acute rejection episodes compared with patients who started with azathioprin and cycosporine. The MMF/tacrolimus patients also had a better $FEV_1$ at the end of the first postoperative year [53].

A large international study recently published by CORRIS *et al.* [54] showed no difference in the incidence of acute rejection and BOS after lung transplantation but a significantly better 1-yr survival for patients treated with a fixed dose of 2 g MMF compared with azathioprin-treated patients (88.1 *versus* 79.1%; p<0.03). Regarding all the published data, a trend towards a reduced acute rejection rate and/or survival rate has been reported for MMF in comparison with azathioprin.

## *Role of tacrolimus*

Tacrolimus, as a comparator to cyclosporin, has been used for basic immunosuppression in lung transplanted patients since 1990. Tacrolimus effectively inhibits lymphokine production, expression of various interleukins and interferon -γ, T-cell activation, cytotoxic T-lymphocyte production, T-helper cell dependent B-cell proliferation and the induction of the proliferation ("priming") of specific T-helper cells [55]. The ratio parent compound/metabolites is 90:10 in tacrolimus and 27:73 in cyclosporin, whose 25 different metabolites are associated with nephrotoxicity [56, 57]. Several studies have addressed the possibility of tacrolimus as initial therapy to reduce the number of acute rejection episodes compared with initial cyclosporin therapy.

Results from a randomised prospective two-centre study involving the University of Vienna and the University of Munich, containing 74 patients, showed a significantly higher freedom from BOS after 3 yrs for patients treated with tacrolimus/MMF in comparison with cyclosporin/MMF (tacrolimus 90% *versus* cyclosporin 59%; p<0.01). There was also a clear trend towards more late rejections in the cyclosporin group (24 *versus* 4% in the tacrolimus group, p=0.07) [58].

KEENAN *et al.* [59] performed a prospective clinical trial to compare the efficacy of tacrolimus *versus* cyclosporin in combination with azathioprin as the primary immunosuppressive agent after lung transplantation. A total of 67 patients were allocated to cyclosporin and 66 to tacrolimus. The 1-yr and 2-yr survival rates were similar. The acute rejection rate per 100 patient-days was lower in the tacrolimus group, although not significantly (0.85 *versus* 1.09, p=0.07). However, fewer patients in the tacrolimus group (21.7%) compared with the cyclosporin-group (38%) developed BO. This difference in BO was significant (p=0.025). A total of 13 cyclosporin based patients needed to switch to tacrolimus, which was significantly more than the opposite switch. In six of the nine patients, a crossover to tacrolimus based therapy controlled persistent acute rejections.

Horning *et al.* [60] looked at the effect of tacrolimus crossover therapy (instead of cyclosporin) for persistent or recurrent acute rejections in 14 lung transplant patients. Tacrolimus switch was performed 238±180 days after transplantation. The number of acute rejection episodes significantly decreased from 4.4±2.1 to 0.4±0.5, whilst the average histological grade of rejection, as well as the incidence of acute rejection, also significantly declined [60].

Since then, numerous authors have reported a reduction in acute rejection and the refractory acute rejection rate, after switching from CsA to tacrolimus [61–64].

In another prospective study using either cyclosporin or tacrolimus as initial therapy, it was demonstrated that the acute rejection rate in the first postoperative year was 1.18 in the tacrolimus group *versus* 1.5 in the cyclosporin group ($p<0.05$), however, there was a higher incidence of diabetes mellitus and renal insufficiency in the tacrolimus group [65]. In a follow-up randomised, prospective two-centre study, it was demonstrated that initial immunosuppressive therapy with tacrolimus resulted in a lower number of acute rejection episodes (0.225 *versus* 0.426 per 100 patient-days, $p<0.05$) compared with cyclosporin based therapy, both in combination with MMF and corticosteroids, although there was no difference in the 6 and 12 months freedom from acute rejection between the two treatments [66].

It seems, therefore, that tacrolimus based initial immunosuppressive therapy may have some beneficial effects over cyclosporin based initial therapy, in addition to the acute rejection rate on the occurrence of BO/BOS. However, most of these studies have too low a power to exclude statistical errors. In that respect, a large multicentre, investigator driven trial has been started to compare tacrolimus *versus* cyclosporin as initial therapy in combination with MMF; however, results are not yet available [67].

## *The role of cytolytic induction therapy*

In a retrospective study comprising of 24 unilateral lung transplant patients, Ross *et al.* [68] investigated the effect of induction therapy with OKT3 (10–14 days) compared with Minnesota Antilymphocyte globulin (MALG, 5–7 days) with regards to the development of BOS. The group found no significant difference in the incidence of BOS, however, the latency until development of BOS stage 1 was significantly longer in the OKT3 group than with the MALG group (354±85 *versus* 962±65 days; $p<0.001$). One patient from the OKT3 group developed an Ebstein Barr virus (EBV)-associated post-transplant lymphoproliferative disease [68]. Another study reported a limited incidence of acute rejections using OKT3 as induction therapy; however since there was no control group these data are difficult to interpret [69].

Reichenspurner *et al.* [70] compared rATG and OKT3 induction therapies in 184 in heart-lung transplant patients. In 68 patients OKT3 ($5\ mg\cdot day^{-1}$) was used for 14 days, whereas 116 patients were treated with rATG for 5 days. The outcome parameter of their study was the acute rejection rate. In fact, the linearised rate of acute rejection per 100 patient-days was significantly higher in the OKT3 group *versus* the rATG group (1.16 *versus* 0.49; $p<0.0002$). At the same time, the incidence of infections was also lower in the rATG group [70].

In a retrospective study by Wiebe *et al.* [71] induction therapy with rATG was compared with no induction with rATG in 147 heart-lung transplant patients. There was no difference in the freedom of BOS between the two groups, although there was a tendency towards a lower incidence of BOS at 2 yrs post-transplantation in the group that had received rATG.

In another single-centre, randomised, prospective study, 44 single and double-lung transplant recipients were included to receive conventional immunosuppressive therapy with or without concomitant rATG induction therapy for 3 days. There was a significant reduction in the number of acute rejections (incidence of 23% *versus* 55%; p=0.03) in the rATG group, with a nonsignificant reduction in the incidence of BO/BOS at the conclusion of the study. There was no difference in the incidence of infections and malignancies, or in the actuarial survival at 6, 12 and 24 months [72].

Comparing daclizumab, an IL-2 receptor blocker, as induction therapy with historical controls, GARRITY *et al.* [73] demonstrated a reduction in the number of grade 2 or higher acute rejection incidences during the first 6 months after transplantation (18% in the daclizumab group *versus* 48% in the control group; p<0.04 ) [73]. In a paediatric lung transplant population, daclizumab increased the 6 months freedom from acute rejection from 43% in the control group to 70% in the daclizumab group, without increasing the incidence of infectious episodes [74].

Only one study has compared the three different induction therapies, rATG, OKT3 and daclizumab, and concluded that in all three drug regimens there was no significant difference in the freedom from acute rejection or BO/BOS [75].

Although it is accepted that the number of acute rejection episodes following transplantation can be reduced by cytolytic therapy, it is still debated whether there is an effect on the prevalence of chronic rejection and it is now accepted that these therapies may increase the rate of infection and might aggravate the reperfusion injury of the transplanted lung. As a consequence, some centres have abolished cytolytic induction therapy. From the present contradictory studies it is therefore not quite clear whether this has a real impact on the acute rejection rate and on the incidence of BO/BOS.

## *Total lymphoid irradiation*

An alternative immunomodulating strategy that has been applied for the management of RAR and BOS is total lymphoid irradiation (TLI). The administration of ionising radiation, in the form of high-dose TLI induced a sustained impairment in cell-mediated immune responses in patients with Hodgkin's disease [76], leading to a prolonged reduction in the lymphocyte proliferative response and the mixed lymphocyte response. Since the initial regimes applied were restricted by unacceptable, severe bone marrow suppression and gastro-intestinal toxicity, TLI regimens have subsequently been optimised, and TLI is currently administered as ten fractions of 0.80-Gy (mid-plane dose), twice weekly for 5 weeks, administered with a 6-million electron volt (MeV) linear accelerator using an anterior-posterior opposed technique per treatment, for a total prescribed dose of 8-Gy. The radiation is administered concurrently in upper (mantle) and lower (inverted Y) fields as described by HUNT *et al.* [77]. The mantle field includes exposure of the middle and lower cervical, supraclavicular, axillary, infraclavicular, mediastinal, and pulmonary hilar lymph nodes, and the thymus. The lower inverted Y field includes exposure of the para-aortic, iliac, and inguinal-femoral lymph nodes and the spleen. In young females, the inverted Y field is truncated, avoiding the inguinal-femoral and most of the iliac nodes, to avoid irradiating the ovaries. Azathioprin, or mycophenolate mofetil are temporarily discontinued during the course of TLI, and reinstituted on completion of therapy once the white blood cell count >3,000 cells·$mm^{-3}$. Individual treatments are postponed if the total white blood cell count falls <3,000·$mm^{-3}$.

TLI has been applied since the 1980s in the management of recurrent acute rejection in heart transplantation [77], and has been noted to be effective in the management of recurrent or persistent rejection after heart transplantation [78] with efficacy equivalent to methotrexate [79] or tacrolimus [80].

VALENTINE *et al.* [81] reported the use of TLI in the management of recurrent acute rejection in heart-lung transplant and lung transplant recipients. Six patients with persistent rejection, unresponsive to high-dose steroid therapy, were treated with 800 cGy of TLI during a 5-week period. TLI was started at a mean of 142 (37–707) days post-transplant. Three patients died between 28 and 457 days after the TLI due to severe rejection or BOS. Two patients have been free from acute rejection with a reversal of the morphological changes, for >4 yrs, and another patient had stable BO some 4 yrs later. The group reported no directly related, serious complications associated with TLI, although one patient developed adult respiratory distress syndrome (ARDS) 1 week following treatment with TLI. Although TLI appeared to confer a degree of protection against cellular rejection in that series, TLI was not associated with a reduction in the subsequent development of BOS.

### *Inhaled corticosteroids*

TAKAO *et al.* [82] investigated the effects of nebulised budesonide on acute and chronic lung function in heart-lung transplant patients. A total of 14 heart-lung transplant patients with three or more episodes of acute rejection within any 3-month period, or who had steroid-resistant acute rejection were included in a prospective, open, randomised, parallel group study. Seven patients received 2 mg inhaled budesonide *b.i.d.* for 1 yr in addition to their current immunosuppressive therapy. The other seven patients received no additional medication and comprised the control group. The number of acute rejection episodes in the budesonide group was lower than in the control group, although this did not reach significance. In the budesonide group, neither BO nor lung function deterioration has been found, whereas three patients from the control group developed BO.

If lymphocytic bronchiolitis is accepted as a manifestation of acute rejection [83], then DE SOYZA *et al.* [84] demonstrated that inhaled budesonide is able to reverse the decrease in $FEV_1$ and the increase in eNO, accompanying lymphocytic bronchiolitis.

### *Extracorporeal photochemotherapy*

In ancient Egypt a plant growing along the Nile called *Ammi majus*, was used for medical purposes. In 1953, LERNER *et al.* [85] showed that the active ingredient of *Ammi majus* is 8-methoxypsoralen (8-MOP) and that the effect is obtained in conjunction with exposure to sunlight [85]. From this observation the concept of psoralen-ultaviolet light-A therapy (oral ingestion of psoralen followed by UV-A irradiation) was developed to treat skin diseases like psoriasis. In 1987, EDELSON *et al.* [86] showed that T-lymphocytes are sensitive to 8-(MOP) and UV-A irradiation [87]. From there, extracorporeal photochemotherapy (ECP) was developed. The first clinical application of ECP was in the treatment of cutaneous T-cell lymphoma or Sezary-syndrome. Due to its low toxicity and its selective effects on pathogenic T-cell clones ECP has also been used in the treatment of nonmalignant immunological disorders. Today, various reports on ECP applied for diseases such as systemic sclerosis [88], rheumatic arthritis [89], systemic lupus erythematosus, atopic dermatitis, multiple sclerosis, rejection and graft *versus* host disease after solid organ and bone marrow transplantation, respectively, do exist.

The technique of ECP is rather simple. A standard apheresis with separation and reinfusion of red blood cells on one hand and a collection of plasma and buffy coat on the other, is performed. The basic procedure has gone through slight modifications since it was first introduced. First, the photoactive substance 8-MOP was given systemically by oral intake. Today, the drug is delivered directly into the collected plasma-buffy coat fraction [90]. In each treatment 140–240 mL of buffy coat is collected, containing enriched lymphocyte solution of 1-6×10$^9$ cells. A total of 200 μg of 8-MOP is injected into the bag with the white cells. The cell solution is then exposed to UV-A light (2 J·cm$^{-1}$·cell$^{-1}$) for 10–90 min depending on the instrument used, and reinfused into the patient. Patients are usually treated on two consecutive days at 2–4 week intervals. Side effects are minimal if at all.

The largest study so far has been performed in cardiac transplant recipients. BARR *et al.* [91] reported on 60 patients treated in 12 centres, randomly assigned after heart transplantation to standard triple immunosuppressive therapy (cyclosporin, azathioprine, prednisone) alone or in conjunction with ECP. The ECP group received a total of 24 ECP treatments, each pair given on two consecutive days during the first 6 months after transplantation. In the ECP group the risk of graft rejection was significantly decreased without increasing the incidence of infection. Moreover, in the nine participating USA centres cytomegalovirus (CMV) DNA in the plasma detected by PCR was significantly reduced in the ECP group compared with the standard therapy group, suggesting that this therapy has a direct antiviral effect [92]

In contrast to this study in which ECP was used in a prophylactic concept *de novo* after transplantation, there are also reports of ECP being applied for the treatment of acute cardiac rejection [93–95], recurrent cardiac rejection [96] and refractory acute cardiac rejection [97]. In addition to the beneficial effects of ECP on acute cardiac rejection, BARR *et al.* [98] also showed that prophylactic ECP was able to decrease chronic allograft dysfunction. The group showed that ECP was able to reduce levels of panel reactive antibodies within the first 6 months and to significantly decrease graft arteriopathy (reduction of graft intimal hyperplasia measured by intracoronary ultrasound) at 1 and 2 yrs post-transplant [98].

The possible role of ECP, in acute lung rejection, has only been documented in one case report. The patient presented with a simultaneous infection and acute rejection and institution of anti-infectious therapy together with ECP, resulting in resolution of the acute rejection [99].

### *Other drug therapy for acute rejection*

In a study by CAHILL *et al.* [100], 12 patients with steroid-resistant acute rejection were treated with methotrexate during 6 weeks. In 82% of the patients there were no more acute rejections during a follow-up of 12.5 months. In two of the patients an acute rejection recurred; however, in both cases they responded to high-dose steroid therapy.

Also ganciclovir prophylaxis has been demonstrated to delay the onset of BO. In this study the development of BO was significantly delayed in the group of heart-lung transplant patients who received ganciclovir prophylaxis (1,072±280 days in the prophylaxis group *versus* 432±189 days in the no prophylaxis group; $p<0.01$) [101]. This has also been confirmed in a rat trachea allograft model, in which ganciclovir prophylaxis inhibited CMV induced tracheal obliteration probably *via* an inhibitory effect on IL-2 and TNF-α release [102].

## Medical treatment of established bronchiolitis obliterans and bronchiolitis obliterans syndrome

As previously discussed, there is a major problem in interpreting studies on the medical treatment of chronic rejection after lung transplantation. Most of the studies have looked at a change of the maintenance immunosuppressive regimen. It had already become apparent in 1987 that augmentation of immunosuppression could lead to an apparent arrest of the BO/BOS evolution. In this particular paper, GLANVILLE *et al.* [103] described the effects of addition of azathioprin in heart-lung transplantation patients with BO. After the institution of azathioprin, the rate of decline in $FEF_{25-75\%}$ improved considerably. Since then, several drugs and experimental therapies have been investigated with regard to their effect on the decline in $FEV_1$ in BO/BOS patients. These different regimens will now be discussed further.

## *Role of tacrolimus*

Several authors have investigated the effect of switching from cyclosporin to tacrolimus in heart-lung transplant patients with progressive BO/BOS [104–110]. All studies were open, nonrandomised and without control groups. They all come to the same conclusion, which was that after the switch, there is an arrest in decline of the $FEV_1$ in about 50–90% of the patients. It is also clear from these papers that the sooner, in the BO/BOS evolution, the conversion is instituted, the better the results might be. In a retrospective study, VERLEDEN *et al.* [34] confirmed the arrest in the decline in $FEV_1$ in lung transplant patients with BO/BOS after conversion from cyclosporin to tacrolimus. However, this was accompanied by a concomitant decrease in the eNO values, suggesting that tacrolimus also has more pronounced anti-inflammatory effects when compared with cyclosporin.

In a retrospective clinical trial in 125 patients from 13 international centres that were switched from CsA to tacrolimus due to RAR (group 1) or BOS (group 2), KLEPETKO *et al.* [64] showed a remarkable reduction in the number of acute rejection episodes (group 1). In patients that were switched due to BOS (group 2) a dramatic effect with a marked reduction in the rate of $FEV_1$ decline was evident. The decline in $FEV_1$ was significantly less in the months after conversion for single lung transplant recipients as well as for bilateral lung transplant recipients ($p<0.01$).

## *Effect of mycophenolate mofetil*

A total of 13 patients with BO were treated with MMF (1.5 g *b.i.d.*) for between 1 week to 24 months. After the initiation of MMF, the $FEV_1$ decline arrested in 10 patients, whereas two patients died of progressive disease. Seven patients experienced gastro-intestinal side effects and one patient developed a fungal infection [111]. SPEICH *et al.* [112] had a similar experience, although they specifically pointed out that the MMF dose seemed to be very important. The group observed that the reduction of MMF from 3 to 2 $g \cdot day^{-1}$ resulted in the deterioration of the lung function, whereas increasing the dose again to 3 $g \cdot day^{-1}$ improved the pulmonary function data. ROMAN *et al.* [113] reported that switching from cyclosporin and azathioprin to tacrolimus and MMF arrested the decline in or improved $FEV_1$ in three out of 12 patients and six out of 12 patients respectively. Only two patients had a progressive decline in $FEV_1$ after switch. DUPONT *et al.* [114] switched 16 lung transplant patients with established BO/BOS from azathioprin to MMF at a mean of 1,348±888 days following lung transplantation and demonstrated a significant reduction of the mean rate of decline of the $FEV_1$ per month after this conversion (from -1.3±1.4% of baseline $FEV_1$/month to +0.4±1.6%, $p<0.05$)

### *Inhaled steroids*

WHITFORD *et al.* [115] performed a 3-month randomised, double blind, placebo controlled trial of 750 µg fluticasone propionate (FP) *b.i.d.* in 30 clinically stable lung transplant recipients, with 20 of the patients completing a 2-yr long-term study of the incidence of BOS. This cohort was without pre-existing airflow limitation and were not selected according to evidence of airway inflammation. There were no beneficial effects of FP treatment on airway inflammation, airflow limitation or incidence of BOS demonstrable. This study followed on from a previous published report, limited to short-term effects of inhaled corticosteroids (ICS) treatment, in the same patient group, which was also negative [116].

In the most recent data from this centre, a parallel group study was performed, in which 3 months treatment with inhaled chlorofluoro carbon (CFC) driven beclomethasone dipropionate 400 µg *b.i.d.*, (CFC-beclomethasone dipropionate: BDP), was compared with a device designed to promote small airway deposition of ICS (HFS driven beclomethasone 200 µg *b.i.d.*: HFS-BDP [117]). In this study allograft recipients were selected on the basis of having a raised eNO or a transbronchial biopsy diagnosis of lymphocytic bronchiolitis. Indices of airway inflammation, airway remodelling and physiology were monitored with serial lung function testing, eNO measurement, transbronchial biopsy and BAL. In this negative study, BAL cell counts and eNO were not significantly changed after 3 months of treatment in either arm. No effect of inhaled steroids was seen on controlling markers of airway inflammation and airway physiology in lung transplant recipients. In addition there was no effect of ICS on small airway reticular basement membrane thickening. In summary there is limited and conflicting data regarding the efficacy of supplementing standard immunosuppression with ICS, with experience to date indicating only equivocal benefit. BOS shares some pathophysiological features with asthma and chronic obstructive pulmonary disease (COPD) and it may be that, as has been postulated for COPD, ICS could be of benefit in a subset of patients. Further randomised controlled trials are required to add to what is at present inadequate literature.

### *Other drug regimens*

Patients suffering from chronic rejection and not showing any improvement after switch of immunosuppression to tacrolimus or MMF based regimens, can hardly be treated sufficiently. Attempts using methotrexate or cyclophosphamide have only been successful in a very few patients, carrying the risk for neoplastic disorders and/or severe infectious complications. DUSMET *et al.* [118] treated 10 patients with persistent or progressive BO/BOS with methotrexate after the failure of conventional therapy (pulse steroids, antilymphocyte products or both) to improve the $FEV_1$. Two patients had no further decline in $FEV_1$, five patients had a reduction of only $\leq 10\%$, and only one patient derived no benefit at all.

VERLEDEN *et al.* [119] treated seven patients who had chronic lung rejection with cyclophosphamide. During a mean follow-up of 21±8 months, the $FEV_1$ increased in five of these patients, whereas there was an arrest in the decline of the $FEV_1$ in another two of the patients. Only one patient died of progressive BO/BOS 18 months after the introduction of cyclophosphamide.

Using commercially available rATG that was initiated at a mean of 657±323 days after lung transplantation in 10 patients with BO/BOS, SNELL *et al.* [120] demonstrated that nine patients responded with a decrease in the decline of their $FEV_1$. This effect was sustained over a follow-up period of 310±110 days. KESTEN *et al.* [121] used antilymphocyte globulin or rATG in 15 patients with BO/BOS. There was an improvement of the $FEV_1$ in only two patients, whereas five remained unchanged and eight deteriorated further [121]. DATE *et al.* [122] treated 48 patients with chronic lung rejection with one of the following: antilymphocyte globulin; antithymocyte globulin; or OKT3. They concluded that the mean decrement in lung function was significantly reduced in the 3 months after the therapy, but the stage of BOS nevertheless progressed over time with only four patients remaining in a lower BOS stage 2 yrs after the treatment.

The potential effect of aerosolised cyclosporin has already been investigated in animal models in the early 1990s where it was shown to prevent and reduce acute allograft rejection [123, 124]. In 1996 the first clinical study in lung transplant patients with chronic rejection was published demonstrating the usefulness of this delivery mode of cyclosporin. From the nine patients with BO/BOS in whom it was used, there were seven responders who experienced a stabilisation in their pulmonary function compared with nine historical control patients who further deteriorated, suggesting that this therapy may be effective for refractory chronic rejection [125]. Later on, it was also demonstrated to be effective in refractory acute rejection. In fact in 14 of the 16 patients who tolerated the treatment (two had to be withdrawn because of side-effects) there was a significant reduction in the acute rejection rate per 100 patient-days after a mean of 37 days of aerosolised cyclosporin treatment (from $2.49 \pm 0.68$ to $0.72 \pm 0.30$ episodes) [126].

Rapamycin as a new antiproliferative drug has successfully been used after liver and kidney transplantation. There is experimental evidence that it may have positive influence on the course of BO [127]. In a recently published study by CAHILL *et al.* [128], sirolimus was utilised in 12 patients with BO/BOS. For this group the decline in pulmonary function was not affected by the addition of sirolimus. However, among individuals with rapidly declining pulmonary mechanics, sirolimus resulted in stabilisation or improvement in pulmonary function. Larger studies and more experience with the use of rapamycin after lung transplantation will reveal the potential effect on BO in the future.

Recently, promising results have been published by using azithromycin, a macrolide antibiotic, as adjunctive treatment to the current immunosuppressive therapy in patients with BOS. In fact five out of six patients in the paper by GERHARDT *et al.* [129] significantly improved their $FEV_1$ (mean increase of 17.1%) after 13.7 weeks treatment. These results have been corroborated by VERLEDEN *et al.* [130] who treated 10 lung transplant patients with established BOS by the addition of azithromycin. The mean improvement of the $FEV_1$ was 16.3% after 12 weeks and remained stable in four patients with a follow up of nine months [130].

## *Other treatment modalities: total lymphoid irradiation and extracorporeal photochemotherapy*

CHACON *et al.* [131] have previously reported the benefits of TLI treatment in 12 subjects with BOS. Although the individual response to TLI was variable, the administration of TLI resulted in a significant slowing in the rate of decline in lung function. A partial recovery of function was noted in certain individuals. An uncontrolled retrospective study by MELVILLE *et al.* [132] compared TLI with a switch from cyclosporin to tacrolimus in the management of BOS. In this series, 11 patients were converted from cyclosporin to tacrolimus as treatment of BOS, leading to a significant reduction in the decline in $FEV_1$ from $-0.13\ L \cdot month^{-1}$ prior to treatment compared to $-0.02\ L \cdot month^{-1}$ afterwards. This compared with a cohort of 20 patients who received treatment with TLI for BOS resulting in a significant median reduction in the fall in $FEV_1$ from -0.13 $L \cdot month^{-1}$ (pre-TLI treatment) to -0.015 (afterwards). Both tacrolimus and TLI were noted to be significantly beneficial in slowing the decline in $FEV_1$ associated with BOS.

FISHER *et al.* [133] have recently reviewed data from a cohort of 37 recipients treated with TLI for progressive BOS between 1988 and 2001 (13 single, 12 bilateral, and 12 heart-lung transplants). BOS was diagnosed at a median of 18 months post-transplant, with BOS grades at the time of TLI being BOS stage 1 (7), BOS stage 2 (14), and BOS stage 3 (16), and a mean $FEV_1$ prior to TLI of 1.32 $L \cdot min^{-1}$. Ten subjects did not complete scheduled TLI treatment: two died early due to respiratory failure; eight were prematurely stopped due to minor marrow suppression or infectious complications; and two patients (5%) had a serious infectious complication. The mean duration of TLI treatment was 62.8 days. The mean rate of decline in $FEV_1$ was -0.123 $L \cdot month^{-1}$ prior to TLI and -0.025 $L \cdot month^{-1}$ following TLI. TLI was well tolerated, with a low incidence of serious side effects, and resulted in a significant reduction in the decline in $FEV_1$ [133]. No immediate life-threatening complications have been described in connection with TLI treatment. The immunosuppressive effects of low dose TLI have been associated with leucopaenia, necessitating adjustments in the maintenance dose of azathioprin. Earlier studies reported an increased incidence of viral infections, including disseminated herpes simplex and CMV pneumonitis. Concerns were raised regarding the risks of increased malignancies; however, this remains anecdotal, although further studies of the potential long-term effects of TLI in the development of malignancy are necessary.

Although the current studies are retrospective and not controlled, the evidence suggests that TLI is safe, well-tolerated and provides effective and prolonged immunosuppression in the management of aggressive BOS. TLI may be of particular benefit in patients suspected of medication noncompliance, assisting the achievement of long-term immunosuppression. Whereas switching from cyclosporin to tacrolimus is a suitable choice in compliant patients, treatment with TLI may be of particular benefit in subjects suspected of medication noncompliance. The proximity of patients to centres specialising in the administration of TLI is another factor that needs to be incorporated into the choice of therapy. As patients receiving treatment with TLI require twice weekly administration of radiotherapy, blood count monitoring, and possible treatment of infectious complications, this may necessitate residing close to the transplant centre for the duration of TLI. Patients living in remote areas, distant from centres experienced in the administration of TLI, may prefer alternative treatment strategies, as discussed above.

Compared with cardiac transplantation experience with ECP in lung transplantation is still scarce. SLOVIS *et al.* [134] described three lung transplant recipients with BO who had stabilisation of airflow obstruction after the use of ECP. SALERNO *et al.* [135] reported on eight patients with BO of whom seven were in BOS grade 3 before start of ECP therapy. In five out of eight patients stabilisation of $FEV_1$ under ECP occurred. In two patients histological reversal of concomittant acute rejection was documented. After a median follow-up of 36 months seven patients were still alive and doing well. VILLANUEVA *et al.* [136] published their experience in 14 patients with BO. Three with concurrent acute rejection responded with resolution of acute rejection. The group demonstrated that seven of the eight patients with lower BOS stages (0 and 1) remained alive (one died from lung cancer), whilst two progressed to BOS stage 2. Conversely, from the six patients with BOS stages 2 or 3, four died of BOS. Here again, it seems that early treatment with ECP provided better results than treatment of higher BOS stages. O'HAGAN *et al.* [137] reported on five paediatric patients with refractory BO of whom four out of five temporarily stabilised their lung function while on ECP.

In the Zürich Lung Transplant Center, ECP has been used since 1998. Current indications include recurrent rejection after acute rejection, onset of BOS, EBV risk constellation (recipient negative, donor positive), and ECP as adjunct therapy in paediatric transplantation. The results so far are encouraging (A. Boehler, Zurich, Switzerland). In brief 21 patients have been treated with ECP from four in 1998 to nine in 2002. Amongst these, five patients were included because of recurrent acute rejection and showed no further rejection after ECP. In three out of the four patients with BOS, $FEV_1$ was stabilised. To date none of the four patients treated for EBV mismatch, has developed lymphoproliferative disease and all three children were in stable conditions with preserved lung function.

### *Retransplantation*

If all other therapeutic options fail, some patients might be considered for retransplantation. This may already pose an ethical problem: because of the donor organ shortage, it is still debated whether retransplantation should be a real therapeutic option in patients with unremitting chronic rejection after lung transplantation [138]. In the recent ISHLT registry, only 1.8% of all lung transplantations are retransplants. Half of these retransplants were performed because of chronic rejection [2].

In the largest cohort so far reported [139], 230 retransplantations from 47 lung transplant programmes have been included. Indications for retransplantations were: chronic rejection in 146 patients; acute graft failure in 52; intractable airway complications in 14; histologically confirmed severe rejection in nine; and miscellaneous conditions in nine. The overall actuarial survival of retransplantation was 47% at 1 yr, which is far beyond the 1-yr survival after a first transplantation, although patients undergoing retransplantation for BO/BOS had a significantly better survival when a centre-adjusted analysis was performed. It also became clear from this data that a longer interval between the first transplantation and the retransplantation operation (especially >2 yrs) was associated with a better survival. The prevalence of chronic rejection after retransplantation for BO/BOS was comparable to the one after a first transplantation, although a higher prevalence of BO/BOS has been demonstrated after a retransplantation in the Hannover experience [140]. It was concluded that the best intermediate-term functional results occurred in more experienced centres, in nonventilated patients and in patients undergoing retransplantation >2 yrs after the first transplantation [141].

## Conclusion

Diagnosis of chronic rejection after lung transplantation still mainly relies on pulmonary function evolution, especially $FEV_1$, nowadays in combination with $FEF_{25-75\%}$ values. The possible role of various surrogate markers for the early diagnosis of chronic rejection is very promising, although more studies are necessary to establish their particular role.

Once chronic rejection has developed, early switch to other immunosuppressive regimens seems imperative, with better results obtained in the lower BOS stages. This can be accompanied by other treatment modalities such as ECP and TLI. Retransplantation may be a valuable option for strictly selected patients in whom other therapeutic modalities fail.

It is hoped, however, that the newer immunosuppressive agents or preventive treatments will be able to reduce the number of acute rejection episodes, which is still the most important risk factor for the development of chronic rejection. With this being achieved, the incidence of chronic rejection might fall in the coming years leading to a better long-term survival and quality of life.

## Summary

Bronchiolitis obliterans (BO) or bronchiolitis obliterans syndrome (BOS) is now regarded as a manifestation of chronic allograft rejection or dysfunction. The patient with BO/BOS presents with increasing symptoms of functional limitation, cough, dyspnoea and recurrent infections. Transbronchial biopsies are not very sensitive for the diagnosis of chronic rejection, that is why the diagnosis is usually based on the flow-volume curve which shows a typical progressive air flow obstruction, for which no other cause can be found.. Recently, several so called surrogate markers for early diagnosis of BO/BOS have been investigated and will be discussed in this chapter. Finally, an overview of the existing treatment modalities for this debilitating condition is given, with specific emphasis on the shift in immunosuppressive drug regimen, which may lead to an arrest in the decline of the pulmonary function parameters. Also some newer (renewed) treatment modalities such as extracorporeal photochemotherapy and total lymphoid irradiation will be discussed.



**Keywords:** Bronchiolitis obliterans syndrome, chronic rejection, bronchiolitis obliterans, treatment.

*Acknowledgements.* Other co-authors of Working Group 1 include: J. Egan, D. Israel-Biet, M. Reynaud-Gaubert, G.C. Riise, L. Sharples, S. Stewart, B. Vanaudenaerde, W. van der Bij, J. Lordan, W. Wuyts.


## References


1. Van den Berg JW, Geertsma A, van der Bij W, *et al.* Bronchiolitis obliterans syndrome after lung transplantation and health-related quality of life. *Am J Respir Crit Care Med* 2000; 161: 1937–1941.
2. Trulock EP, Edwards LB, Taylor DO, *et al.* The registry of the International Society for Heart and Lung Transplantation: twentieth official adult heart-lung report – 2003. *J Heart Lung Transplant* 2003; 22: 625–635.
3. Valentine VG, Robbins RC, Berry GJ, *et al.* Actuarial survival of heart-lung and bilateral lung transplant recipients with bronchiolitis obliterans. *J Heart Lung Transplant* 1996; 15: 371–383.
4. Reichenspurner H, Girgis RE, Robbins RC, *et al.* Obliterative bronchiolitis after lung and heart-lung transplantation. *Ann Thorac Surg* 1995; 60: 1845–1853.
5. Pomerance A, Madden B, Burke MM, Yacoub MH. Transbronchial biopsy in heart and lung transplantation: clinicopathologic correlations. *J Heart Lung Transplant* 1995; 14: 761–763.
6. Kramer MR, Stoehr C, Wang JL, *et al.* The diagnosis of obliterative bronchiolitis after heart-lung and lung transplantation: low yield of transbronchial biopsies. *J Heart Lung Transplant* 1993; 12: 675–681.
7. Cooper JD, Billingham M, Egan T, *et al.* A working formulation for the standardisation of nomenclature and for clinical staging of chronic dysfunction in lung allografts. *J Heart Lung Transplant* 1993; 12: 713–716.
8. Verleden GM, Egan J, Israel-Biet D, *et al.* Chronic lung allograft rejection: prevalence, pathology, risk factors and pathophysiology. *Eur Respir Monograph* 2004; 29: 1–18.
9. Estenne M, Maurer J, Boehler A, *et al.* Bronchiolitis obliterans syndrome 2001: an update of the diagnostic criteria. *J Heart Lung Transplant* 2002; 21: 297–310.
10. Patterson GM, Wilson S, Whang JL, *et al.* Physiologic definitions of obliterative bronchiolitis in heart-lung and double lung transplantation: a comparison of the forced expiratory flow between

25% and 75% of the forced vital capacity and forced expiratory volume in one second. *J Heart Lung Transplant* 1996; 15: 175–181.

11. Reynaud-Gaubert M, Thomas P, Badier M, Cau P, Giudicelli R, Fuentes P. Early detection of airway involvement in obliterative bronchiolitis after lung transplantation. Functional and bronchoalveolar lavage findings. *Am J Respir Crit Care Med* 2000; 161: 1924–1929.
12. Ouwens JP, van der Mark TW, Koëter GH, de Boer J, Grevink RG, van der Bij W. Bronchiolar airflow impairment after lung transplantation: an early and common manifestation. *J Heart Lung Transplant* 2002; 21: 1056–1061.
13. Kelly K, Hertz MI. Obliterative bronchiolitis. *Clin Chest Med* 1997; 18: 319–337.
14. Ikonen T, Kivisaari L, Taskinen E, Piilonen A, Harjula AL. High-resolution CT in long-term follow-up after lung transplantation. *Chest* 1997; 111: 370–376.
15. Worthy SA, Park CS, Kim JS, Muller NL. Bronchiolitis obliterans after lung transplantation: high-resolution CT findings in 15 patients. *Am J Roentgenol* 1997; 169: 673–677.
16. Leung AN, Fisher K, Valentine V, *et al.* Bronchiolitis obliterans after lung transplantation: detection using expiratory HRCT. *Chest* 1998; 113: 365–370.
17. Bankier AA, Van Muylem A, Knoop C, Estenne M, Gevenois PA. Bronchiolitis obliterans syndrome in heart-lung transplant recipients: diagnosis with expiratory CT. *Radiology* 2001; 218: 533–539.
18. Knollmann FD, Ewert R, Wundrich T, Hetzer R, Felix R. Bronchiolitis obliterans syndrome in lung transplant recipients: use of spirometrically gated CT. *Radiology* 2002; 225: 655–662.
19. Lee E-S, Gotway MB, Reddy GP, Golden JA, Keith FM, Webb WR. Early bronchiolitis obliterans follwing lung transplantation. *Radiology* 2000; 216: 472–477.
20. Millet WT jr, Kotlof RM, Blumenthal NP, Aronchick JM, Gefter WB, Miller WT. Utility of high resolution computed tomography in predicting bronchiolitis obliterans syndrome following lung transplantation: preliminary findings. *J Thorac Imaging* 2001; 16: 76–80.
21. Bankier AA, Van Muylem A, Scillia P, De Maertelaer V, Estenne M, Gevenois PA. Air trapping in heart lung transplant recipients: variability of anatomical distribution and extent on sequential expiratory thin-section CT. *Radiology* 2003; 229: 737–742.
22. Buist AS, Ross BB. Quantitative analysis of the alveolar plateau in the diagnosis of early airway obstruction. *Am Rev Respir Dis* 1973; 108: 1078–1087.
23. Cosio MH, Ghezzo JC, Hogg R, *et al.* The relations between structural changes in small airways and pulmonary-function tests. *N Engl J Med* 1978; 298: 1277–1281.
24. Paiva M, Engel LZA. Theoretical studies of gas mixing and ventilation distribution in the lung. *Physiol Rev* 1987; 67: 750–796.
25. Verbanck S, Schuermans A, Van Muylem A, *et al.* Conductive and acinar lung zone contribution to ventilation inhomogeneity in COPD. *Am J Respir Crit Care Med* 1998; 157: 1573–1577.
26. Estenne M, Van Muylem A, Knoop C, Antoine M. Detection of obliterative bronchiolitis after lung transplantation by indexes of ventilation distribution. *Am J Respir Crit Care Med.* 2000; 162: 1047–1051.
27. Reynaud-Gaubert M, Thomas P, Badier M, Cau P, Giudicelli R, Fuentes P. Early detection of airway involvement in obliterative bronchioltiis after lung transplantation. Functional and bronchoalveolar lavage cell findings. *Am J Respir Crit Care Med* 2000; 161: 1924–1929.
28. Arens R, McDonough M, Zhao H, Blumenthal NP, Kotloff RM, Grunstein MM. Altered lung mechanics after double-lung transplantation. *Am J Respir Crit Care Med* 1998; 158: 1403–1409.
29. Fisher AJ, Gabbay E, Small T, Doig S, Dark JH, Corris PA. Cross sectional study of exhaled nitric oxide levels following lung transplantation. *Thorax* 1998; 53: 454–458.
30. Verleden GM, Dupont LJ, Lamont J, *et al.* Is there a role for measuring exhaled nitric oxide in lung transplant recipients with chronic rejection? *J Heart Lung Transplant* 1998; 17: 231–232.
31. Gabbay E, Walters EH, Orsida B, *et al.* Post-lung transplant bronchiolitis obliterans syndrome is characterized by increased exhaled nitric oxide levels and epithelial inducible nitric oxide synthase. *Am J Respir Crit Care Med* 2000; 162: 2182–2187.
32. Verleden GM, Dupont LJ, Delcroix M, *et al.* Exhaled nitric oxide after lung transplantation: impact of the native lung. *Eur Respir J* 2003; 21: 429–432.

33. Verleden GM, Delcroix M, Buyse B, Dupont L and the Leuven Lung Transplant Group. Exhaled NO after lung transplantation: a prospective study. *J Heart Lung Transplant* 2001; 20: 208.
34. Verleden GM, Dupont LJ, Van Raemdonck D, Vanhaecke J. The effect of switching cyclosporine A to tacrolimus on exhaled nitric oxide and pulmonary function in patients with chronic rejection after lung transplantation. *J Heart Lung Transplant* 2003; 22: 908–913.
35. Verleden GM, Dupont LJ, Delcroix M, Van Raemdonck DE and the Leuven lung Transplant Group. Accuracy of exhaled NO measurements for the diagnosis of chronic rejection after lung transplant. *J Heart Lung Transplant* 2003; 22: Suppl. 1, S182–S183.
36. Otulana BA, Higenbottam T, Ferrari L, Scott J, Igboaka G, Wallwork J. The use of home spirometry in detecting acute lung rejection and infection following heart-lung transplantation. *Chest* 1990; 97: 353–357.
37. Bjortuft O, Johansen B, Boe J, Foerster A, Holter F, Geiran O. Daily home spirometry facilitates early detection of rejection in single lung transplant recipients with emphysema. *Eur Respir J* 1993; 6: 705–708.
38. Finkelstein SM, Snyder M, Stibbe CE, *et al.* Staging of bronchioitis obliterans using home spirometry. *Chest* 1999; 116: 120–126.
39. Wagner FM, Weber A, Park JW, *et al.* New telemetric system for daily pulmonary function surveillance of lung transplant recipients. *Ann Thorac Surg* 1999; 68: 2033–2038.
40. Morlion B, Knoop C, Pavia M, Estenne M. Internet-based home monitoring of pulmonary function after lung transplantation. *Am J Respir Crit Care Med* 2002; 165: 694–697.
41. Stanbrook MB, Kesten S. Bronchial hyperreactivity after lung transplantation predicts early bronchiolitis obliterans. *Am J Respir Crit Care Med* 1999; 160: 2034–2039.
42. Dupont LJ, Rochette F, Demedts MG, Verleden GM. Exhaled nitric oxide correlates with airway hyperresponsiveness in steroid-naïve patients with mild asthma. *Am J Respir Crit Care Med* 1998; 157: 894–898.
43. Reynaud-Gaubert M, Marin V, Thirion X, *et al.* Upregulation of chemokines in bronchoalveolar lavage fluid as a predictive marker of post-transplant airway obliteration. *J Heart Lung Transplant* 2002; 21: 721–730.
44. Jonosono M, Fang KC, Keith FM, Finkbeiner WE, Golden JA, *et al.* Measurement of fibroblast proliferative activity in bronchoalveolar laage fluid in the analysis of obliterative bronchiolitis among lung transplant recipients. *J Heart Lung Transplant* 1999; 18: 972–985.
45. Henke JA, Golden JA, Yelin EH, Keith FA, Blanc PD. Persistent increases of BAL neutrophils as a predictor of mortality following lung transplant. *Chest* 1999; 115: 403–409.
46. Beeh KM, Kornmann O, Lill J, Buhl R. Induced sputum cell profiles in lung transplant recipients with or without chronic rejection: correlation with lung function. *Thorax* 2001; 56: 557–560.
47. Beeh KM, Beier J, Kornmann O, Micke P, Buhl R. Sputum levels of metalloproteinase-9 and tissue inhibitor of metalloproteinase-1, and their ratio correlate with airway obstruction in lung transplant recipients: relation to tumour necrosis factor-alpha and interleukin-10. *J Heart Lung Transplant* 2001; 20: 1144–1151.
48. Reichenspurner H, Kur F, Treede H, *et al.* Optimization of an immunosuppressive protocol after lung transplantation. *Transplantation* 1999; 68: 67–71.
49. O'Hair DP, Cantu E, McGregor C, *et al.* Preliminary experience with mycophenolate mofetil used after lung transplantation. *J Heart Lung Transplant* 1998; 17: 864–868.
50. Ross DJ, Waters PF, Levine M, Kramer M, Ruzevich S, Kass RM. Mycophenolate mofetil versus azathioprine immunosuppressive regimens after lung transplantation: preliminary experience. *J Heart Lung Transplant* 1998; 17: 768–774.
51. Zuckermann A, Birsan T, Taghavi S, *et al.* Mycophenolate mofetil in lung transplantation. *Transplant Proc* 1998; 30: 1514–1516.
52. Palmer SM, Baz MA, Sanders L, *et al.* Results of a randomised, prospective, multicenter trial of mycophenolate mofetil and azathioprine in the prevention of acute rejection. *Transplantation* 2001; 71: 1772–1776.
53. Gerbase MW, Spiliopoulos A, Fathi M, Nicod LP. Low doses of mycophenolate mofetil with low

doses of tacrolimus prevent acute rejection and long-term function loss after lung transplantation. *Transplant Proceedings* 2001; 33: 2146–2147.

54. Corris P, Glanville A, McNeil K, *et al.* One year analysis of an ungoing international randomized study of mycophenolate mofetil (MMF) vs azathioprine (AZA) in lung transplantion. *J Heart Lung Transplant* 2001; 20: Suppl. 1, 149–150.
55. Spencer CM, Goa KL, Gillis JC. Tacoliumus. An update of its pharmacology and clinical efficacy in the management of organ transplantation. *Drugs* 1997; 54: 925–975.
56. Christians U, Braun F, Sattler M, Almeidal VM, Linck A, Sewing KF. Interaction of FK506 and cyclosporine metabolism. *Transplant Proc* 1991, 23. 2794–2796.
57. Undre NA, Meiser BM, Uberfuhr P, *et al.* Pharmacokinetics of tacrolimus (FK506) in primary orthotopic heart transplantation. *Transplant Proc* 1998; 30: 1112–1115.
58. Zuckermann A, Reichenspurner H, Jaksch P, *et al.* Long term follow up of a prospective randomised trial comparing tacrolimus versus cyclosporine in combination with MMF after lung transplantation. *J Heart Lung Transplant* 2003; 22: Suppl. 1, S76–S77.
59. Keenan RJ, Konishi H, Kawai A, *et al.* Clinical trial of tacrolimus versus cyclosporine in lung transplantation. *Ann Thorac Surg* 1995; 60: 580–585.
60. Horning NR, Lynch JP, Sundaresan SR, Patterson GA, Trulock EP. Tacrolimus therapy for persistent or recurrent acute rejection after lung transplantation. *J Heart Lung Transplant* 1998; 17: 761–767.
61. Onsager DR, Canver CC, Jahania MS, *et al.* Efficacy of tacrolimus in the treatment of refractory rejection in heart and lung transplant recipients. *J Heart Lung Transplant* 1999; 18: 448–455.
62. Vitulo P, Oggionni T, Cascina A, *et al.* Efficacy of tacrolimus rescue therapy in refractory acute rejection after lung transplantation. *J Heart Lung Transplant* 2002; 21: 435–439.
63. Sarahrudi K, Carretta A, Wisser W, *et al.* The value of switching from cyclosporine to tacrolimus in the treatment of refractory acute rejection and obliterative bronchiolitis after lung transplantation. *Transplant Int* 2002; 15: 24–28.
64. Klepetko W, Estenne M, Glanville A, *et al.* A multicenter study to assess outcome following a switch in the primary immunosuppressant from cyclosporine to tacrolimus in lung recipients. *J Heart Lung Transplant* 2003; 20: Suppl. 1, 208.
65. Kur F, Reichenspurner H, Meiser BM, *et al.* Tacrolimus (FK506) as primary immunosuppressant after lung transplantation. *J Thorac Cardiovasc Surg* 1999; 47: 174–178.
66. Treede H, Klepetko W, Reichenspurner H, *et al.* Tacrolimus versus cyclosporine after lung transplanation: a prospective, open, randomised two-center trial comparing two different immunosuppressive protocols. *J Heart Lung Transplant* 2001; 20: 511–517.
67. Reichenspurner H, Glanville A, Klepetko W, *et al.* Prospective randomised internatinal multicenter investigator driven study comparing TAC and CSA (+MMF/Steroids) after lung transplantation – Interim analysis of 110 patients. *J Heart Lung Transplant* 2003; 22: Suppl. 1, S77.
68. Ross DJ, Jordan SC, Nathan SD, Kass RM, Koerner SK. Delayed development of obliterative bronchiolitis syndrome with OKT3 after unilateral lung transplantation. A plea for multicenter immunosuppressive trials. *Chest* 1996; 109: 870–873.
69. Wain JC, Wright CD, Ryan DP, Zorb SL, Mathisen DJ, Ginns LC. Induction immunosuppression for lung transplantation with OKT3. *Ann Thorac Surg* 1999; 67: 187–93.
70. Reichenspurner H, Robbins R, Miller J, *et al.* RATG-induction therapy significantly reduces incidence of acute pulmonary rejection compared to OKT3 treatment. *J Heart Lung Transplant* 1996; 15: Suppl. 1, S103.
71. Wiebe K, Harringer W, Wahlers T, *et al.* ATG induction therapy and the incidence of bronchiolitis obliterans after lung transplantation: does it make a difference? *Transplant Proc* 1998; 30: 1517–1518.
72. Palmer SM, Miralles AP, Lawrence CM, Gaynor JW, Davis RD, Tapson VF. Rabbit antithymocyte globulin decreases acute rejection after lung transplantation. *Chest* 1999; 116: 127–133.
73. Garrity ER, Villanueva J, Bhorade SM, Husain AN, Vigneswaran WT. Low rate of acute lung

allograft rejection after the use of daclizumab, an interleukin 2 receptor antibody. *Transplantation* 2001; 71: 773–777.

74. Sweet SC, De La Morena MT, Shapiro SD, Mendeloff EN, Huddleston CB. Interleukin-2-receptor blockade with daclizumab decreases the incidence of acute rejection in pediatric lung transplant recipients. *J Heart Lung Transplant* 2001; 20: 221–222.
75. Brock MV, Borja MC, Ferber L, *et al.* Induction therapy in lung transplantation: a prospective, controlled clinical trial comparing OKT3, anti-thymocyte globulin and daclizumab. *J Heart Lung Transplant* 2001; 20: 1282–1290.
76. Fuks Z, Strober S, Bobrove AM, Sasazuki T, McMichael A, Kaplan HS. Long term effects of radiation of T and B lymphocytes in peripheral blood of patients with Hodgkin's disease. *J Clin Invest* 1976; 58: 803–814.
77. Hunt SA, Strober S, Hoppe RT, Stinson EB. Total lymphoid irradiation for treatment of intractable cardiac allograft rejection. *J Heart Lung Transplant* 1991; 10: 211–216.
78. Keogh AM, Morgan GW, Macdonald P, Spratt P, Mundy J, McCosker C. Clinical heart transplantation. Total lymphoid irradiation for persistant rejection after heart transplantation: only moderate success medium-term. *J Heart Lung Transplant* 1996; 15: 231–233.
79. Ross HJ, Gullestad L, Pak J, Slauson S, Valantine HA, Hunt SA. Methotrexate or total lymphoid radiation for treatment of persistant or recurrent allograft cellular rejection: a comparative study. *J Heart Lung Transplant* 1997; 16: 179–189.
80. Keogh AM, Arnold RH, Macdonald PS, Hawkins RC, Morgan GW, Spratt PM. A randomised trial of tacrolimus (FK506) versus total lymphoid irradiation for the control of repetitive rejection after cardiac transplantation. *J Heart Lung Transplant* 2001; 20: 1331–1334.
81. Valantine VG, Robbins RC, Wehner JH, Patel HR, Berry GJ, Theodore J. Total lymphoid irradiation for refractory acute rejection in heart-lung and lung allografts. *Chest* 1996; 109: 1184–1189.
82. Takao M, Higenbottam TW, Audley T, Otulana BA, Wallwork J. Effects of inhaled nebulized steroids (budesonide) on acute and chronic lung function in heart-lung transplant recipients. *Transplant Proc* 1995; 27: 1284–1285.
83. Ross DJ, Marchevsky A, Kramer M, Kass RM. Refractoriness of airflow obstruction associated with isolated lymphocytic bronchiolitis/bronchitis in pulmonary allografts. *J Heart Lung Transplant* 1997; 16: 832–838.
84. De Soyza A, Fisher AJ, Small T, Corris P. Inhaled corticosteroids and the treatment of lymphocytic bronchiolitis following lung transplantation. *Am J Respir Crit Care Med* 2001; 164: 1209–1212.
85. Lerner AB, Denton CR, Fitzpatrick TB. Clinical and experimental studies with 8-methoxypsoralen in vitiligo. *J Invest Dermatol* 1953; 20: 229–314.
86. Edelson R, Berger C, Gasparro F, *et al.* Treatment of cutaneous T-cell lymphoma by extracorporeal photochemotherapy. Preliminary results. *N Engl J Med* 1987; 316: 297–303.
87. Khavari PA, Edelson RL, Lider O, Gasparro FP, Weiner HL, Cohen IR. Specific vaccination against photoinactivated cloned T cells. *Clin Res* 1988; 36: 662A.
88. Krasagakis K, Dippel E, Ramaker J, Owsianowski M, Orfanos CE. Management of severe scleroderma with long-term extracorporeal photopheresis. *Dermatology* 1998; 196: 309–315.
89. Holbrook MR, Powell RJ. Is there a future for extracorporeal photochemotherapy in the treatment of the rheumatological diseases. *Ann Rheum Dis* 1997; 56: 339–340.
90. Knobler RM, Trautinger F, Graninger W, *et al.* Parenteral administration of 8-methoxypsoralen in photopheresis. *J Am Acad Dermatol* 1993; 28: 580–584.
91. Barr ML, Meiser BM, Eisen HJ, *et al.* Photopheresis for the prevention of rejection in cardiac transplantation. Photopheresis transplantation study group. *N Engl J Med* 1998; 339: 1744–1751.
92. Goodrich RP, Yerram NR, Tay-Goodrich BH, *et al.* Selective inactivation of viruses in the presence of human platelets: UV sensitization with psoralen derivatives. *Proc Natl Acad Sci USA* 1994; 91: 5552–5556.
93. Costanzo-Nordin MR, Hubbell EA, O'Sullivan EJ, *et al.* Photopheresis versus corticosteroids in the therapy of heart transplant rejection. *Circulation* 1992; 86: II-242–II-250.

94. Macey WH, DeNardo B, Rook AH, Singh A, Bromley P. Use of extracorporeal photochemotherapy in heart transplant recipients during acute rejection: a case study. *Am J Crit Care* 1994; 3: 452–456.
95. Wieland M, Thiede VL, Strauss RG, *et al.* Treatment of severe cardiac allograft rejection with extracorporeal photochemotherapy. *J Clin Apheresis* 1994; 9: 171–175.
96. Dall'Amico R, Livi U, Milano A, *et al.* Extracorporeal photochemotherapy as adjuvant treatment of heart transplant recipients with recurrent rejection. *Transplantation* 1995; 60: 45–49.
97. Lehrer MS, Rook AH, Tomaszewski JE, DeNofrio D. Successful reversal of severe refractory cardiac allograft rejection by photopheresis. *J Heart Lung Transplant* 2001; 20: 1233–1236.
98. Barr ML, Baker CJ, Schenkel FA, *et al.* Prophylactic photopheresis and chronic rejection: effects on graft intimal hyperplasia in cardiac transplantation. *Clin Transplant* 2000; 14: 162–166.
99. Andreu G, Achkar A, Couetil JP, *et al.* Extracorporeal photochemotherapy treatment for acute lung rejection episode. *J Heart Lung Transplant* 1995; 14: 793–796.
100. Cahill BC. Methotrexate for lung transplant recipients with steroid-resistant acute rejection. *J Heart Lung Transplant* 1996; 15: 1130–1137.
101. Soghikian MV, Valentine VG, Berry GJ, Patel H, Robbins RC, Theodore J. Impact of ganciclovir prophylaxis on heart-lung and lung transplant recipients. *J Heart Lung Transplant* 1996; 15: 881–887.
102. Tikkanen JM, Kallio EA, Bruggeman CA, Koskinen PK, Lemstrom KB. Prevention of cytomegalovirus infection-enhanced experimental obliterative bronchiolitis by antiviral prophylaxis or immunosuppression in rat tracheal allografts. *Am J Respir Crit Care Med* 2001; 15: 672–679.
103. Glanville AR, Baldwin JC, Burke CM, Theodore J, Robin ED. Obliterative bronchiolitis after heart-lung transplantation: apparent arrest by augmented immunosuppression. *Ann Int Med* 1987; 107: 300–304.
104. Ross DJ, Lewis MI, Kramer M, Vo A, Kass RM. FK 506 rescue immunosuppression for obliterative bronchiolitis after lung transplantation. *Chest* 1997; 112: 1175–1179.
105. Kesten S, Chaparro C, Scavuzzo M, Gutierrez C. Tacrolimus as rescue therapy for bronchiolitis obliterans syndrome. *J Heart Lung Transplant* 1997; 16: 905–912.
106. Reichenspurner H, Meiser BM, Kur F, *et al.* First experience with FK 506 for treatment of chronic pulmonary rejection. *Transplant Proc* 1995; 27: 2009.
107. Knoop C, Antoine M, Vachiery JL, Yernault JC, Estenne M. FK 506 rescue therapy for irreversible airway rejection in heart-lung transplant recipients: report on five cases. *Transplant Proc* 1994; 26: 3240–3241.
108. Wiebe K, Harringer W, Franke U, *et al.* FK506 rescue therapy in lung transplantation. *Transplant Proc* 1998; 30: 1508–1509.
109. Lipson DA, Palevsky HI, Kotloff RM, Edelman J. Conversion to Tacrolimus (FK506) from cyclosporine after orthotopic lung transplantation. *Transplant Proc* 1998; 30: 1505–1507.
110. Revell MP, Lewis ME, Llewellyn-Jones CG, Wilson IC, Bonser RS. Conservation of small-airway function by Tacrolimus/Cycosporine conversion in the management of bronchiolitis obliterans following lung transplantation. *J Heart Lung Transplant* 2000; 19: 1219–1223.
111. Whyte RI, Rossi SJ, Mulligan MS, *et al.* Mycophenolate mofetil for obliterative bronchiolitis syndrome after lung transplantation. *Ann Thorac Surg* 1997; 64: 945–948.
112. Speich R, Boehler A, Thurnheer R, Weder W. Salvage therapy with mycophenolate mofetil for lung transplant bronchiolitis obliterans: importance of dosage. *Transplantation* 1997; 15: 533–535.
113. Roman A, Bravo C, Monforte V, Reyes L, Canela M, Morell F. Preliminary results of rescue therapy with tacrolimus and mycophenolate mofetil in lung transplanted patients with bronchiolitis obliterans. *Transplant Proc* 2002; 34: 146–147.
114. Dupont LJ, Delcroix M, Vanhaecke J, Van Raemdonck D, Verleden GM. Azathioprine/mycophenolate conversion in the management of bronchiolitis obliterans syndrome (BOS) following (heart)-lung transplantation. *J Heart Lung Transplant* 2003; 22: Suppl. 1, S123.
115. Whitford H, Walters EH, Levvey B, *et al.* Addition of inhaled corticosteroids to systemic

immunosuppression after lung transplantation: a double-blind, placebo-controlled trial. *Transplantation* 2002; 73: 1793–1799.
116. Whitford H, Orsida B, Kotsimbos T, *et al.* Bronchoalveolar lavage cellular profiles in lung transplantation: the effect of inhaled corticosteroids. *Annals of Transplantation.* 2000; 5: 31–37.
117. Ward C, De Soyza A, Fisher A, Pritchard G, Corris P. Small airway reticular basement membrane (Rbm) thickening in clinically stable lung transplant recipients is not affected by three months treatment with inhaled corticosteroids. *Eur Respir J* 2002; 20: 347s.
118. Dusmet M, Maurer J, Winton T, Kesten S. Methotrexate can halt the progression of bronchiolitis obliterans syndrome in lung transplant recipients. *J Heart Lung Transplant* 1996; 15: 948–954.
119. Verleden GM, Buyse B, Delcroix M, *et al.* Cyclophosphamide rescue therapy for chronic rejection after lung trannsplantation. *J Heart Lung Transplant* 1999; 18: 1139–1142.
120. Snell GI, Esmore DS, Williams JW. Cytolytic therapy for the bronchiolitis obliterans syndrome complicating lung transplantation. *Chest* 1996; 109: 874–878.
121. Kesten S, Rajagopalan N, Maurer J. Cytolytic therapy for the treatment of bronchiolitis obliterans syndrome following lung transplantation. *Transplantation* 1996; 61: 427–430.
122. Date H, Lynch JP, Sundaresan S, Patterson GA, Trulock EP. The impact of cytolytic therapy on bronchiolitis obliterans syndrome. *J Heart Lung Transplant* 1998; 17: 869–875.
123. Dowling RD, Zenati B, Burckart GJ, *et al.* Aerosolized cyclosporine as single-agent immunotherapy in canine lung allografts. *Surgery* 1990; 108: 198–204.
124. Zenati M, Duncan AJ, Burckart GJ, *et al.* Immunosuppression with aerosolised cyclosporine for prevention of lung rejection in a rat model. *Eur J Cardiothorac Surg* 1991; 5: 266–271.
125. Iacono AT, Keenan RJ, Duncan SR, *et al.* Aerosolized cyclosporine in lung recipients with refractory chronic rejection. *Am J Respir Crit Care Med* 1996; 153: 1451–1455.
126. Keenan RJ, Iacono A, Dauber JH, *et al.* Treatment of refractory acute allograft rejection with aerosolised cyclosporine in lung transplant recipients. *J Thorac Cardiovasc Surg* 1997; 113: 335–340.
127. Reichenspurner H, Adams B, Morris RE, *et al.* Obliterative airway disease after heterotopic tracheal xenotransplantation in a concordant rodent model – pathogenesis and treatment. *Transplant Proc* 1996; 28: 740–741.
128. Cahill BC, Somerville T, Karwande SW, *et al.* Early experience with sirolimus in lung transplant recipients with chronic allograft rejection. *J Heart Lung Transplant* 2003; 22: 169–176.
129. Gerhardt SW, McDyer JF, Girgis RE, Conte JV, Yang SC, Orens JB. Maintenance azithromycin therapy for bronchiolitis obliterans syndrome. Resuls of a pilot study. *Am J Respir Crit Care Med* 2003; 168: 121–125.
130. Verleden GM, Dupont LJ, Delcroix M, Van Raemdonck DE. Azithromycin treatment for chronic allograft dysfunction after lung transplantation. *Eur Respir J* 2003; 22: Suppl. 45, 202s.
131. Chacon RA, Corris PA, Dark JH, Gibson GJ. Tests of airway function in detecting and monitoring treatment of obliterative bronchiolitis after lung transplantation. *J Heart Lung Transplant* 2000; 19: 263–269.
132. Melville A, Wardle J, Parry G, Corris P, Dark J. Comparison of total lymphoid irradiation (TLI) versus tacrolimus for the treatment of obliterative bronchiolitis (OB) in lung transplants. *J Heart Lung Transplant* 2001; 20: Suppl. 1, S208.
133. Fisher AJ, Bozzino JM, Rutherford RM, Parry G, Dark JH, Corris PA. The tolerability and efficacy of total lymphoid irradiation (TLI) in the control of rapidly progressive bronchiolitis obliterans syndrome. *J Heart Lung Transplant* 2003; 22: Suppl. S151.
134. Slovis BS, Loyd JE, King LE jr. Photophoresis for chronic rejection of lung allografts. *N Engl J Med* 1995; 332: 962.
135. Salerno CT, Park SJ, Kreykes NS, *et al.* Adjuvant treatment of refractory lung transplant rejection with extracorporeal photopheresis. *J Thorac Cardiovasc Surg* 1999; 117: 1063–1069.
136. Villanueva J, Bhorade SM, Robinson JA, Husain AN, Garrity ER jr. Extracorporeal photopheresis for the treatment of lung allograft rejection. *Ann Transplant* 2000; 5: 44–47.
137. O'Hagan AR, Stillwell PC, Arroliga A, Koo A. Photopheresis in the treatment of refractory bronchiolitis obliterans complicating lung transplantation. *Chest* 1999; 115: 1459–1462.

138. Shennib H, Novick R, Mulder D, *et al.* Is lung retransplantation indicated? Report on four cases. *Eur Respir J* 1993; 6: 354–357.
139. Novick R, Stitt LW, Al-Kattan K, *et al.* Pulmonary retransplantation: predictors of graft function and survival in 230 patients. *Ann Thorac Surg* 1998; 65: 227–234.
140. Schäfers HJ, Hausen B, Walters T, Fieguth HG, Jurmann M, Borst HG. Retranspantation of the lung. A single center experience. *Eur J Cardiothorac Surg* 1995; 9: 291–295.
141. Novick RJ, Stitt L. Pulmonary retransplantation. *Semin Thorac Cardiovasc Surg* 1998; 10: 227–236.

*CHAPTER 3*

# Infection and bronchiolitis obliterans syndrome in lung transplant recipients

*C.W. Ward*, T. DeSouza*, D.T. Keating#, J. Lordan*, J.J. Egan#*

**Freeman Hospital, Newcastle, UK, and #Mater Misericordiae Hospital, Dublin Ireland.*

*Correspondence: J.J. Egan, National Heart and Lung Transplant Program, Mater Misericordiae Hospital, Eccles St, Dublin 7, Ireland.*

Since the advent of effective immunosuppression lung transplantation has gained wide acceptance for treatment of advanced lung diseases. Survival rates following transplantation is limited by the onset of chronic graft failure affecting up to 50% of long-term survivors. The term bronchiolitis obliterans syndrome (BOS) is applied to describe chronic graft failure [1]. Early acute cellular rejection is associated with the development of BOS, consequently BOS is frequently referred to as chronic rejection. However, nonalloimmune injury, especially infection, is increasingly recognised as a potential factor in the development of BOS. The aim of this chapter is to review the potential influence of infection on the cause and progression of BOS.

## The impact of infection on lung transplant recipients

Infection and chronic rejection (BOS) are the major causes of mortality and morbidity in lung allografts [2]. Viral, bacterial and fungal lower-respiratory infections are common in the lung transplant population [3–7]. A total of 70% of deaths following lung transplantation are associated with infection [2]. Compared with other solid organ transplants the lung allograft is unique, due to its interface with the environment. This interaction, in the presence of systemic immunosuppression, leaves it vulnerable to a variety of infections.

## Why are lung allografts at particular risk of infection?

In the context of lung transplantation the host is frequently colonised with multiresistant bacterial organisms as a consequence of their primary disease. This is classically the case in patients with cystic fibrosis or bronchiectais and to a lesser extent emphysema. Therefore, irrespective of immunosuppression the host is a risk factor for the development of infection. Unlike other solid organ transplants the lung is constantly exposed to the environment. Thousands of litres of air travel through the lung every hour containing varying levels of contaminants which include particulates and microorganisms. Recently, it has been shown that there are deficiencies in lung lining fluid constituents, which protect against infection and airway-oxidant damage, these include decreased levels of glutathione and secretory leucocyte protease inhibitor [8, 9]. A sterile environment suitable for gas exchange is normally maintained by pulmonary macrophages. Macrophages which deal with the majority of microbiological challenges are

Eur Respir Mon, 2004, 29, 44–54. Printed in UK - all rights reserved. Copyright ERS Journals Ltd 2004; European Respiratory Monograph; ISSN 1025-448x. ISBN 1-904097-33-2.

matched and complimented by an efficient mucociliary escalator that clears particulates and cells from the airways in a thin stream of extracellular epithelial lining fluid. Video photomicroscopy has demonstrated impaired mucocilliary clearance which also contributes to a risk of infection. Finally a fundamental characteristic in lung allografts is that they are denervated, thereby causing an resulting in an impaired cough reflex. In animal models the loss of neurally controlled mechanisms leads to the modulation of inflammation (table 1) [10].

## Specific organisms and bronchiolitis obliterans

Cytomegalovirus (CMV), a DNA herpes virus, is second only to bacterial infections as an opportunistic pathogen in lung transplant recipients. There appears to be a particularly higher prevalence in lung transplant recipients (in excess of 60%) as compared with other solid organ transplants [16]. Although prophylactic regimens are now widely used, CMV infections remain as major causes of morbidity. Once CMV infection occurs the virus has the ability to enter into a latent phase. Although there is a greater concern over the CMV naive recipient receiving a transplant from a CMV positive donor, infections can also occur after blood transfusion from a CMV positive blood donor or a recrudescence of a latent infection.

The immunomodulatory effects of CMV are important when considering the risk of BOS. CMV viral infections are directly associated with alterations in the biphasic alveolar macrophage cytokine production with an initial increased interlekin (IL)-6, and subsequent transforming growth factor-β secretion [17]. CMV can induce a similar cytokine profile that is observed in acute rejection, which included elevated mRNA expression of IL-2, interferon-γ, IL-10 and intracellular adhesion molecule (ICAM)-1 in clinical bronchoalveolar lavage (BAL) specimens [18]. Further data supporting the plausibility of the causal relationship between CMV and BOS have been seen in experimental models of renal allografts. In these instances CMV infection caused increased collagen I and III deposition in addition to causing myofibroblast accumulation [19]. Rat lung transplant models of CMV infection also show an association between infection and enhanced cell proliferation and histological changes of BO [20]. An association between CMV infection and major histocompatibility complex class II expression has been demonstrated in experimental lung transplantation, but interestingly not in clinical specimens [21, 22].

CMV infection appears to be an important risk factor for the development of fungal [23] and bacterial super infection [24], acute vascular rejection [25, 26], which in themselves, may contribute to the risk of BOS. However, the link between CMV and acute vascular rejection has not been seen in all studies [27]. Despite data from *in vitro* studies supporting the role of CMV in the development of BOS, assessment of CMV as a

**Table 1. – Normal homeostatic mechanisms for dealing with infection compromised in lung allografts**

| Mechanism | Finding |
|---|---|
| Abnormal mucociliary clearance (denervated lung) | Decreased ciliary beat frequency [11] |
| Abnormal cough reflex (denervated lung) | Depressed [2] |
| Abnormal lymphatic drainage | Interrupted (especially in first weeks) [2] |
| Depressed alveolar macrophages (front line phagocytes), due to immunosuppression | Depressed expression of a wide range of functional receptors [12] |
| Alteration in constituents of lung lining fluid | Loss of antioxidants, loss of protection against proteases and overall compromise of microbiological defences, [8, 9, 13, 14, 15] |
| Disturbance of neural control of inflammation | Loss of neural control [16] |

risk factor for the development of BOS in clinical studies has yielded conflicting results. CMV infection was noted to have a hazard ratio of 1.62 in one study, whereas in another CMV pneumonitis was associated with a relative risk of 2.3 [28]. An association between CMV and BOS has been observed in a number of studies [24, 25, 29] but the absence of an association has also been reported [11, 26]. One negative study did not demonstrate a higher risk for developing BO or BOS with donor CMV seropositive/recipient CMV seronegative (CMV D+/R-) [30]. Notably in this study there was no association between CMV D+/R- and recurrent acute vascular rejection which conflicts with data from the renal transplant literature [14, 15]. These conflicting data are, in part, related to difficulties in defining what constitutes CMV infection. These disparities are probably related to different diagnostic techniques and the application of different definitions of CMV. In certain studies CMV seroconversion has been used to define a CMV illness where as in other studies CMV pneumonitis was used to define illness.

## Community respiratory viral infections

Community respiratory viral (CRV) infections, including respiratory syncytial virus (RSV), influenza, para-influenza, and adenovirus are a common cause of seasonal respiratory tract infections in children and adults. Although these viruses predominantly involve the upper airways, lower respiratory tract infection in the immunocompromised host is also described. It has increasingly been recognised that CRVs are a significant cause of acute infection involving the lower respiratory tract in lung transplant recipients [31, 32].

The majority of studies investigating the involvement of CRV infections in lung transplantation have been retrospective. In an analysis of 200 infectious complications involving 73 heart-lung transplant recipients, infections with: RSV, influenza, or adenovirus, were confirmed in only 3% of the cases [33]. Holt *et al.* [34] reviewed CRV infections in 137 lung or heart-lung transplant recipients and noted that RSV, adenovirus, influenza, and parainfluenza accounted for only 9% of infections. Four cases of adenovirus infection were detected in an analysis of 308 paediatric and adult lung and heart-lung transplant recipients [35]. In contrast, 18 out of 84 (21%) patients were infected with RSV or para-influenza in a series of paediatric and adult lung or heart-lung transplant recipients [36]. However, the varying incidence of CRV infections recorded in these studies is likely to reflect the variable sensitivities of the techniques applied to detect viral infections. Direct fluorescence antibody testing, which has an increased sensitivity compared with viral culture for CRV detection, has only been available in certain units since 1995 [37]. Advances in diagnostic techniques for viral infections including: rapid antigen detection, nucleic acid hybridisation, and gene amplification, may facilitate the earlier diagnosis of viral infection compared with traditional cell culture methods. The recent application of testing with indirect fluorescent antibody testing of naso-pharyngeal and throat swabs has been shown to increase the detection of influenza viral infection in lung transplant recipients [38].

A seasonal variation in the onset of BOS has been reported by some investigators in lung transplant recipients, with a peak in late winter, which corresponds with the peak incidence of respiratory viral infections in the community [39]. Vilchez *et al.* [40] noted a higher incidence of human para-influenza virus-3 infection in the summer months. However, another study has noted that the diagnosis of BO/BOS occurred throughout the year and was not associated with the seasonal variation in CRV infections [41]. Infection with para-influenza and adenovirus has been recorded throughout the year in immunosuppressed patients [42].

The question has been posed at to whether occult or subclinical infection with CRVs may have persistent adverse effects on lung allograft function, predisposing a patient to the development of BO [43, 44]. An increased high rate of BO has been observed in lung transplant recipients with previous CRV infections [44]. Viral infections in the development of bronchiolitis are well recognised, even in immune-competent hosts [45]. Adenoviral infection has been linked with the development of BO in children [46]. RSV induced bronchiolitis is characterised by: neutrophilic infiltration [47], increased airway fluid IL-8, neutrophil elastase, activity [48], epithelial damage and increased expression of ICAM-1 for neutrophils on airway epithelial cells *in vitro* [49]. Studies have shown that experimental infections in airway epithelial cells or leucocytes *in vitro* with a rhinovirus [50], RSV [51], adenovirus [47], or influenza [52] lead to an increased production of pro-inflammatory cytokines relevant to the airway remodelling process of BOS. The ability of viral infections to activate immunological mechanisms in lung allografts is also supported by a study demonstrating a high association of para-influenza infection in 18 out of 22 lung allograft recipients (82%) with histological confirmation of acute cellular rejection [42]. In addition, 32% of the allograft recipients affected by para-influenza infection in that study subsequently developed active BO which was confirmed using histology [42].

Viral infections with RSV and other paramyxoviruses have also been linked with increased airway damage in animal models of lung transplantation. Infection of a rat-model lung transplantation with sendai virus, a para-influenza type virus similar to human RSV, led to progressive lymphocytic submucosal infiltration of large airways and bronchioles of the lung allograft, with histological changes similar to those seen in human BO [53, 54]. Thus, a unifying hypothesis has been proposed that viral infection may have a direct cytopathic effect on the bronchial epithelium, increasing the allogenicity of the airway epithelium, leading to enhanced cell mediated immune damage to the small airways of allografts and the subsequent development of BO.

# Bacteria

Pneumonia is common in the first month after a transplant, in part reflecting nonimmune factors such as reduced cough, post-surgical atelectasis and delayed mucociliary clearance. Interest in the role of bacterial infections and an association with either acute or chronic rejection has attracted less interest than CMV. This is surprising given the prevalence of bacterial infections in other solid organ transplant recipients [55, 56]. In renal transplant recipients an association has been observed between renal graft failure and urinary tract infections as far back as the late 1970s. In heart transplant recipients acute graft rejection coincided with systemic infection was associated with a prolongation of inflammatory cells in follow up biopsies [57]. Cardiac transplant patients who were infected with *Helicobacter pylori* are noted as having increased immunosuppressant requirements as compared with seronegative patients [58].

A rat renal transplant model has demonstrated a role for bacterial lipopolysaccharide (LPS) in the genesis of renal allograft failure [59]. In these experiments, rats were administered purified LPS but not viable bacteria. The host response to the LPS resulted in accelerated graft loss, in the absence of an active infective process, suggesting dysregulated immune responses [59]. Clinical lung transplant studies have demonstrated that bacterial infections of human lung allografts are associated with similar pro-inflammatory cytokine induction to that of acute vascular rejection [18]. Other data have demonstrated that bacterial infections in 19 lung transplant recipients were associated with raised endothelin-1 levels in BAL and that five out of seven patients, with the highest endothelin-1 levels, subsequently developed BOS [60]. Little data is available regarding the role of bacterial infections in the development of BOS. However, bacterial infections have been associated with potentiating the effect of acute rejection on subsequent developments of BOS [8, 61].

An area of great difficulty in evaluating the impact of infection in lung transplantation is the definition of infection. The presence of new infiltrates, a fall in lung function, leucocytosis, pyrexia and hypoxia associated with positive BAL or sputum cultures makes bacterial infection probable. The presence of possible pathogens in a clinically stable patient's sputum, in the absence of the above criteria, leaves a diagnostic and therapeutic dilemma. Although perceived to be the gold standard BAL cultures that have a bacterial pathogen isolated from them may still reflect some contamination of the bronchoscope with oropharyngeal flora. Recent data has suggested that Gram-negative bacterial cell-to-cell signalling molecules (acyl homoserine lactones) are present in the lavages of stable lung transplant recipients, even in those which were culture negative, suggesting infection with viable unidentified bacteria [62]. This data is consistent with observations that intracellular pathogens are capable of infecting airway cells [63] and that bacteria can enter dormant phases which can be culture negative but still viable [64, 65].

## Pseudomonas

Isolation of *Pseudomonas* sp. from lung allografts are very common and can be a result of *de novo* establishment of this opportunistic organism, or a consequence of the previous suppurative lung pathology that led to the transplantation. The latter scenario, where treatment resistant bacteria may be found, is an unambiguous threat, and drives the rigorous antibiotic [1] and bactericidal prophylaxes [66] used at most centres.

In contrast clinically insignificant culture of *Pseudomanas* sp. are often ignored. It is perhaps surprising, and a deficiency, that in contrast to recommendations in chronic obstructive pulmonary disease (COPD), and promising work in other chronic lung disease [3, 65], that most lung transplant centres do not have quantitative cultures available [67–70]. There is increasing evidence that the decline of lung function in COPD is related to bacterial load [4–7]. In the setting of COPD a cut-off point of $10^3$ colony forming units·$mL^{-1}$ of BAL has been proposed as clinically significant with nonquantitative data being regarded as not worthwhile. In contrast, there is no information regarding lung allografts and quantitative cultures are not generally used or available.

## *Burkholderia cepacia*

SNELL *et al.* [71] were the first to describe an association between *Burkholderia cepacia* and an increased death rate in organ transplantation reject. However, it has been shown that there are different genomovar strains (I-VII) of *B. cepacia*. Emerging data illustrates the vital necessity of having such detailed microbiological information available with excessive mortality detected in patients infected with *Burkholderia cenocepacia* (genomovar III) prior to transplantation, but not in those infected with other genomovars [72]. Notably there was a persistence of non *B. cenocepacia* in lavages taken up to 1-yr after the transplant operation in the absence of obvious clinical infections. The long-term outcomes of these patients are not yet known and are eagerly awaited with interest.

## Fungal infections

Fungal infections are a significant cause of postoperative morbidity and mortality in lung transplant recipients [73]. The risk factors and course of fungal infections in lung transplant recipients are similar to those seen in other solid organ transplants. However, higher rates of fungal infection as compared with other transplant recipients with infection rates of up to 44% have been reported [23]. Lung transplant recipients also appear to have more severe (invasive) fungal disease; invasive rates in 13% of lung transplant recipients have been noted as compared with 0.4% of heart transplant recipients [74]. An association between fungal infection with CMV or bacterial co-infection has been noted [23], although some studies have failed to show any such associations with more invasive fungal infections [75]. Early fungal infections are generally related to surgical complications or pre-existing fungal infections in either the donor or the recipient [76]. Fungal infections, 1 yr after organ transplantation, are often associated with augmented immunosuppressive treatment for BOS or bronchial anastomotic abnormalities [77]. Although a wide variety of fungal pathogens have been described, most infections involve *Aspergillus* sp. Other prominent pathogens include Candida, Pneumocystis, Cryptococcus [78], and endemic fungi [79]. Although fungi are a relatively prominent pathogen group in lung transplantation, the data regarding the role of fungal infections in the subsequent development of BOS are scarce. However, there does appear to be a synergistic effect of fungal infections with CMV and acute vascular rejection for subsequent BOS [8].

## Mycobacteria in lung allografts

Mycobacterial infections have been reported relatively rarely with most concerning *Mycobacterium tuberculosis*. Tuberculosis, though uncommon in lung allografts, is a serious infection which may elude diagnosis and lead to significant patient morbidity, although patients do respond to treatment [2], as confirmed in an extensive review of the spectrum of mycobacterial infection by WIEBE *et al.* [12], which indicated that

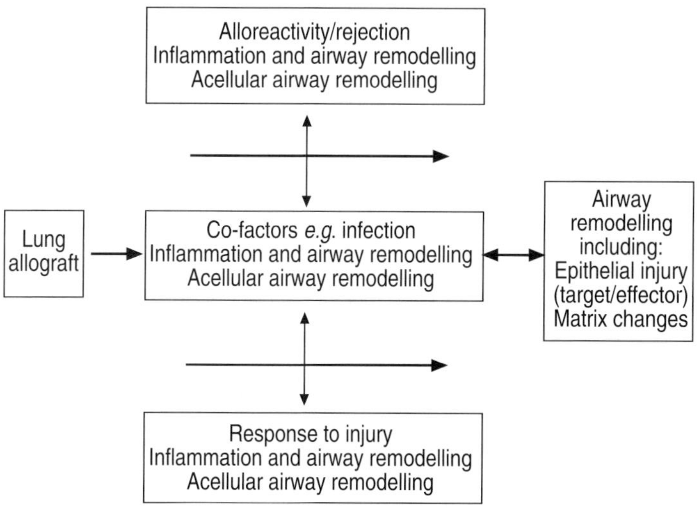


Fig. 1. – A paradigm for bronchiolitis obliterans syndrome aetiology.

mycobacteria were potentially an under-recognised problem, with most of the organisms isolated not being *M. tuberculosis* (*e.g. Mycobacterium avium, Mycobacterium abscessus, Mycobacterium kanasii*, and *Mycobacterium haemophilum*). This retrospective study found mycobacterial infection in 23 out of a series of 261 patients (9%) and that this relatively common complication responded to therapy but was potentially associated with permanent graft dysfunction [12].

## Conclusions

Although this chapter reviews the possible pathways in which various infectious agents may contribute to chronic rejection, directly or indirectly, it remains unclear as to what the precise role of infections is in BOS. Much of this relates to a current lack of standardisation in respect to methodology, particularly with regards the definition of infection. If low-grade infections are enough to alter immunogenicity are current surveillance programmes adequate enough to detect these? Many facets of the complex interaction between the innate and adaptive immunity are emerging, and it is likely that infection contributes to this paradigm (fig. 1).

## Summary

Infection and chronic rejection are the major causes of mortality and morbidity in lung allografts. The host for lung transplantation is frequently colonised with multiresistant bacterial organisms as a consequence of their primary disease; therefore, irrespective of immunosuppression, the host is at risk of infection. The cytomegolavirus appears to be an important risk factor for fungal and bacterial super infection, and possibly for acute vascular rejection, which in themselves may all contribute to the risk of bronchiolitis obliterans syndrome (BOS). The precise role of bacterial infection in the development of BOS remains unclear; much of this relates to a current lack of standardisation of the definition of infection.

**Keywords:** Bronchiolitis obliterans, cytomegalovirus, infection, lung transplant.

## References

1. Estenne M, Maurer JR, Boehler A, *et al.* Bronchiolitis obliterans syndrome 2001: an update of the diagnostic criteria. *J Heart Lung Transplant* 2002; 21: 297–310.
2. Hosenpud JD, Bennett LE, Keck BM, Edwards EB, Novick RJ. Effect of diagnosis on survival benefit of lung transplantation for end-stage lung disease. *Lancet* 1998; 351: 24–27.
3. Alexander BD, Tapson VF. Infectious complications of lung transplantation. *Transpl Infect Dis* 2001; 3: 128–137.
4. Riise GC, Andersson BA, Kjellstrom C, *et al.* Persistent high BAL fluid granulocyte activation marker levels as early indicators of bronchiolitis obliterans after lung transplant. *Eur Respir J* 1999; 14: 1123–1130.
5. Chaparro C, Kesten S. Infections in lung transplant recipients. *Clin Chest Med* 1997; 18: 339–351.
6. Riise GC, Kjellstrom C, Ryd W, *et al.* Inflammatory cells and activation markers in BAL during

acute rejection and infection in lung transplant recipients: a prospective, longitudinal study. *Eur Respir J* 1997; 10: 1742–1746.
7. Brooks RG, Hofflin JM, Jamieson SW, Stinson EB, Remington JS. Infectious complications in heart-lung transplant recipients. *Am J Med* 1985; 79: 412–422.
8. Girgis RE, Tu I, Berry GJ, *et al.* Risk factors for the development of obliterative bronchiolitis after lung transplantation. *J Heart Lung Transplant* 1996; 15: 1200–1208.
9. Siddiqui MT, Garrity ER, Martinez R, Husain AN. Bronchiolar basement membrane changes associated with bronchiolitis obliterans in lung allografts: a retrospective study of serial transbronchial biopsies with immunohistochemistry [corrected]. *Mod Pathol* 1996, 9. 320–328.
10. King MB, Pedtke AC, Levrey-Hadden HL, Hertz MI. Obliterative airway disease progresses in heterotopic airway allografts without persistent alloimmune stimulus. *Transplantation* 2002; 74: 557–562.
11. Sharples LD, Tamm M, McNeil K, Higenbottam TW, Stewart S, Wallwork J. Development of bronchiolitis obliterans syndrome in recipients of heart-lung transplantation-- early risk factors. *Transplantation* 1996; 61: 560–566.
12. Wiebe K, Wahlers T, Harringer W, vd. Hardt H, Fabel H, Haverich A. Lung transplantation for cystic fibrosis--a single center experience over 8 years. *Eur J Cardiothorac Surg* 1998; 14: 191–196.
13. Alho HS, Inkinen KA, Salminen US, *et al.* Expression of proalpha1(I)- and proalpha1 (III) collagen mRNA in chronic allograft rejection in a porcine heterotopic bronchial transplantation model. *Transplant Proc* 2001; 33: 2478.
14. Sageda S, Nordal KP, Hartmann A, *et al.* The impact of cytomegalovirus infection and disease on rejection episodes in renal allograft recipients. *Am J Transplant* 2002; 2: 850–856.
15. McLaughlin K, Wu C, Fick G, Muirhead N, Hollomby D, Jevnikar A. Cytomegalovirus seromismatching increases the risk of acute renal allograft rejection. *Transplantation* 2002; 74: 813–816.
16. Duncan SR, Paradis IL, Dauber JH, Yousem SA, Hardesty RL, Griffith BP. Ganciclovir prophylaxis for cytomegalovirus infections in pulmonary allograft recipients. *Am Rev Respir Dis* 1992; 146: 1213–1215.
17. Magnan A, Mege JL, Escallier JC, *et al.* Balance between alveolar macrophage IL-6 and TGF-beta in lung-transplant recipients. Marseille and Montreal Lung Transplantation Group. *Am J Respir Crit Care Med* 1996; 153: 1431–1436.
18. Ross DJ, Moudgil A, Bagga A, *et al.* Lung allograft dysfunction correlates with gamma-interferon gene expression in bronchoalveolar lavage. *J Heart Lung Transplant* 1999; 18: 627–636.
19. Inkinen K, Soots A, Krogerus L, Bruggeman C, Ahonen J, Lautenschlager I. Cytomegalovirus increases collagen synthesis in chronic rejection in the rat. *Nephrol Dial Transplant* 2002; 17: 772–779.
20. Tikkanen JM, Kallio EA, Bruggeman CA, Koskinen PK, Lemstrom KB. Prevention of cytomegalovirus infection-enhanced experimental obliterative bronchiolitis by antiviral prophylaxis or immunosuppression in rat tracheal allografts. *Am J Respir Crit Care Med* 2001; 164: 672–679.
21. Steinmuller C, Steinhoff G, Bauer D, *et al.* Analysis of leukocyte activation during acute rejection of pulmonary allografts in noninfected and cytomegalovirus-infected rats. *J Leukoc Biol* 1997; 61: 40–49.
22. Arbustini E, Morbini P, Grasso M, *et al.* Human cytomegalovirus early infection, acute rejection, and major histocompatibility class II expression in transplanted lung. Molecular, immunocytochemical, and histopathologic investigations. *Transplantation* 1996; 61: 418–427.
23. Ruffini E, Baldi S, Rapellino M, *et al.* Fungal infections in lung transplantation. Incidence, risk factors and prognostic significance. *Sarcoidosis Vasc Diffuse Lung Dis* 2001; 18: 181–190.
24. Duncan AJ, Dummer JS, Paradis IL, *et al.* Cytomegalovirus infection and survival in lung transplant recipients. *J Heart Lung Transplant* 1991; 10: 638–644.
25. Keller CA, Cagle PT, Brown RW, Noon G, Frost AE. Bronchiolitis obliterans in recipients of single, double, and heart-lung transplantation. *Chest* 1995; 107: 973–980.

26. Bando K, Paradis IL, Komatsu K, *et al.* Analysis of time-dependent risks for infection, rejection, and death after pulmonary transplantation. *J Thorac Cardiovasc Surg* 1995; 109: 49–57.
27. Flint A, Frank TS. Cytomegalovirus detection in lung transplant biopsy samples by polymerase chain reaction. *J Heart Lung Transplant* 1994; 13: 38–42.
28. Heng D, Sharples LD, McNeil K, Stewart S, Wreghitt T, Wallwork J. Bronchiolitis obliterans syndrome: incidence, natural history, prognosis, and risk factors. *J Heart Lung Transplant* 1998; 17: 1255–1263.
29. Keenan RJ, Lega ME, Dummer JS, *et al.* Cytomegalovirus serologic status and postoperative infection correlated with risk of developing chronic rejection after pulmonary transplantation. *Transplantation* 1991; 51: 433–438.
30. Luckraz H, Sharples L, McNeil K, Wreghitt T, Wallwork J. Cytomegalovirus antibody status of donor/recipient does not influence the incidence of bronchiolitis obliterans syndrome in lung transplantation. *J Heart Lung Transplant* 2003; 22: 287–291.
31. Palmer SM, Jr., Henshaw NG, Howell DN, Miller SE, Davis RD, Tapson VF. Community respiratory viral infection in adult lung transplant recipients. *Chest* 1998; 113: 944–950.
32. Billings JL, Hertz MI, Wendt CH. Community respiratory virus infections following lung transplantation. *Transpl Infect Dis* 2001; 3: 138–148.
33. Kramer MR, Marshall SE, Starnes VA, Gamberg P, Amitai Z, Theodore J. Infectious complications in heart-lung transplantation. Analysis of 200 episodes. *Arch Intern Med* 1993; 153: 2010–2016.
34. Holt ND, Gould FK, Taylor CE, *et al.* Incidence and significance of noncytomegalovirus viral respiratory infection after adult lung transplantation. *J Heart Lung Transplant* 1997; 16: 416–419.
35. Ohori NP, Michaels MG, Jaffe R, Williams P, Yousem SA. Adenovirus pneumonia in lung transplant recipients. *Hum Pathol* 1995; 26: 1073–1079.
36. Wendt CH, Fox JM, Hertz MI. Paramyxovirus infection in lung transplant recipients. *J Heart Lung Transplant* 1995; 14: 479–485.
37. Matar LD, McAdams HP, Palmer SM, *et al.* Respiratory viral infections in lung transplant recipients: radiologic findings with clinical correlation. *Radiology* 1999; 213: 735–742.
38. Hopkins PM, Plit ML, Carter IW, Chhajed PN, Malouf MA, Glanville AR. Indirect fluorescent antibody testing of nasopharyngeal swabs for influenza diagnosis in lung transplant recipients. *J Heart Lung Transplant* 2003; 22: 161–168.
39. Hohlfeld J, Niedermeyer J, Hamm H, Schafers HJ, Wagner TO, Fabel H. Seasonal onset of bronchiolitis obliterans syndrome in lung transplant recipients. *J Heart Lung Transplant* 1996; 15: 888–894.
40. Vilchez RA, McCurry K, Dauber J, *et al.* The epidemiology of parainfluenza virus infection in lung transplant recipients. *Clin Infect Dis* 2001; 33: 2004–2008.
41. Billings JL, Hertz MI, Savik K, Wendt CH. Respiratory viruses and chronic rejection in lung transplant recipients. *J Heart Lung Transplant* 2002; 21: 559–566.
42. Zahradnik JM. Adenovirus pneumonia. *Semin Respir Infect* 1987; 2: 104–111.
43. Massad MG, Ramirez AM. Influenza pneumonia in thoracic organ transplant recipients: what can we do to avoid it ? *Chest* 2001; 119: 997–999.
44. Palmer SM Jr, Henshaw NG, Howell DN, Miller SE, Davis RD, Tapson VF. Community respiratory viral infection in adult lung transplant recipients. *Chest* 1998; 113: 944–950.
45. Elssner A, Vogelmeier C. The role of neutrophils in the pathogenesis of obliterative bronchiolitis after lung transplantation. *Transpl Infect Dis* 2001; 3: 168–176.
46. Penn CC, Liu C. Bronchiolitis following infection in adults and children. *Clin Chest Med* 1993; 14: 645–654.
47. Bruder JT, Jie T, McVey DL, Kovesdi I. Expression of gp19K increases the persistence of transgene expression from an adenovirus vector in the mouse lung and liver. *J Virol* 1997; 71: 7623–7628.
48. Abu-Harb M, Bell F, Finn A, *et al.* IL-8 and neutrophil elastase levels in the respiratory tract of infants with RSV bronchiolitis. *Eur Respir J* 1999; 14: 139–143.

49. Wang SZ, Xu H, Wraith A, Bowden JJ, Alpers JH, Forsyth KD. Neutrophils induce damage to respiratory epithelial cells infected with respiratory syncytial virus. *Eur Respir J* 1998; 12: 612–618.
50. Subauste MC, Jacoby DB, Richards SM, Proud D. Infection of a human respiratory epithelial cell line with rhinovirus. Induction of cytokine release and modulation of susceptibility to infection by cytokine exposure. *J Clin Invest* 1995; 96: 549–557.
51. Arnold R, Humbert B, Werchau H, Gallati H, Konig W. Interleukin-8, interleukin-6, and soluble tumour necrosis factor receptor type I release from a human pulmonary epithelial cell line (A549) exposed to respiratory syncytial virus. *Immunology* 1994; 82: 126–133.
52. Skoner DP, Gentile DA, Patel A, Doyle WJ. Evidence for cytokine mediation of disease expression in adults experimentally infected with influenza A virus. *J Infect Dis* 1999; 180: 10–14.
53. Frost AE. Role of infections, pathogenesis, and management in lung transplantation. *Transplant Proc* 1999; 31: 175–177.
54. Winter JB, Gouw AS, Groen M, Wildevuur C, Prop J. Respiratory viral infections aggravate airway damage caused by chronic rejection in rat lung allografts. *Transplantation* 1994; 57: 418–422.
55. Green M, Wald ER, Fricker FJ, Griffith BP, Trento A. Infections in pediatric orthotopic heart transplant recipients. *Pediatr Infect Dis J* 1989; 8: 87–93.
56. Ascher NL, Stock PG, Bumgardner GL, Payne WD, Najarian JS. Infection and rejection of primary hepatic transplant in 93 consecutive patients treated with triple immunosuppressive therapy. *Surg Gynecol Obstet* 1988; 167: 474–484.
57. Durham JR, Nakhleh RE, Levine A, Levine TB. Persistence of interstitial inflammation after episodes of cardiac rejection associated with systemic infection. *J Heart Lung Transplant* 1995; 14: 774–780.
58. Hruby Z, Myszka-Bijak K, Gosciniak G, *et al.* Helicobacter pylori in kidney allograft recipients: high prevalence of colonization and low incidence of active inflammatory lesions. *Nephron* 1997; 75: 25–29.
59. Heemann UW, Azuma H, Tullius SG, Schmid C, Philipp T, Tilney NL. Infections and reduced functioning kidney mass induce chronic rejection in rat kidney allografts. *Clin Nephrol* 1996; 46: 34–38.
60. Charpin JM, Stern M, Lebrun G, Aubin P, Grenet D, Israel-Biet D. Increased endothelin-1 associated with bacterial infection in lung transplant recipients. *Transplantation* 2001; 71: 1840–1847.
61. Heng D, Sharples LD, McNeil K, Stewart S, Wreghitt T, Wallwork J. Bronchiolitis obliterans syndrome: incidence, natural history, prognosis, and risk factors. *J Heart Lung Transplant* 1998; 17: 1255–1263.
62. Ward C, Camara M, Forrest I, *et al.* Quorum signals are present in clinically stable lung allograft recipients. *Thorax* 2003; 58: 444–446.
63. von HL. Role of persistent infection in the control and severity of asthma: focus on Chlamydia pneumoniae. *Eur Respir J* 2002; 19: 546–556.
64. Nystrom T. Nonculturable bacteria: programmed survival forms or cells at death's door? *Bioessays* 2003; 25: 204–211.
65. Gabriel R, Selwyn S, Brown D, *et al.* Virus infections and acute renal transplant rejection. *Nephron* 1976; 16: 282–286.
66. Vilchez RA, Dauber J, Kusne S. Infectious etiology of bronchiolitis obliterans: the respiratory viruses connection - myth or reality? *Am J Transplant* 2003; 3: 245–249.
67. Husain S, Singh N. Bronchiolitis obliterans and lung transplantation: evidence for an infectious etiology. *Semin Respir Infect* 2002; 17: 310–314.
68. Billings JL, Hertz MI, Wendt CH. Community respiratory virus infections following lung transplantation. *Transpl Infect Dis* 2001; 3: 138–148.
69. Cainelli F, Vento S. Infections and solid organ transplant rejection: a cause-and-effect relationship? *Lancet Infect Dis* 2002; 2: 539–549.

70. Ward C, Whitford H, Snell G, *et al.* Bronchoalveolar lavage macrophage and lymphocyte phenotypes in lung transplant recipients. *J Heart Lung Transplant* 2001; 20: 1064–1074.
71. Snell GI, de Hoyos A, Krajden M, Winton T, Maurer JR. Pseudomonas cepacia in lung transplant recipients with cystic fibrosis. *Chest* 1993; 103: 466–471.
72. De Soyza, Archer L, McDowell A, *et al.* Lung transplantation for cystic fibrosis; the effect of *B. cepacia* genomovars on post transplant outcomes. *J Heart Lung Transplant* 2001; 20: 158.
73. Kubak BM. Fungal infection in lung transplantation. *Transpl Infect Dis* 2002; 4: Suppl 3, pp. 24–31.
74. Minari A, Husni R, Avery RK, *et al.* The incidence of invasive aspergillosis among solid organ transplant recipients and implications for prophylaxis in lung transplants. *Transpl Infect Dis* 2002; 4: 195–200.
75. Helmi M, Love RB, Welter D, Cornwell RD, Meyer KC. Aspergillus infection in lung transplant recipients with cystic fibrosis: risk factors and outcomes comparison to other types of transplant recipients. *Chest* 2003; 123: 800–808.
76. Nunley DR, Ohori P, Grgurich WF, *et al.* Pulmonary aspergillosis in cystic fibrosis lung transplant recipients. *Chest* 1998; 114: 1321–1329.
77. Nunley DR, Gal AA, Vega JD, Perlino C, Smith P, Lawrence EC. Saprophytic fungal infections and complications involving the bronchial anastomosis following human lung transplantation. *Chest* 2002; 122: 1185–1191.
78. Wu G, Vilchez RA, Eidelman B, Fung J, Kormos R, Kusne S. Cryptococcal meningitis: an analysis among 5,521 consecutive organ transplant recipients. *Transpl Infect Dis* 2002; 4: 183–188.
79. Tamm M, Malouf M, Glanville A. Pulmonary scedosporium infection following lung transplantation. *Transpl Infect Dis* 2001; 3: 189–194.

*CHAPTER 4*

# Bronchiolitis obliterans syndrome and bronchiolitis obliterans in lung transplantation: will a pathologist and a physician ever meet?

*E.K. Verbeken, S. Stewart*

*Dept of Pathology, Katholieke Universiteit Leuven, Belgium. #Papworth Hospital, Cambridge, UK.*

*Correspondence: E.K. Verbeken, Dept of Pathology, University Hospital St. Rafaël, Minderbroedersstraat 12, B-3000, Leuven, Belgium.*

In pathology, there is the obvious and the not so obvious. Bronchiolitis obliterans syndrome (BOS) and bronchiolitis obliterans (BO) belong to the not so obvious, with regards to their aetiology, interrelationship, evolution and responsiveness to therapy.

BOS is a severe clinical syndrome that occurs in lung transplanted patients. It is characterised by a persistent decrease in expiratory flow as measured by the forced expiratory volume in 1 second (FEV1) [1]. BOS is potentially life threatening, and ongoing decline of lung function necessitates re-transplantation.

BO on the contrary, is only a nonspecific pathological lesion of the small conducting airways which is repaired by proliferation of granulation tissue. BO is not uncommonly encountered by pulmonary pathologists as it occurs in a wide variety of conditions, including organ transplantation (not only of lungs), infections, auto-immune diseases, after inhalation of toxic agents, allergic diseases, drugs, radiation and distally to a bronchial obstruction and, if no cause can be found, then BO remains cryptogenic [2].

The confrontation between a potentially life threatening syndrome and a nonspecific pathological lesion is a traditional source of commotion. Such a condition indeed is ranked among the "pitfalls in pathology". Opinions differ between specialists, however; for the physician the pitfall is the pathologist, for the pathologist, the pitfall is the pathology. The friendly *modus vivendi* is that the discordance between severe symptoms in BOS and disappointing or inconclusive findings on fibreoptic biopsy are due to insufficient sampling, patchy distribution of early lesions, or to the fact that older fibrous lesions may impede the collection ofadequate specimens. Some inexperience of the pathologist is also mentioned, as the lesions, in particular the early ones, may be subtle. All this is true, however, the discrepancies between BOS and BO are more complicated than sampling errors or missing subtle lesions by light microscopy.

The clinical term BOS suggests an intimate link between inflammation, fibrosis and the decline in FEV1. However, the relationship between the insult, the inflammatory infiltrate and the proliferation of fibroblasts with subsequent collagen deposition are not fully understood. The insult leading to BOS is still unidentified. Histologically, only the repair reaction is observed. Furthermore, in recent years new paradigms have been proposed for the pathogenesis of fibrosis, that more or less dissociate the fibrosis from the inflammation, key observations in the repair process. Also, the extent and progression of the lesions and the correlation with the decline of FEV1 are largely unknown, as are the morphological predictors of the latter progression. In spite of this,

Eur Respir Mon, 2004, 29, 55–65. Printed in UK - all rights reserved. Copyright ERS Journals Ltd 2004; European Respiratory Monograph; ISSN 1025-448x. ISBN 1-904097-33-2.

the pathologist on duty is not supposed to stare into the microscope at a nonspecific lesion, but merely urged to explore the whole BOS in the ever too small endobronchial biopsy.

The present chapter firstly gives an overview of the histological and anatomical spectrum of BO lesions as they are clearly observed in open lung biopsies (OLB) or autopsy specimens. Secondly, the pathology will be briefly discussed in view of some basic pathogenetic paradigms with regard to inflammation and fibroproliferation.

## Overview of the anatomical distribution and histology of bronchiolitis obliterans lesions

The human airway tree consists, in consecutive order, of the following: central cartilaginous bronchi (B), membranous bronchioles (MBs), respiratory bronchioles (RBs), and peripheral alveolar ducts (ADs). The alveoli do not contribute to the bifurcating tree, (also called a "fractal tree"), as they are only outpouchings of the distal airway walls [3]. Alveoli progressively increase in number and density from the RB onwards. Conversely, the cartilaginous support of bronchi progressively disappears from a continuous layer in the central bronchi to discontinuous spots in the most distal bronchial generation. In MBs and the first generation of RBs, cartilage and glands are lacking, but these airways preserve a well developed muscular wall. RBs bear, in addition, some alveolar outpouchings. Thus the morphological characteristics of the airways wall only gradually changes from one type to another, *i.e.* B to MB, from MB to RB, from RB to AD. The respective anatomical disposition is presented in figure 1, in which Weibel's original generation numbers [4] are adjusted to more recent histological reconstructions [3]. Corresponding average diameters are also indicated. MBs are <1 mm, and correspond to generation number 12–14. The conventional "small airways >2 mm in diameter" corresponds in fact to the seventh generation of bronchi. It is also noteworthy that the first generation of RBs are likely to figure as an MB on a histological transsection, because the alveolar outpouchings in their walls are discontinuous [3].

Consequent to its name, BO histologically involves only the MBs or first generation of RBs. Therefore, it is only the "pure" type of BO that is being dealt with. In contrast to the other causes of BO, mentioned previously, where BO figures merely as a proximal extension of a basically parenchymal ("distal") disease, BO in lung allografts appears to involve primarily the bronchiolar bifurcations of the fractal tree. Pure BO is very frequently encountered as the predominant site in a transplant biopsy. Almost always, however, BO lesions extend into a distal direction of the fractal tree, into the RBs and the first generation of ADs. This is the extended type of BO. This extended type results in a histological involvement of the centriacinar area (fig. 1). Indeed, the more distal the extension, the more the centrilobular area is involved and the more the lesion resembles bronchiolitis obliterans organising pneumonia (BOOP) or cryptogenic organising pneumonia (COP). Also, the more distal the extension of the disease, the more the lung function is restrictive. A restrictive lung function is confined to interstitial lung diseases at the parenchymal level. The decline of $FEV_1$, however, may be due to a disease along the entire tree. This is a weakness of the definition of BOS.

BO represents proximal disease, whereas BOOP and, even more, COP are more distally located in the fractal tree [5]. Rarely, BO may extend proximal to the MBs into the cartilaginous bronchi. Partial or complete obstruction of an airway may result in postobstructive phenomena including alveolar accumulation of foamy macrophages, and fibrosis and atelectasis distally to the obstruction.

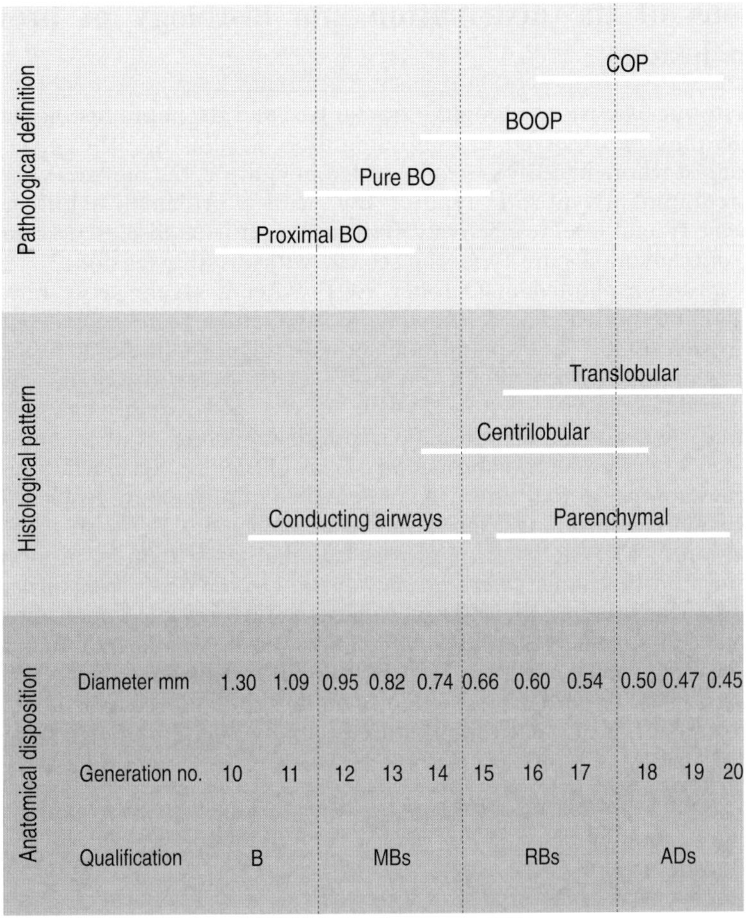


Fig. 1. – Correlation between anatomical disposition, definition of pathological terms and histological pattern. COP: cryptogenic organising pneumonia; BOOP: bronchiolitis obliterans organising pneumonia; BO: bronchiolitis obliterans; B: bronchus; MB: membranous bronchiole; RB: respiratory bronchiole; AD: alveolar duct.

Histologically a spectrum of BO lesions is also observed. The spectrum ranges from a predominantly inflammatory (BOi) to an almost exclusively fibrotic type (BOf). The inflammatory type is characterised by a prominent mononuclear infiltrate in association with fibromyxoid or collagenous connective tissue within the bronchiolar lumen (or more distal alveolar in case of a distal extension). The fibrotic type is characterised by collagenous scarring of the bronchiolar wall with absent or minimal inflammation.

Both the inflammatory type and the fibrotic type may figure either as a pure or as an extended form, and both types may affect the tree only very focally. On transsection, the lesions may be excentric or concentric, or may completely obliterate the lumen. However, both types will finally result in complete fibrous scarring of the bronchiolar lumen.

Experience shows that asynchronous lesions are not observed in one biopsy. The spectrum between predominantly inflammatory and predominantly collagenous lesions is mainly observed between biopsies or between patients. According to the working formulation [6], the lesion is considered active if inflammation is present; if not, BO is considered inactive.

## Illustrations of the distribution and histology of bronchiolitis obliterans lesions

All the anatomic extensions along the fractal tree and the entire histological spectrum of BO lesions may be observed in lung allografts. To illustrate this, five patients are presented, four of whom had BOS. As illustrated in figure 2, the biopsies of three patients showed a predominantly fibrotic type of BO, with a proximal, a pure and a distal extension in the fractal tree, respectively. Two other patients disclosed an inflammatory type of BO, one having a pure type, the second with distal extension.

Patient 1 was transplanted in October 2001. After a severe acute rejection in the summer of 2003 the patient was re-transplanted in October 2003 because of developing rapidly progressive BOS. The explant lung shown in figure 3 disclosed a fibrotic type of BO, with a remarkably centripetal extension into several bronchi, whereas distal extension was minimal.

Patient 2 was transplanted in August 2002. In January 2003 the patient suffered an acute severe rejection confirmed by transbronchial biopsy (TBB). BOS, clinically suspected, was not confirmed on biopsy at that time. The patient died of progressive BOS in August 2003. Autopsy specimens of the lung (fig. 4) showed almost pure BO with total or subtotal fibrotic occlusion of MBs and RBs, and with minimal infiltration by mononuclear cells. Atelectatic and fibrotic changes were present distally to the obstructed airways.

Patient 3 was transplanted in 1995. In August, a TBB revealed dense fibrotic strands lining thin walled airspaces, presumably ADs. There was no significant inflammation. MBs in the biopsy were normal. A diagnosis of BO/BOOP was made, which was confirmed in OLB in January 1996. The latter biopsy (fig. 5) remarkably showed a distal presentation of BO with involvement of the centrolobular areas, and with only minimal pure BO lesions.

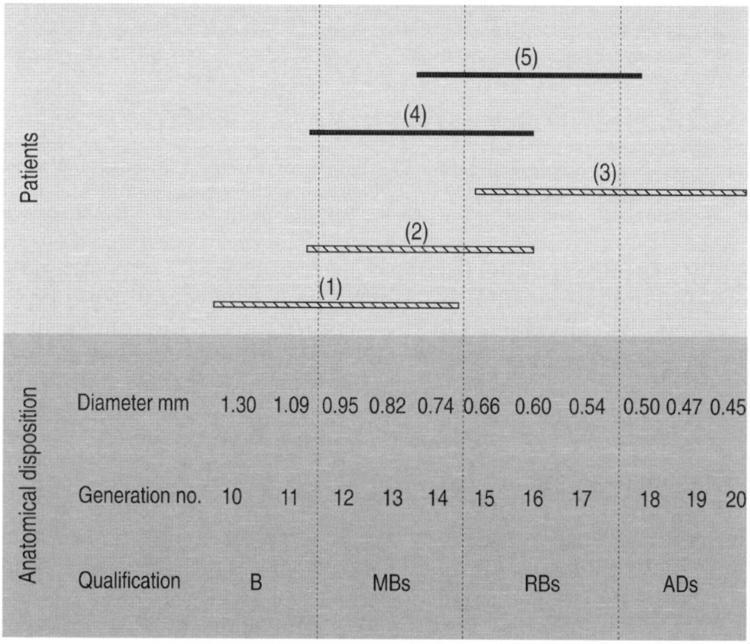


Fig. 2. – Bronchiolitis obliterans (BO) lesions in five patients with different anatomical extensions and histological subtypes. (■): inflammatory type BO; (▧): fibrotic type BO; B: bronchus; MB: membranous bronchiole; RB: respiratory bronchiole; AD: alveolar duct.

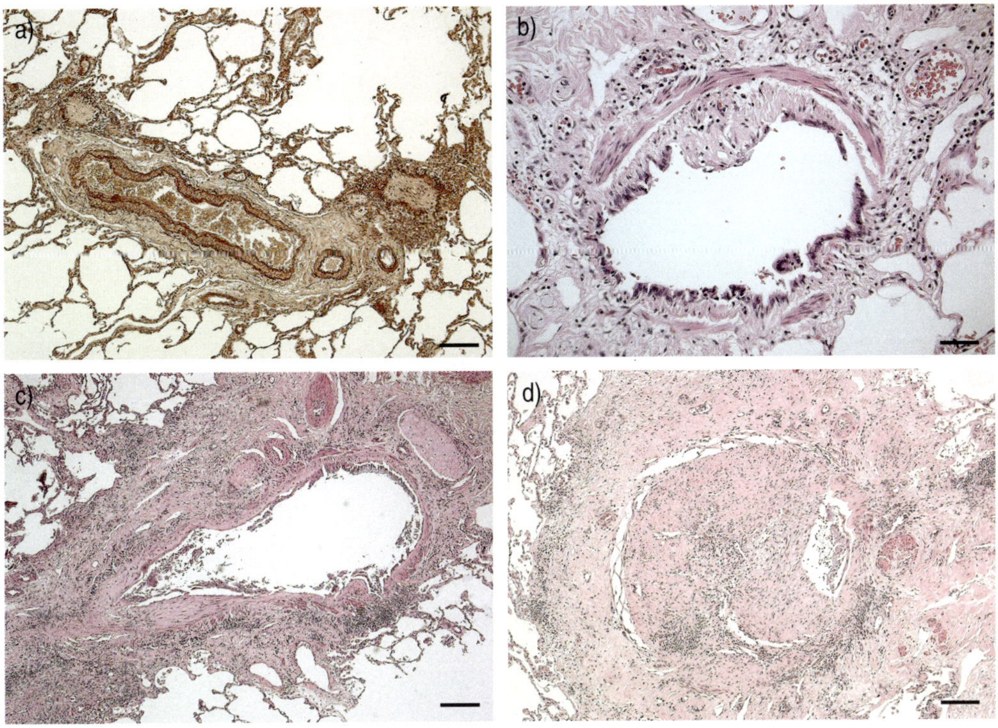


Fig. 3. – Open lung biopsy of patient 1 with bronchiolitis obliterans syndrome showing bronchiolitis obliterans (BO) of the fibrotic type with proximal extension. a) Typically in BO, the lumen of membranous bronchioles (MBs) are narrowed or occluded by granulation tissue or fibrous plugs. Present elastic stain shows a longitudinal and oblique transsection through two normal pulmonary arteries. The accompanying MBs are totally occluded. The surrounding parenchyma is normal. No distal extension of the disease into the alveolated parenchyma was observed in this case (elastic stained, scale bar=50 cm). b) The luminal occlusion may be very focal, limited to a single small fibrous polyp protruding into the bronchiolar lumen (haematoxylin and eosin stained: H&E, scale bar=200 cm). c) The "proximal extension" of BO consists of bronchial involvement. The airway shown here is a cartilaginous bronchus (diameter 1.15 mm, not incorporating collapse due to tissue processing). An excentric mucosal fibrous plaque is present (H&E stained, scale=50 cm). d) Another larger airway, diameter 1.38 mm, is totally obliterated by a fibrous plug. The airway wall also is almost entirely sclerotic (H&E stained, scale=50 cm).

The accompanying inflammatory infiltrate was only mild. BOOP lesions were obviously contaminated by an endogenous or postobstructive lipid pneumonia. The patient died from BOS a few months later in March 1996, with identical histological findings at autopsy.

Patient 4 underwent lung transplantation in March 1992. Two years later, an OLB disclosed BO with rather selective involvement of MBs. Remarkably, fibroproliferation was intimately linked with a dense inflammatory infiltrate (fig. 6). The patient died of slowly progressive BOS in November 2000. The autopsy specimen, also shown in figure 6, revealed total fibrous obliteration of MBs, almost no residual inflammation, and postobstructive fibrosis and atelectasis. This patient developed identical lesions, in 6.5 yrs, as patient 2 did in <8 months.

Finally, patient 5 had no clinical BOS. After double lung transplantation in August 1998 a severe bronchial stenosis and bronchomalacia developed in the right lung, for which the patient was finally re-transplanted. The patient has done well since. Histology of the explant lung is presented in figure 7. It shows fibromyxoid polyps protruding into bronchiolar lumina, corresponding to pure BO, together with distally extending BOOP lesions in the centrilobular areas, and associated with a dense inflammatory infiltrate.

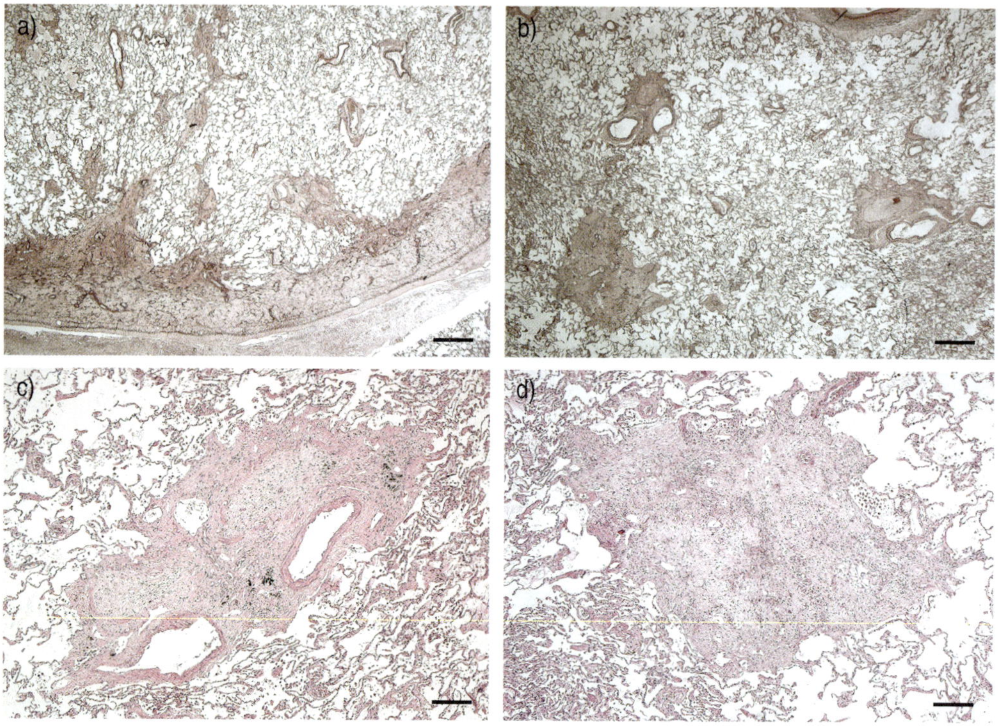


Fig. 4. – Autopsy specimen of patient 2 with bronchiolitis obliterans syndrome, showing fibrotic obliteration of membranous bronchioles (MBs) and proximal respiratory bronchioles. a) Overview of a subpleural area of the lung. A peripheral rim of collapsed and fibrotic parenchyma is seen underneath a normal pleura; the intact elastic lamina is clearly seen. At least three MBs supplying the subpleural parenchyma are present. Their lumen is completely obliterated by fibrous plugs. No extension of bronchiolitis obliterans (BO) in the surrounding parenchyma is seen (elastic stained, scale bar=12.5). b) Low power view of the same lung. Three BO lesions are present: two of the pure type, and one showing some extension into the surrounding parenchyma, thus representing bronchiolitis obliterans organising pneumonia (BOOP). Most cases of "pure BO" have few such BOOP areas (elastic stained, scale bar=12.5). c) Two MBs, accompanied by their normal pulmonary arteries, have just bifurcated. Their lumina are totally obliterated without extension of the disease into the surrounding parenchyma. This is pure BO (haematoxylin and eosin stained: H&E, scale bar=50 cm). b) BOOP extension, in the same case. The lesion is well circumscribed and sharply demarcated from the surrounding alveoli. Only the centrilobular area is affected in these cases (H&E scalebar=50 cm).

The patients illustrated represent almost all OLBs performed for BOS in lung allografts in the University Hospital of Leuven. This fact illustrates the histological and anatomical variability of BO lesions. Intriguingly, the three BOf patients had rapidly progressive BOS with re-transplantation after 6 months, or fatal outcome at ~7 and 8 months respectively. The BOi patient fared better, having slowly progressive disease, but died nevertheless from BOS 6.5 yrs later. Clinically, two types of BOS have been identified [8], namely an acute onset BOS of with poor prognosis, and a chronic onset BOS, characterised by a slow decline of lung function. However little information was revealed on the underlying pathology of these different patterns, As TBBs are mostly unreliable for the identification of the BO lesions, and as OLBs are only rarely obtained, it is believed that only multicentre studies can further clarify the structure-function analysis with regard to BOS and BO.

In summary, anatomically, a pure and an extended type of BO are distinguished and both types are seen at the same time in a biopsy, although one single type is prevailing. Histologically, a spectrum is found between a predominantly inflammatory type and a

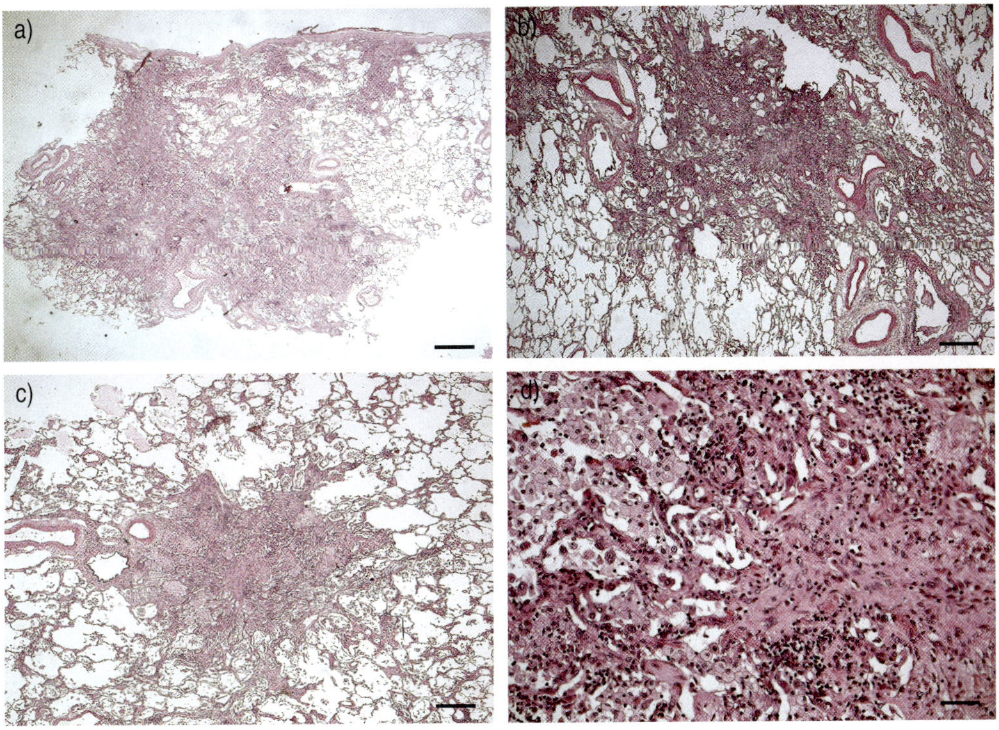


Fig. 5. – Autopsy specimen of Patient 3 with bronchiolitis obliterans syndrome. The lungs represent bronchiolitis obliterans (BO) of the fibrotic type and mainly involve the distal respiratory bronchioles (RBs) and alveolar ducts (ADs), without significant involvement of the membranous bronchioles (MBs). a) The low power view shows a lobulated pattern of the parenchyma. Diseased areas involve the lobular centre from which they extend more peripherally into the lobule. The more peripheral the extension, the larger the diseased area and the more the lesion resembles cryptogenic organising pneumonia. Note that the diseased areas are mostly separated from each other by interpositioned normal alveolated parenchyma (haematoxylin and eosin stained: H&E, scale bar=12.5 cm. b) At closer inspection, the MBs, seen here along their accompanying pulmonary arteries, which supply the diseased areas, are normal and their lumen is patent. The fibrous obliteration occurs more distally in the tree, namely in RBs and ADs. This is typical for distal BO (H&E scale bar=25 cm). c) The MB figuring along the diseased area is normal. The obliteration is more distal in the airway tree and thus adjacent to the supplying MB. The latter topographic relation is a direct consequence of lung anatomy [7]. The obliteration is centrilobular as a rim of alveolated parenchyma persists between the BO lesion and the interlobular septum, seen at the bottom and at the right. (H&E scale bar=25). d) Elements of a postobstructive or endogenous lipid pneumonia (ELP) are often seen in BO. It consists of some mononuclear cell infiltrate into the thickened alveolar septa, and, more importantly, accumulation of foamy macrophages in the alveolar lumina. They are waiting in vain for the mucociliary escalator. The lymphocytic infiltrate in this case is probably mainly related to the ELP, rather than to the BO (H&E scalebar=200 cm).

predominantly collagenous type. Only one type prevails in one biopsy. The morphology remains nonspecific, even in a lung transplant setting. BO may be secondary to allograft rejection or to other causes including infection. The finding of BO does not necessarily predispose the patient to chronic rejection [9].

## Bronchiolitis obliterans and paradigms of inflammation and fibrosis

It is beyond the scope of this chapter to go in depth into the aetiopathogenetic mechanisms of post-transplant BO. Suffice to say that, today, the evolving concept is that

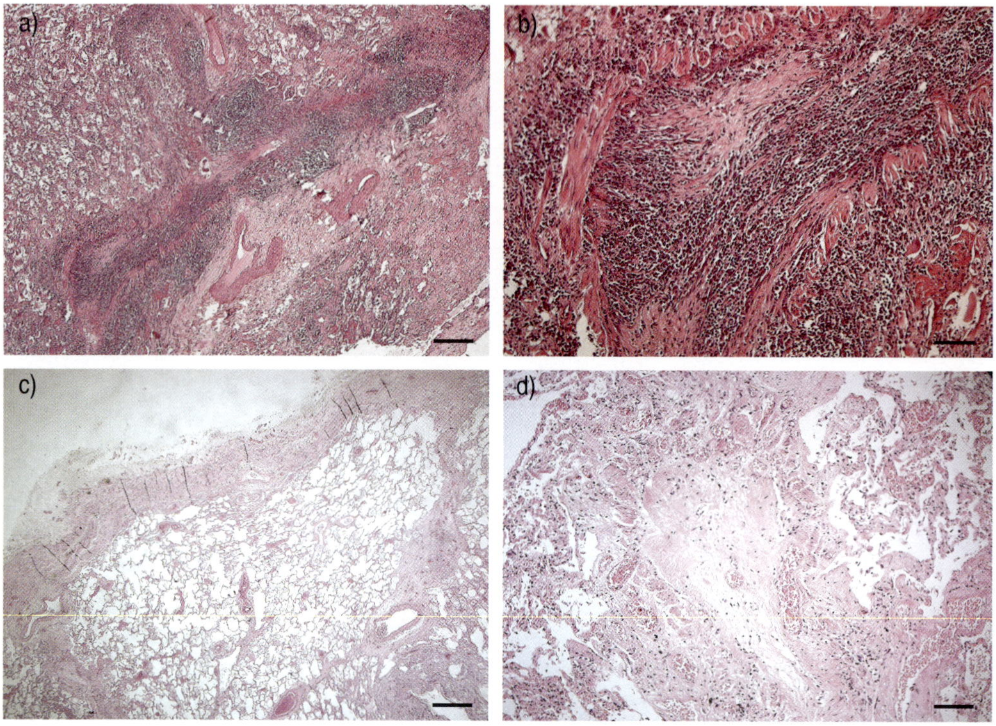


Fig. 6. – "Pure bronchiolitis obliterans (BO)" of the inflammatory type in a patient with bronchiolitis obliterans syndrome. Both the open lung biopsy and the autopsy specimen, >6 yrs later, are shown. a) Bifurcating membranous bronchioles (MBs) are massively infiltrated by mononuclear inflammatory cells. Their walls can only be discerned by their elastic fibres and smooth muscle cells. The lumen is partially obliterated by a fibrous plug. The surrounding parenchyma shows a severe rejection in this particular case (haematoxylin and eosin stained: H&E, scale bar=25 cm). b) Detail of the fibrous plugging in the bronchiolar lumen seen in a (H&E scale bar=100 cm). c) Subpleural area of a *post mortem* specimen of the same patient, 6.5 yrs later. The low power view shows a fibrotic type of pure BO, associated with collapse and fibrosis of the peripheral lung tissue. The supplying bronchioles are obliterated by a fibrous plug. However, the picture is identical to figure 5a. The latter patient had an evolution of <8 months (H&E scale bar=12.5 cm). d) Detail of c, showing the fibrous obliteration of the MB supplying the subpleural parenchyma (H&E scale bar=100 cm).

BO represents a "final common pathway" lesion in which various insults can lead to a similar histological result [10]. Therefore, post-transplant BO can be dealt with as one of the idiopathic interstitial pneumonias (IIPs) including cellular and fibrotic NSIP (nonspecific interstitial pneumonia), UIP (usual interstitial pneumonia), and idiopathic BOOP/COP. Indeed, all the latter IIPs are characterised by an analogous spectrum of morphological nonspecific elements dominated either by inflammation, by young connective tissue or fibroblast foci, or by collagenous scars. Each of these elements is relevant for prognosis and responses to therapy. As is well documented for NSIP and UIP, the prognosis worsens with the amount of fibrosis, and steroid responsiveness increases with inflammatory activity [11–13]. For idiopathic BOOP/COP, collagenous fibrosis is also a predictor of unfavourable outcome despite steroid therapy [14].

Irrespective of the primary injury, the final common pathway lesion of post-transplant BO results in inflammation and fibroproliferation. Their interrelation is subject to several hypotheses giving rise to an equal number of paradigms of airway remodelling. Regardless of the primary injury site, four basic mechanisms must be considered.

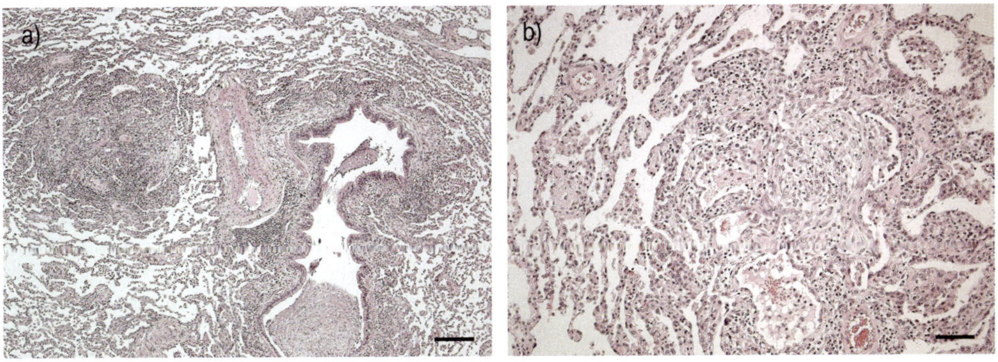


Fig. 7. – Distal bronchiolitis obliterans (BO) of the inflammatory type in a patient without bronchiolitis obliterans syndrome. a) Representative overview showing an association of fibromyxoid polyps in the lumen of membranous bronchioles (MBs), accompanied by a moderate mononuclear infiltrate. To the left a centrilobular area is involved with young granulation tissue proliferating in a respiratory bronchiole (which is partially surrounded by a smooth muscle wall) and in some adjacent alveolar ducts. This area represents a "distal" or bronchiolitis obliterans organising pneumonia extension (haematoxylin and eosin stained: H&E, scale bar=50 cm). b) Detail of the BOOP area. Also in the latter extension, a moderate lymphocytic infiltrate is present (H&E scale bar=100 cm).

***Hypothesis I.*** This hypothesis dominated in the 1970s and the 1980s and suggests that an unidentified insult initiates a smouldering chronic inflammation that ultimately leads to chronic injury with subsequent fibrosis. The corresponding "direct inflammatory paradigm" has therapeutic implications; anti-inflammatory medication should prevent fibrosis.

***Hypothesis II.*** In the 1990s, a new hypothesis was formulated according to which a still unidentified repeated stimulus causes a sequential injury with epithelial cell damage and loss of basement membrane integrity. This is followed by an aberrant wound healing through direct epithelial-mesenchymal interactions without inflammation and, finally, with subsequent fibrosis. This is the direct fibroplastic paradigm, basically propagating an inflammatory independent fibrogenesis. According to this model, therapy should focus on inhibitors of fibrogenesis [15].

***Hypothesis III.*** A recently formulated mechanism of chronic lung disease is based on models using antigens that trigger a profound immune response [16]. In this model inflammation is again an integral part of the fibrogenetic process. In brief an injury (antigen or pathogen) activates an initial foreign challenge with a type I cascade of cytokines that activates neutrophils and macrophages but inhibits fibrogenesis. If the agent is not cleared, a switch to a more sophisticated type 2 immune response occurs. The type 2 cascade of cytokines activates fibroblasts and collagen deposition. The balance between normal tissue repair and excess collagen deposition is thus dictated by the cytokine phenotype. This model is "the type 1/type 2 paradigm of tissue remodelling" according to which therapeutic targeting should focus on the cytokine 2 cascade and inhibition of fibrogenesis.

***Hypothesis IV.*** The frequent occurrence of pure BO in post-transplant BO remains intriguing. From a mechanical viewpoint, MBs have been shown to be particularly prone to compression, due to overexpansion of the surrounding airspaces. This is related to the anatomic disposition of MBs [7]. These, indeed, follow an intraseptal course and are encroached by acini they supply themselves with air. The influence of compressive mechanical stresses on fibrotic airway remodelling is not explored extensively. TSCHUMPERLIN and DRAZEN [17] who reviewed the data, promote a "mechanotransduction paradigm" of fibrotic airway remodelling, linking inflammatory and mechanical stimuli exerted on the bronchiolar wall. In this paradigm, the signals for airway remodelling are derived from the effects of mechanical stress on the airway epithelium. One of the key observations is that foetal lung fibroblast respond to mechanical stimulation of the epithelium by increasing collagen synthesis in a pressure-dependent manner.

Each of these paradigms has diagnostic, prognostic and therapeutic consequences. As suggested by the direct inflammatory paradigm, fibrosis in a biopsy should not necessarily be regarded as inactive or older lesions. Some cases of post-transplant BO may exhibit a predominant fibrotic reaction, whereas others are mainly inflammatory. Comparable to what is observed in UIP *versus* NSIP, the type of BO should be specified in the biopsy report.

Furthermore, what matters as a prognostic indicator is the amount of fibrosis; there are no asynchronous lesions. Consequently, one can expect that, if the biopsy shows a fibrotic type of BO, re-transplantation is the option. In contrast, if a predominant inflammatory type is observed in an OLB of a patient with BOS, an anti-inflammatory therapy may be helpful, albeit to slow down deterioration of the lung function. In this respect, a surgical biopsy is recommended in patients with early BOS.


## Summary

Bronchiolitis obliterans (BOS) syndrome is a severe clinical syndrome in lung transplanted patients. The corresponding morphological lesion is bronchiolitis obliterans (BO). The correlation between BOS and BO is far from clear.

The presented chapter gives an overview of BO in open lung biopsies and autopsy specimens of lung allografts, both with regard to their anatomical localisation and their histology. Anatomically, BO may present either in a pure type, involving mainly membranous and proximal respiratory bronchioles (RBs), in a "proximal" type, involving also bronchi, or in a distal type, involving mainly distal RBs and alveolar ducts. The latter type overlaps with bronchiolitis obliterans organising pneumonia or cryptogenic organising pneumonia. In a biopsy, one of these types prevails with a wide range, though.

Histologically, BO lesions consist of a spectrum between a predominantly inflammatory and a predominantly fibrotic type. In a single biopsy, one type prevails with only a very narrow range. Asynchronous lesions are not observed.

Finally, the pathology is briefly discussed in view of some basic pathogenetic paradigms recently formulated regarding inflammation and fibroproliferation. Parallels are drawn between inflammatory and fibrotic and other idiopathic interstitial pneumonias such as non-specific interstitial pneumonia and usual interstitial pneumonia.

The aim of this chapter is to promote a good understanding between Physician and Pathologist, and between bronchiolitis obliterans syndrome and bronchiolitis obliterans.


**Keywords:** Bronchiolitis obliterans, bronchiolitis obliterans syndrome, lung transplantation, morphology, pathology.

## References

1. Cooper J, Billingham M, Egan T, *et al.* A working formulation for the standardization of nomenclature and for clinical staging of chronic dysfunction in lung allografts. International Society for Heart and Lung Transplantation. *J Heart Lung Transplant* 1993; 12: 713–716.

2. Schlesinger C, Meyer CA, Veeraraghavan S, Koss MN. Constrictive (obliterative) bronchiolitis: diagnosis, etiology and a critical review of the literature. *Ann Diagn Pathol* 1998; 2: 321–334.
3. Verbeken EK, Cauberghs M, Lauweryns JM, Van de Woestijne KP. Anatomy of membranous bronchioles in normal, senile, and emphysematous human lungs. *J Appl Physiol* 1992; 72: 2343–2353.
4. Weibel ER. Morphometry of the Human Lung. Berlin, Springer Verlag, 1963; p.139.
5. Verbeken EK. Classifying interstitial lung disease in a fractal lung: a morphologist's view "anno Domini 2000". *Eur Respir J* 2001; 18: Suppl. 32, 17s–29s.
6. Yousem SA, Berry GJ, Gagle PT, *et al.* Revision of the 1990 working formulation for the classification of pulmonary allograft rejection: lung rejection study group. *J Heart Transplant* 1996; 15: 1–15.
7. Verbeken EK, Cauberghs M, Van de Woestijne KP. Membranous bronchioles and connective tissue network of normal and emphysematous lungs. *J Appl Physiol* 1996; 81: 2468–2480.
8. Jackson CH, Sharples LD, McNeil K, Stewart S, Wallwork J. Acute and chronic onset of bronchiolitis obliterans syndrome (BOS): are they different entities? *J Heart Lung Transplant* 2002; 21: 658–666.
9. Siddiqui MT, Garrity ER, Husain AN. Bronchiolitis obliterans organizing pneumonia-like reactions: a non-specific response or an atypical form of rejection or infection in lung allograft recipients? *Hum Pathol* 1996; 27: 714–719.
10. Boehler A, Estenne M. Post-transplant bronchiolitis obliterans. *Eur Respir J* 2003; 22: 1007–1018.
11. Bjoraker JA, Ryu JH, Edwin MK, *et al.* Prognostic significance of histopathological subsets in idiopathic pulmonary fibrosis. *Am J Respir Crit Care Med* 1998; 157: 199–203.
12. Travis WD, Matsui K, Moss J, Ferrans VJ. Idiopathic non-specific interstitial pneumonia: prognostic significance of cellular and fibrosing patterns: survival comparison with usual interstitial pneumonia and desquamative interstitial pneumonia. *Am J Surg Pathol* 2000; 24: 19–33.
13. Daniil ZD, Gilchrist FC, Nicholson AG, *et al.* A histologic pattern of non-specific interstitial pneumonia is associated with a better prognosis than usual interstitial pneumonia in patients with cryptogenic fibrosing alveolitis. *Am J Respir Crit Care Med* 1999; 160: 899–905.
14. Yousem SA, Lohr RH, Colby TV. Idiopathic bronchiolitis obliterans organizing pneumonia/cryptogenic organizing pneumonia with unfavourable outcome: pathologic predictors. *Mod Pathol* 1997; 10: 864–871.
15. Gross TJ, Hunninghake GW. Idiopathic pulmonary fibrosis. *N Engl J Med* 2001; 345: 517–525.
16. Kunkel SL, Chensue SW, Lukacs N, Hogaboam C. Cytokine phenotypes serve as a paradigm for experimental immune-mediated lung diseases and remodeling. *Am J Respir Cell Mol Biol* 2003; 29: S63.
17. Tschumperlin DJ, Drazen JM. Mechanical stimuli to airway remodeling. *Am J Respir Crit Care Med* 2001; 164: 90–94.

CHAPTER 5

# Strategies in the prevention and the treatment of ischaemia-reperfusion injury after lung transplantation

*D. Van Raemdonck*, M. Strüber#, F. Venuta¶, D. Vlasselaers+, W. Wisser§, M.E. Erasmus f, and other co-authors of Working Group 2*

**Dept of Thoracic Surgery, +Dept of Intensive Care Medicines, University Hospital Gasthuisberg, Leuven, Belgium, #Dept of Thoracic, Cardiac and Vascular Surgery, Medical High School, Hannover, Germany, ¶Dept of Thoracic Surgery Umberto I Hospital, Rome, Italy, §Dept of Cardiothoracic Surgery, University Hospital, Vienna, Austria, and f Dept of Cardiothoracic Surgery, University Hospital, Groningen, the Netherlands.*

*Correspondence: D. Van Raemdonck, Dept of Thoracic Surgery, University Hospital Gasthuisberg, Herestraat 49, B-3000, Leuven, Belgium.*

Over the last 20 yrs, lung transplantation has become the mainstay of therapy for selected patients suffering from many varieties of end-stage lung disease refractory to medical management. This form of surgical treatment has enjoyed increasing success with better early and late survival rates [1]. Despite its success, lung transplantation is still hampered by persisting problems *e.g.* donor organ shortage, early graft dysfunction (ischaemia-reperfusion injury), late graft dysfunction (bronchiolitis obliterans syndrome: BOS), and morbidity related to long-term immunosuppression [2].

Ischaemia-reperfusion-induced lung injury (IRI) is the term commonly used to summarise the insult that leads to acute and severe dysfunction of the allograft early (<24–72 h) after transplantation [3]. The insult is a combination of cell alterations that occur during the ischaemic period and the damage that occurs during the subsequent reperfusion phase. Other synonyms, frequently used in the literature, to describe this specific organ damage are: reimplantation oedema; reimplantation response; reperfusion oedema; noncardiogenic pulmonary oedema; early graft dysfunction; and primary graft failure. The situation is in many ways comparable with that of acute respiratory distress syndrome (ARDS) or acute lung injury (ALI) [4–6].

Clinically, the injury is characterised by the following: poor oxygenation (arterial oxygen tension/inspiratory oxygen fraction: $P_{a,O_2}/F_{I,O_2}$; high alveolar-arterial partial pressure ($P_{O_2}$) gradient); decreased lung compliance; increased pulmonary vascular resistance with intrapulmonary shunting and protein-rich fluid loss *via* the endotracheal tube (alveolar oedema) or chest drains (interstitial oedema); patchy perihilar pulmonary infiltrates on radiographs (fig. 1); and nonspecific diffuse alveolar damage on biopsy [7]. The diagnosis becomes apparent after attempts are made to exclude secondary causes of allograft dysfunction as there are hyperacute rejection [8, 9], early infection [10], venous anastomotic compromise [11, 12], fluid overload and cardiogenic pulmonary oedema as a result of left ventricular failure [13].

The purpose of this chapter is to describe current strategies in the prevention and the treatment of early graft dysfunction, based on current, scientific knowledge.

Eur Respir Mon, 2004, 29, 66–88. Printed in UK - all rights reserved. Copyright ERS Journals Ltd 2004; European Respiratory Monograph; ISSN 1025-448x. ISBN 1-904097-33-2.

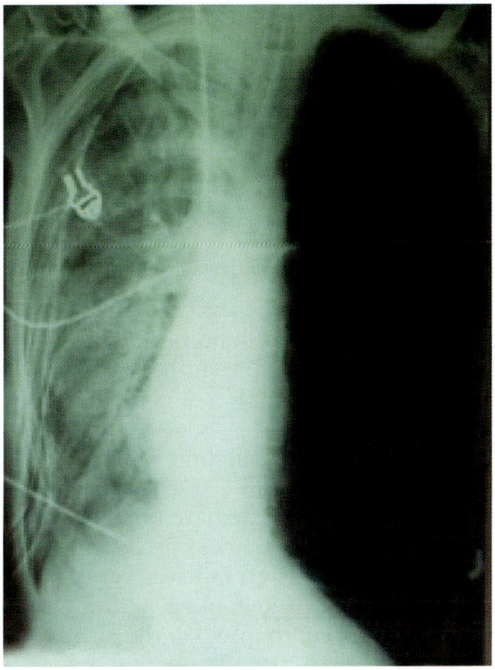

Fig. 1. – Chest radiograph on the second postoperative day following right single-lung transplantation in a 56-yr old male with pulmonary emphysema. Note the whitening of the allograft on the right side and the hyper-inflation of the native left lung.

# Ischaemia-reperfusion injury: the problem

Up to 97% of transplanted lungs will have some degree of perihilar oedema during the immediate postoperative period [14]. Many of these patients will develop mild, transient, and clinically insignificant reimplantation pulmonary oedema. Severe graft dysfunction occurs in 10–20% of lung transplant recipients with a significant impact on clinical outcome with prolonged ventilation, prolonged intensive care unit (ICU) and hospital stay, increased morbidity and mortality, and increased costs. IRI has been identified as the main cause of primary graft failure resulting in a post-transplant mortality of 2–5% [1, 2].

Comparison between different transplant centres is difficult, since there is currently no consensus on the exact definition of this entity. In a retrospective study by CHRISTIE *et al.* [15] looking at 100 consecutive lung transplant recipients, the incidence of primary graft failure (PGF) was 15%. In-hospital mortality was 60% in this subgroup compared with 8.2% in the other subgroup ($p<0.005$). Duration of mechanical ventilatory support in patients with PGF was 36±43 days compared with 4±6 days in the others ($p<0.0001$). Hospital stay was also significantly longer (75±105 *versus* 27±38 days, respectively; $p<0.005$). A 1-yr actuarial survival was 40 *versus* 69%, respectively ($p<0.005$). In another retrospective study by KING *et al.* [16] also looking at 100 consecutive lung transplantations, the incidence of significant reperfusion injury was 22%. In-hospital mortality (40.9 *versus* 11.7%; $p<0.02$), postoperative ventilation (393.5 *versus* 56.8 h; $p<0.001$), ICU stay (22.2 *versus* 10.5 days; $p<0.01$), and hospital stay (48.8 *versus* 25.6 days; $p<0.03$) were all significantly greater in the 22 patients with IRI compared with the 78 others without IRI, respectively. In a third retrospective study including

**Table 1. – Retrospective clinical studies on ischaemia-reperfusion injury**

| First author [Ref.] | Total number of tranplants | IRI | Patients n | Vent days | ICU days | Hospital days | Mortality % | 1-yr survival % |
|---|---|---|---|---|---|---|---|---|
| CHRISTIE [15] | 100 | Yes | 15 | 36# | N.S. | 75* | 60* | 40# |
| | | No | 82 | 4 | N.S. | 27 | 8 | 69 |
| KING [16] | 100 | Yes | 22 | 16# | 22# | 49# | 41# | N.S |
| | | No | 78 | 2 | 11 | 26 | 12 | N.S |
| KHAN [17] | 99 | Yes | 24 | 5 | N.S. | 35 | N.S | N.S |
| | | No | 75 | 2 | N.S. | 20 | N.S. | N.S. |

IRI: ischaemia-reperfusion injury; ICU: intensive care unit; #: excluding mild type; N.S.: not stated.

99 patients transplanted at the Cleveland Clinic Foundation, the incidence of PGF was calculated to be 57% [17]. In that study, the authors combined all patients with mild (n=33), moderate (n=13) and severe (n=11) IRI. A comparison between the three studies mentioned above is presented in table 1.

Several authors have tried to predict the outcome in recipients developing severe IRI in an attempt to alter the clinical course [18]. In a study from Pittsburgh looking at a group of single-lung transplant recipients, the immediate postoperative oxygenation expressed as the $P_{a,O_2}/F_{I,O_2}$ ratio was found to be the best predictor of prolonged ICU length of stay [19]. Recently, an ischaemia/reperfusion injury severity score (IRISS) based on four variables (graft ischaemic time, recipient age, oxygenation index ($P_{a,O_2}/F_{I,O_2}$), and early haemodynamic failure) was proposed to predict the probability of ICU death after pulmonary transplantation [20]. Measuring extravascular lung water using the thermal dye dilution technique may have a prognostic value in these critically ill patients [21] although its routine use is currently not recommended outside selected clinical research studies [22]. Measurement of alveolar fluid clearance may also be useful to predict the outcome when pulmonary oedema develops after lung transplantation [23].

In addition to the increased risk for early mortality, severe reperfusion injury can also be associated with an increased risk of acute rejection [24]. It is still unclear, however, whether IRI may also lead to chronic rejection and graft dysfunction in the long term [25, 26].

## Pathophysiology of ischaemia-reperfusion injury

The mechanism of lung damage during IRI is extremely complex and all components of injury have yet to be fully elucidated. There is a myriad of cellular and molecular events that occur during ischaemia, hypothermia, hypoxia and subsequent reoxygenation and reperfusion. Better insight in the individual points of impact may allow for intervention at specific points in this process. Current knowledge on the pathophysiological mechanism of IRI have been recently published in several excellent review papers [27–29]. A detailed description of these events if beyond the scope of this chapter. Mechanisms can be briefly summarised as follows. During ischaemia and reperfusion oxygen free radicals are produced resulting in damage of the endothelial cell membrane leading to increased permeability and oedema. Attracted neutrophils will interact with the injured pulmonary endothelium at the onset of reperfusion *via* a complex system of adhesion molecules resulting in rolling, binding and extravasation of the neutrophils into the interstitium. Further damage will occur not only at the level of the endothelium but also at the level of the epithelium, especially the alveolar type II cells. This will lead to alterations in surfactant resulting in alveolar instability and damage. An important strategy in lung preservation, therefore, is to preserve the integrity of both the endothelial and epithelial cells in the face of ischaemia and reperfusion [27].

## Risk factors for ischaemia-reperfusion injury

Risk factors for development of IRI may be donor, preservation, procedure or recipient-related.

The lung injury occurring during ischaemia and reperfusion may be aggravated by a number of events already occurring in the donor before lung retrieval: mechanical ventilation, pneumonia, aspiration, trauma, hypotension, and brain death [29]. SOMMERS *et al.* [30] demonstrated that early lung allograft function was influenced by donor age, length of donor hospitalisation, and donor cause of death. In another study by CHRISTIE *et al.* [31] donor age, gender and race have also been identified as risk factors. The cause of donor brain death was further investigated in two studies, one from Newcastle, UK [32] and the other from St Louis, USA [33]. No difference in early outcome was observed when comparing recipients receiving donor lungs from traumatic *versus* nontraumatic brain injury groups. However, recipients of organs from donors who died of traumatic brain injury had a higher severity and frequency of rejection episodes during the first year after transplantation and a lower freedom from BOS at 5 yrs (34.5 *versus* 50.8%) [33]. An enhanced pulmonary inflammation was noticed in organ donors following nontraumatic brain injury [34].

Controversy persists over whether prolonged graft ischaemia time is an independent risk factor for primary graft failure. In some retrospective studies no difference was found in graft-ischaemia-time between recipients who developed IRI and those who did not [15–17, 31]. However, other studies have demonstrated an increased risk of developing IRI with longer ischaemia times [20, 35, 36]. KSHETTRY *et al.* [37] conducted a retrospective analysis in 83 recipients comparing different graft ischaemia times, <4 h, 4–6 h, or >6 h. No difference was seen in ICU and hospital stay, forced expiratory volume in one second (FEV1) at 1 month or the number of acute rejection episodes and long-term survival. UENO *et al.* [38] also compared three different ischaemic periods (<5 h, 5–8 h, >8 h) in 74 double-lung-transplant recipients. Immediate postoperative oxygenation was worse ($p<0.01$) in the group with long (>8 h) ischaemia, but no differences in the early outcome were found. GAMMIE *et al.* [39] from Pittsburgh also compared three different time periods (<4 h, 4–6 h, >6 h) in 352 recipients which also showed no difference in outcome. FISER *et al.* [40] reported no difference in early and late mortality in a group of 136 patients comparing graft-ischaemia-times of <6 *versus* >6 h. In a study by NOVICK *et al.* [41], based on data from the Registry of the International Society for Heart and Lung Transplantation, an interaction between a long graft-ischaemia-time (>7 h) and higher donor age (>55 yrs) increased the risk of early mortality. Recent data from the same registry indicate that ischaemia time is a continuous risk factor for 1-yr mortality after lung transplantation with odds ratio (OR)>1 after 2 h of cold ischaemia [42]. An Australian study reported worse survival after 1 month in 106 recipients if ischaemia succeeded >5 h [35]. Finally, in a French multicentre study including 259 recipients, graft-ischaemia-time alone was an independent risk factor (OR 2.6) for poor outcome [20].

The type of solution used for hypothermic lung preservation may well influence the incidence of IRI. This will be discussed in details further in this article.

The use of cardiopulmonary bypass is known to mediate an inflammatory cascade resulting in a capillary leak syndrome with an increase in extravascular lung water. Several studies have reported a deleterious effect of cardiopulmonary bypass on early graft function [15, 17, 43–47]. The presence of moderate-to-severe right ventricular dysfunction necessitating the use of cardiopulmonary bypass in itself, was shown to be an independent prognostic factor for the development of IRI [47].

Some studies have found that the recipient diagnosis of pretransplant pulmonary hypertension was predictive of early graft dysfunction and a need for longer post-operative mechanical ventilation, especially in single-lung recipients subjecting the newly implanted allograft to virtually the entire cardiac output [1, 16, 17, 30, 31, 48, 49]. In other studies, no difference in pretransplant pulmonary artery pressures was found between recipients developing IRI and those who did not [15, 17].

Recently, a simple clinical predictive model for primary lung graft failure following transplantation was proposed by Christie *et al.* [31]. The model is based on four independent variables which are: donor age, race, sex and recipient diagnosis.

## Markers of ischaemia-reperfusion injury

Several mediators correlating with IRI have been identified over the last few years. In a dog, lung transplant model, Serrick *et al.* [50] found that cytokines (interleukin (IL)-2, tumour necrosis factor-α and interferon-γ) could play an important role in the development of early allograft dysfunction. Pham *et al.* [51] were the first to demonstrate in humans that serum levels of the cytokine IL-6 in the immediate postoperative period (4 h) are a useful marker of preservation injury in clinical lung transplantation. Fisher *et al.* [52] reported that elevated donor lung levels of IL-8, a potent chemokine promoting neutrophil migration and activation, was associated with early graft failure after lung transplantation [52]. The authors concluded that attenuation of the donor's inflammatory response before organ retrieval might improve early outcome after lung transplantation, and help maximise lung use from the existing donor pool. de Perrot *et al.* [53] showed that IL-8 release in the transplant recipient, early after reperfusion, correlated well with oxygenation, airway pressure, and length of ICU stay after transplantation. Longer ischaemic-time was associated with significantly higher levels of IL-8 before reperfusion; older donors had significantly lower levels of IL-10 after reperfusion. They concluded that IL-8 levels could predict early graft function after human lung transplantation and that donor age and ischaemic-time may influence release of specific cytokines during ischaemia-reperfusion. In a rat model of hilar occlusion, Eppinger *et al.* [54] could demonstrate that endogenous IL-10, an anti-inflammatory cytokine, was beneficial in protecting the lung from IRI. More studies are currently under way to investigate the possibility of adenoviral-mediated human IL-10 gene transfection of donor lungs [55].

Beside cytokines, the role of other mediators such as platelet activating factor (PAF), complement, and endothelin have been investigated; mainly in animal models, over the past few years [27–29]. Two randomised, double-blinded, placebo-controlled clinical trials have been reported. A multicentre group investigated the role of a complement inhibitor in 59 patients and found that a greater proportion of patients in the treated group was extubated within 24 h [56]. In a small series of 24 patients, Wittwer *et al.* [57] looked at the effect of a PAF antagonist. The group reported a trend towards better alveolar-arterial oxygen gradient during the initial 32 h of reperfusion.

In the future, methods to rapidly assess the degree of inflammation in the donor lung, for instance by measuring the levels of pro-inflammatory cytokines or adhesion molecules, may be useful to determine the type of lung suitable for transplantation and the potential tolerance to prolonged ischaemia.

## Strategies to prevent ischaemia-reperfusion injury

### *The role of new preservation solutions*

When lung transplantation was clinically established, grafts were preserved by means of autoperfusion with extracorporeal circulation [58], topical cooling [59] or donor core-cooling [60]. The standard procedure used most often became single pulmonary artery flush perfusion using Euro-Collins (EC) solution at 4°C [61, 62]. However, reperfusion injury remained a significant factor for morbidity and early mortality after lung preservation. Therefore, acceptance of grafts for transplantation was highly selective and the number of lung transplants remained low. Several dozen papers were published reporting experimental results on modified EC solution. None of the suggested improvements were introduced into clinical practice, except for adding vasodilative prostacyclin derivatives to the flush solution. With the introduction of University of Wisconsin solution (UW) [63] hopes were raised for improvement of lung preservation; however, significant advantages were not shown clinically [64]. According to the latest survey published in 1998 [65], 93% of the transplant centres were using a cold crystalloid solution, either EC solution in 78% or UW in 15%. The remaining transplant centres (7%) preferred a colloid solution based on donor blood (Papworth solution) [66].

After >10 yrs of research, extra-cellular type solutions such as low-potassium dextran glucose (LPDG) [67, 68] or Perfadex® (Vitrolife, Göteborg, Sweden) [69] and Celsior® (Sangstat, Lyon, France) [70] have now been introduced clinically replacing the intra-cellular type solutions such as EC and UW solution (table 2). This recent switch to extra-cellular type solutions was based on the observations that the high potassium content in the intracellular type is not only responsible for reduced endothelium dependent vasorelaxation [71, 72], but can also directly cause endothelial damage [73–75]; resulting in an increased risk of hydrostatic as well as permeability oedema, upon reperfusion. In

**Table 2. – Composition of crystalloid solutions used for pulmonary preservation**

| | EC | UW | Celsior® | LPDG |
|---|---|---|---|---|
| Na | 10 | 28 | 100 | 138 |
| K | 115 | 125 | 15 | 6 |
| Cl | 15 | 0 | 41,5 | 142 |
| Mg | 0 | 0 | 13 | 0.8 |
| $SO_4$ | 0 | 4 | 0 | 0.8 |
| $PO_4$ | 57.5 | 25 | 0 | 0.8 |
| Ca | 0 | 0 | 0.26 | 0.3 |
| $HCO_3$ | 10 | 5 | 0 | 0 |
| Dextran 40 $g{\cdot}L^{-1}$ | 0 | 0 | 0 | 50 |
| Glucose | 20 | 0 | 0 | 5 |
| Raffinose | 0 | 30 | 0 | 0 |
| Lactobionate | 0 | 100 | 80 | 0 |
| Glutathione | 0 | 3 | 3 | 0 |
| Adenosine | 0 | 5 | 0 | 0 |
| Allopurinol | 0 | 1 | 0 | 0 |
| Pentafraction $g{\cdot}L^{-1}$ | 0 | 50 | 0 | 0 |
| Glutamate | 0 | 0 | 20 | 0 |
| Histidine | 0 | 0 | 30 | 0 |
| Mannitol | 0 | 0 | 60 | 0 |

Data presented as $mM{\cdot}L^{-1}$ unless otherwise stated. EC: Euro-Collins; UW: University of Wisconsin solution; LPDG: low-potassium dextran glucose.

addition, experimental work by the group of R. Novick demonstrated alterations in surfactant function and composition of lungs preserved with EC solution [76]. Later HOHLFELD *et al.* [77] was able to show that this finding holds true also for clinical lung transplantation. Surfactant function was better preserved in lungs flushed with LPDG solution in experimental lung transplantation [78]. Also, *in vitro* metabolic activity of type II pneumocytes were better preserved with LPDG compared with EC [79].

In LPDG, the presence of the dextran 40 and the low potassium content are critical components of the solution improving pulmonary microcirculation and preserving the endothelial-epithelial barrier [67]. Celsior® [70], in contrast to LPDG, contains high amounts of antioxidants such as reduced glutathione, histidine, and lactobionate, which may play an important role in the prevention of free radical injury (table 2).

Numerous experimental studies in various animal models comparing the effect of different preservation solutions on early graft function, have been reported in the literature [80–83]. However, only a few clinical trials comparing different preservation solutions in humans have been reported so far. HARDESTY *et al.* [64] in 1993 compared two intracellular solutions (EC: n=30 *versus* UW: n=70). They reported an increased incidence of reperfusion oedema that were noticed on chest radiographs on day 1 with EC but with no difference in gas exchange and early mortality. Clinical reports from four centres have compared the effect of LPDG with an historical group of lungs preserved with EC [84–87]. All four reports showed significantly better graft function on arrival in the intensive care unit and a trend towards a lower 30-day mortality with LPDG (table 3). In a French multicentre study involving 170 patients, early outcome was compared between two intracellular solutions (EC: n=61; UW: n=24) and two extra-cellular solutions (Celsior®: n=21; Papworth: n=64) [88]. The use of extra-cellular solutions was associated with a lower incidence of reperfusion oedema with no difference in 1-month mortality. D'ARMINI *et al.* [89] have reported on a small prospective randomised clinical study comparing Celsior® (n=10) *versus* UW (n=10) solution in double-lung transplants [89]. The arterial-alveolar oxygen tension ($P_{A\text{-}a,O_2}$) gradient was significantly better in UW up to 24 h. No differences, however, were observed in primary graft failure, length of ventilation, ICU stay and long-term survival. Finally, one French study in 44 cystic fibrosis transplant recipients reported on a retrospective comparison between the use of Celsior® solution (n=18) *versus* the modified blood Wallwork solution (n=26) [90]. No difference in early outcome was noticed. The authors concluded that the use of a crystalloid solution like Celsior® is preferred, as this solution does not need to be prepared on site.

In summary, although no prospective clinical trial has been carried out so far to prove the superiority of one solution over another, clinical and experimental evidence suggests that an extra-cellular solution is currently the preservation solution of choice for lung transplantation.

**Table 3. – Studies comparing low-potassium dextran glucose (LPDG) and Euro-Collins (EC) in clinical lung transplantations**

| First author [Ref.] | Number of transplants | | 30-day mortality | | | Initial graft function | | |
|---|---|---|---|---|---|---|---|---|
| | LPDG | EC | LPDG % | EC % | p-value | LPDG | EC | p-value |
| MÜLLER [84] | 32 | 48 | 6 | 12 | 0.36 | 159±145# | 242±265# | 0.028 |
| STRÜBER [85] | 57 | 63 | 8 | 14.2 | 0.35 | 34±11¶ | 30±10¶ | 0.04 |
| FISCHER [86] | 46 | 48 | 6.5 | 10.4 | 0.82 | 370±133+ | 310±134+ | 0.017 |
| REGA [87] | 50 | 50 | 2 | 10 | 0.04 | 168±14# | 249±22# | 0.001 |

#: Alveolar-arterial oxygen gradient (mmHg); ¶: lung compliance (mL·$mmHg^{-1}$); +: arterial oxygen tension/inspiratory oxygen fraction ratio.

### *The role of retrograde left atrial and antegrade bronchial flush*

The route of administration of the perfusate may also have an impact on IRI. Use of cold antegrade flush perfusion combined with a vasodilating agent such as prostaglandin (PG)$E_1$ or $PGI_2$ to counteract temperature and potassium-induced vasoconstriction, was the routine in many transplant teams, until recently [65]. This technique, however, presents a number of drawbacks. Flushing the pulmonary artery leaves the bronchial tissue to be preserved by topical cooling alone. Clots and fat or brain tissue emboli, especially in donors with major trauma and multiple bone fractures, may also hamper uniform flushing and cooling and therefore impair graft function upon reperfusion [91, 92].

An entirely new approach to enhance the uniform distribution of the solution and cooling of the graft, involves the technique of retrograde flush, where the preservation solution is administered *via* the left atrial appendage into the pulmonary venous system and drained through the pulmonary artery, as previously described in both, experimental [93–96] and clinical, lung preservation [97–100]. Compared to the classic antegrade flush *via* the pulmonary artery, this technique has the potential of flushing not only pulmonary vessels but also the bronchial network, contributing to the adequate perfusion of the tracheobronchial submucosa and therefore better airway healing. Preserving the small but important bronchial component might be valuable as this is responsible for the blood flow of the visceral pleura, pulmonary interstitium, lymphatic nodes and the vessels of the pulmonary wall [101]. Retrograde flush will also limit the effect of hypothermic pulmonary arterial vasoconstriction. Also, less ventilated areas, such as the posterior segments of lower lobes, are better flushed. An additional advantage of this technique is the washing out of residual blood and harmful constituents and any possible micro-thrombi that may obstruct the pulmonary vessels. This technique is certainly an advantage when lung retrieval is considered from non-heart-beating donors [102].

In a canine left-unilateral transplant model, the retrograde flush was found to improve lung preservation after 6 h with less oedema, decreased airway resistance, and improved oxygenation [95]. In a subsequent study using the same animal model and retrograde UW flush prior to 24 h cold preservation, the authors could demonstrate that the addition of $PGE_1$ to the flush solution was still helpful in reducing pulmonary vascular resistance, airway resistance and in improving lung compliance [103]. In an extracorporeal rat model, Celsior® flush provided better lung preservation than Perfadex® when administered in an antegrade fashion. Retrograde application of Perfadex® resulted in significant functional improvement as compared with antegrade perfusion [104]. More recently, STRÜBER *et al.* [105] showed in a pig lung transplant model that retrograde flush perfusion with LPDG for a 24-h lung preservation, lead to better initial graft function, with less vascular leakage and inflammatory response in the pulmonary circulation compared with the standard antegrade flush technique. A moderate impairment of surfactant function was found in both groups, which was more pronounced in the antegrade perfusion group. Evidence from clinical series, however, is more limited. No comparative studies are available at the moment. VARELA *et al.* [98, 99] have described their experience with retrograde flush in a series of 23 patients that resulted in satisfactory early graft function.

Many transplant teams have now adopted a combined technique with an antegrade flush through the pulmonary artery, followed by a retrograde flush through each of the pulmonary veins while the lung is still being ventilated inside the cadaver [98, 100]. ALVAREZ *et al.* [100] has reported their clinical experience with this combined technique using EC solution in a series of 55 consecutive lung transplants. The authors believe that this technique has contributed to their improved results with less early graft dysfunction, less bronchial complications and better long-term outcome as compared with their historical experience.

Pre-implantation retrograde flush refers to the administration of a second flush immediately prior to implantation of the graft. This technique was recently described by VENUTA *et al.* [106]. The rationale behind this second flush is to wash out post-ischemic inflammatory agents thereby improving post-transplant graft function. In a small, randomised clinical series of 14 patients, they compared a group with antegrade flush only *versus* a group with antegrade and pre-implantation retrograde flush. Oxygenation index, extravascular lung water, time to extubation and length of ICU stay did not differ significantly between both groups. Intrapulmonary shunt fraction, $P_{A-a,O_2}$ gradient, mean airway pressure and chest radiograph scores were significantly improved in the group with the combined flush.

Other teams have advocated antegrade bronchial artery flushing using a catheter (or cardioplegic pin) that is put into the aortic arch, distal to the ascending aortic clamp. The three supra-aortic branches are clamped as is the distal descending thoracic aorta (often already clamped by the liver team). One to two litres of the same perfusion solution is delivered under pressure (7.98–13.30 kPa: 60–100 mmHg) into the isolated aortic segment containing the bronchial arteries, by means of a pressure cuff around the perfusion bag [107]. The advantage of antegrade perfusion of the bronchial arteries (as compared with retrograde flush *via* the pulmonary veins) is that it can be done at physiological pressure without causing pulmonary oedema. In a canine isolated perfused working lung model, LOCICERO *et al.* [101] compared three different groups of lung preservation: pulmonary artery flush, bronchial artery flush or simultaneous pulmonary-bronchial artery flush. Graft function was superior in the combined group indicating that a crystalloid flush of the bronchial circulation contributes to lung preservation.

However, no large prospective clinical studies in humans, comparing all the above mentioned flushing techniques, are available.

## *The role of controlled reperfusion*

Reperfusion of the lung graft following hypothermic preservation is a critical moment in the process of lung transplantation and should therefore be executed with special attention. Conditions for reperfusion can be controlled in two ways: by regulating the pulmonary artery pressure and by modifying the composition of the perfusate.

In several small and large animal studies, it was pointed out that a key component in the prevention of IRI is the maintenance of low pulmonary artery pressures during the first 10 min of reperfusion because of the elevated endothelial permeability following ischaemia [108–116]. Special attention is necessary in patients with pulmonary hypertension. Many teams have adopted a technique of slowly releasing the pulmonary artery clamp in order to gradually increase blood flow through the cold graft over a 10-min period. When a transplant is carried out on a cardiopulmonary bypass patient, the rate of perfusion can be controlled with the pump. In the high risk cohort of patients with severe pretransplant pulmonary hypertension, the use of intra-operative extracorporeal membrane oxygenation (ECMO) [117,118], and even prolonged postoperative ECMO [119, 120], support have been advocated to achieve both controlled reperfusion and nonaggressive ventilation. This results in excellent initial organ function and improved outcome even in advanced forms of pulmonary hypertension.

HALLDORSSON *et al.* [112] demonstrated in a pig lung model of *in situ* warm ischaemia that modifying the reperfusate, by mixing the recipients blood with a modified crystalloid solution in a 4:1 ratio or by extracting the white blood cells using a filter, attenuates IRI. Reperfusion using both a modified reperfusate and a white blood cell filter completely eliminated IRI [112]. Removing white blood cells in the perfusate may ameliorate IRI as neutrophils are well recognised as one of the most important injurious elements in the pathophysiological cascade of events during reperfusion [121–124]. Further research combining both techniques of pulmonary artery pressure control and modified reperfusate resulted in better outcome of the graft after *ex vivo* cold [113] and *in situ* warm ischaemia [115]. This new reperfusion technique was applied for the first time in humans by LICK *et al.* [125]. In a small series of five transplant patients, the lung was reperfused for 10 min at a controlled rate (200 $mL \cdot min^{-1}$) and pressure (<2.66 kPa: <20 mmHg) using an extracorporeal perfusion circuit filled with a 4:1 mixture of white cell-filtered autologous blood (1,500 mL) and modified Buckberg solution. All recipients had excellent gas exchange and were extubated on the first postoperative day. This study was criticised by Halldorsson's group for the large volume (1,500 mL) of autologous blood withdrawn from the recipient leading to hypotension, haemodynamic instability, and the need for blood transfusion [126]. Others have questioned the benefit of this complex set up of a bypass machine [127]. More transplant teams have now reported their clinical experience with controlled reperfusion [123, 128, 129].

However, no prospective clinical studies in humans, comparing all the above mentioned reperfusion techniques, are available

### *The role of controlled reventilation*

There have been a large number of experiments suggesting that preservation of the lung is improved when they are inflated with oxygen. The mechanism may be three-fold: 1) aerobic metabolism continues, 2) integrity of pulmonary surfactant is maintained, and 3) epithelial fluid transport is preserved [29]. Conversely, hyperinflation during lung preservation may increase IRI [130].

It is well known that ventilation in itself may induce lung injury [131]. Recent experimental data have suggested that ventilation of the cold ischaemic graft during initial reperfusion should also be executed in a controlled fashion [132, 133]. In a rat lung transplant model, DE PERROT *et al.* [132] demonstrated that a protective ventilatory strategy with low tidal volumes to minimise pulmonary mechanical stress can lead to improved lung function. Oxygenation was better, the morphological signs of injury were lower, and there was less production of inflammatory markers. In a porcine isolated lung reperfusion model following combined warm and cold ischaemia, REGA *et al.* [133] pointed out that the cold pulmonary allograft should be rewarmed to ~32°C prior to the start of ventilation. Airway pressures, pulmonary vascular resistance and oedema were lower compared with a group with simultaneous onset of ventilation and reperfusion of the graft (28°C). This study is in contrast with a lung reperfusion study in rats reported by DECAMPOS *et al.* [134], suggesting that alveolar collapse, in the cold implanted graft, should be overcome firstly by inflation or ventilation prior to the onset of reperfusion in order to protect the lung from mechanical-stress induced injury

## Strategies in the treatment of ischaemia-reperfusion injury

### *Protective mechanical ventilation*

Mechanical ventilation is a lifesaving and necessary medical intervention in the immediate postoperative period after lung transplantation. In patients with severe IRI the period of mechanical ventilatory support can be prolonged to overcome the phase of hypoxia.

Recent publications have focused on lung protective mechanical ventilation in patients with ALI and ARDS [135, 136]. This protective approach is simplified as low tidal volumes (5–7 $mL \cdot kg^{-1}$ body weight), higher frequency and high positive end-expiratory pressure (PEEP) instead of the more traditional tidal volumes ($\geq 10$ mL·kg$^{-1}$) with lower frequencies and lower PEEP. This technique diminishes the overdistention of lung units or shear forces generated during repetitive opening and closing of atelectatic lung units and causes less ventilator-induced lung injury or barotrauma and the accompanied inflammatory response. This technique is now recommended as beneficial for patients with ALI and ARDS.

IRI resembles ALI and ARDS [4, 6] and it could be questioned if the applied mode of mechanical ventilation can trigger or worsen the pulmonary damage in the phase of reperfusion. Unfortunately, there are no studies available to discuss the effect of the mechanical ventilatory strategy on the development or the outcome of IRI. A cautious conclusion could be that, in view of the available data, a protective mechanical ventilatory strategy together with the lowest acceptable $F_{I,O_2}$ is preferred in the setting of postoperative management of lung transplant recipients.

### *Fluid management*

There is an old adage in the intensive care world that says "a dry lung is a happy lung". This is especially so in the setting of lung transplantation and IRI with severe capillary leakage, fluid restriction is advised in the first 48 h after surgery. Maintenance fluid requirements are set at 1 mL·kg$^{-1}$ body weight and fluid losses *via* the pleural drains or *via* the endotracheal tube are cautiously replaced by albumin solutions or fresh frozen plasma in case of clotting factor deficiency to prevent acute hypovolaemia and postoperative bleeding. The haematocrit level is kept between 25 and 30% and diuretics are used liberally to excrete excessive extravascular fluid. Unfortunately, there is no evidence or consensus in the current literature for the optimal fluid regime.

Tight glycaemia control (range 80–110 mg·dL$^{-1}$) with an insulin infusion is highly recommended to reduce mortality and morbidity in surgical intensive care patients [137].

### *Circulatory support*

The circulatory management of the postoperative patient after lung transplantation is primarily focused on preventing the formation of pulmonary oedema due to the increased vascular permeability. For this reason cardiac output is kept in the low-normal range and overstimulation with inotropes is avoided. When IRI develops with severe pulmonary arterial hypertension and increased afterload for the right ventricle leading to right ventricular failure, circulatory support consists of two principles, which are: pulmonary vasodilatation to decrease the right ventricular afterload; and optimising the right ventricular contractility and coronary perfusion pressure. Early and repeated transoesophageal echocardiography is an indispensable tool for an accurate management. It can exclude pulmonary venous obstruction [11] and provides an assessment of the ventricular function and the filling state of the heart. Various catecholamines or phosphodiesterase-inhibitors are currently used to stimulate right ventricular contractility. Again, no evidence exists on the optimal therapeutic regimen to support the circulation in the setting of severe IRI.

### *Vasodilatory therapy*

Pulmonary vasodilatation to reduce right ventricular afterload can be achieved with inhaled nitric oxide (iNO), inhaled or intravenous prostaglandins, or other intravenous vasodilators (nitrates, phosphodiesterase-inhibitors, *etc.*) or a combination.

NO is a signal transduction molecule involved in many processes of cell homeostasis, cell protection and cell injury. It is involved in vasoregulation by smooth muscle relaxation *via* the cyclic 3', 5' guanosine monophosphate (cGMP)-pathway, it inhibits blood platelet aggregation and adherence to the endothelium and it modulates the host defense mechanism (immunomodulation) by decreasing leukocyte chemotaxis and sequestration. Due to its very short half-life, iNO has the unique property to reduce pulmonary vascular resistance without altering systemic vascular resistance and to exert its effect only in the lungs. In selected patients, iNO can also improve oxygenation because it ameliorates ventilation/perfusion ($V'/Q'$) matching, thereby reducing the shunt fraction. These vascular, immunological, and respiratory properties of iNO make it an attractive agent in the setting of IRI after lung transplantation [138]. Multiple strategies have been developed to compensate for the fall in endogenous NO that is noticed after ischaemia and reperfusion of the lung. Exogenous NO has been given directly by inhalation or indirectly by: infusion of an NO donor such as FK 409, nitroprusside, nitroglycerin; increasing the activity of the enzyme NO synthase (NOS) with cofactors; or by transfecting the donor with an adenovirus containing endothelial NOS before lung retrieval [29]. Several studies in humans have reported a beneficial effect of inhaled NO in the treatment of IRI by improving ventilation-perfusion mismatch and gas exchange and by decreasing pulmonary artery pressure without affecting systemic pressures [139–141]. However, the role of inhaled NO in preventing IRI during clinical lung transplantation remains controversial [142, 143]. Two clinical prospective trials in adult lung transplant recipients showed that prophylactic inhaled NO does not prevent IRI [144, 145]. A third, comparative study showed that the administration of inhaled NO in combination with pentoxyfylline at the time of reperfusion, reduced the incidence of IRI when compared with an historical group [146]. Finally, side-effects such as methemoglobinaemia should be carefully monitored in these patients [139, 140].

The continuous intravenous administration of $PGE_1$ to the recipient during the early phase of reperfusion has been shown to reduce IRI of the lung in animal transplant models [29]. This effect is partially attributed to its vasodilatory effect and partially to its anti-inflammatory and anti-aggregant effect. On the basis of experimental evidence, some centres routinely use an infusion of $PGE_1$ during the post-transplant period whereas others reserve $PGE_1$ infusion for the treatment of severe IRI [147, 148]. However, randomised trials in humans, to demonstrate any beneficial effect of routine administration of prostaglandins are lacking. The use of aerosolised prostacyclin (epoprostenol) has been studied as an alternative to inhaled NO [149]. Novel vasodilatory agents such as prostacyclin-analogues (iloprost, beraprost) and phosphodiesterase inhibitors (zaprinast) will also be tested for this indication. Further, well conducted, clinical trials in humans are needed to define the role of these newer agents.

## *Surfactant therapy*

Pulmonary surfactant, secreted by type II pneumocytes, reduces the surface tension of the fluid that lines the alveolar surface. The main surfactant phospholipid class phosphatidylcholine, in particular its saturated form dipalmitoylphosphatidylcholine, has the unique property to form a stable monolayer. Due to the formation of this monolayer, surfactant stabilises the alveoli at end-expiration, preventing atelectasis and alveolar oedema and secures an optimal surface area for gas exchange [150].

Surfactant dysfunction has been shown to occur during IRI of the lung [75, 76, 151–153] and the grade of dysfunction is correlated with the degree of IRI [151]. This will result in a decrease in lung compliance, alveolar collapse, $V'/Q'$ mismatch and lung oedema. Most of the alterations have been shown to progressively increase during ischaemic storage and to be significantly less with extra-cellular-type preservation solutions [78] and with the technique of retrograde flush [105].

Experimental studies [151, 153–156] and clinical observations [157] have found that exogenous surfactant therapy can improve pulmonary function after lung transplantation and has a beneficial effect on endogenous surfactant metabolism, up to one week after transplantation [158]. Exogenous surfactant given to the donor before retrieval has been associated with better and more reliable results than when it was administered just before or immediately after reperfusion [153, 155]. STRÜBER *et al.* [157] have successfully used a nebulised synthetic surfactant in six patients with reperfusion injury after lung transplantation. They observed rapid improvement in pulmonary compliance and in $P_{A-a,O_2}$ gradient, leading to extubation within a few days of application. The key issues that need to be further considered, prior to widespread application of this treatment modality, include: the type of exogenous surfactant used (synthetic *versus* natural); the optimal dose (high or low) [157]; its preferred delivery technique (instillation *versus* nebulisation); and the optimal timing of administration (in the donor, in the recipient, or in both) [159]. Further confirmation of the benefit of exogenous surfactant administration in a prospective, randomised trial is mandatory before this expensive drug therapy can be administered on a routine basis.

## *Extracorporeal membrane oxygenation*

If ventilatory and pharmacological support fails in the treatment of IRI following lung transplantation, then the next step is mechanical extracorporeal support. In the setting of poor oxygenation due to reperfusion oedema, ECMO is the preferred mechanical assistance device [117–120, 160–165]. This technique can be applied *via* the femoral vessels in the groin. In the case of poor ventricular function or haemodynamic instability, as might be the case in patients with severe pretransplant pulmonary hypertension and uncontrolled reperfusion of the graft post-transplant and sometimes transient left ventricular failure [13], veno-arterial cannulation is preferred to provide simultaneous respiratory and circulatory support.

The primary aim of ECMO is to overcome the life-threatening situation and to avoid aggressive ventilation, which may further damage the lungs. Implantation of an ECMO system in such a critical situation has to be carried out as early as possible to maintain adequate oxygenation and to avoid complications of prolonged hypoxia [164–166]. The use of the oxygenation index (mean airway pressure multiplied by % $F_{I,O_2}/P_{a,O_2}$) has been advocated as a predictor for the need of ECMO [166]. An increase in the index >30 was an early predictor of primary graft failure requiring acute intervention. In a small series of eight patients in whom ECMO was instituted for primary graft failure ZENATI *et al.* found a mortality of 25% [161]. Nguyen *et al.* [164] reported on a series which included 14 patients, nine of whom had early (<24 h) graft failure with a hospital mortality of 44% and five of whom had late (>7 days) graft failure, with a 100% mortality. Investigators from the Pittsburgh group, showed similar data [160]. In a retrospective study from the St Louis group, twelve out of 444 (2.7%) isolated transplant recipients required ECMO after failure of conventional therapy [165]. The mean length of support was 4.2 days. Five patients (41.6%) died in hospital. All survivors had begun receiving ECMO support by post-transplantation day 1.

Observations and good results, especially with prolonged ECMO support, suggest its potential usage in marginal donor lungs. In some instances, if clear signs of pulmonary oedema are present on the chest radiographs, donor lungs are rejected. In such a situation, it may be beneficial to use prolonged ECMO to dry out the lungs after transplantation [167]. Further studies are needed to clarify if ECMO support is beneficial in these circumstances.

Complications related to the procedure and the use of an extracorporeal circuit for several days are frequent and include: local bleeding at the site of cannulation, vessel injury; dislocation of cannulas and tubing, mechanical pump failure, renal failure, spontaneous intracranial bleeding, stroke, coagulopathy, and sepsis [165]. The duration of this support should therefore be as short as possible. It is estimated that ~60–80% of these patients can be successfully weaned off ECMO support [160, 164, 165].

### *Early retransplantation*

In patients who cannot be weaned from bypass, ECMO may ultimately serve as a bridge to retransplantation.

In an international survey on retransplantation in North America and Europe, early graft failure was the indication in 14 out of 63 cases (22.2%) with a mean interval of 9±1 days between both procedures [168]. Survival was ~30%, 9 months after the second transplant. In a single centre report from the Vienna Lung Transplant Group, nine out of 20 (45%) retransplants were performed in patients while still being in ICU for the first transplant; with a 1-yr survival of only 22.2%. Seven of the procedures were performed because of primary graft failure [169]. In contrast, the Hannover Lung Transplant Group reported better results in a series of 14 retransplant procedures including five for early graft failure, with a 1-yr survival of 60% [170, 171]. Reports from other distinguished transplant centres also reveal high (>50%) mortality in early retransplantation [160, 165].

In summary, overall results of retransplantation for primary graft failure are very poor as reported anecdotally. Therefore, a very restricted approach towards early retransplantation is recommended.

## Conclusions

Better understanding of the mechanisms and risk factors of ischaemia-reperfusion injury have lead to the introduction of new preservation techniques and solutions, and of new methods to better control the critical moment of reperfusion and reventilation of the vulnerable graft.

Over the last decade, new strategies have also become available for the treatment of severe lung ischaemia-reperfusion injury and primary graft failure with a beneficial impact on the outcome in these patients, who are at high risk for early death.

## Summary

Ischaemia-reperfusion-induced lung Injury (IRI) remains an important problem after lung transplantation occurring in 10–20% of the recipients with a significant impact on clinical outcome. IRI has been identified as the main cause of primary graft failure resulting in a post-transplant mortality of 2–5%. This syndrome occurs within 72 h after transplantation and is characterised by impaired gas exchange, fluid loss *via* endotracheal tube and chest drains, pulmonary infiltrates on chest radiographs, elevated pulmonary vascular resistance, decreased pulmonary compliance, and diffuse alveolar damage on biopsy. Risk factors that have been identified are related to the donor, the preservation, the transplant procedure, and the recipient. Better

understanding of the complex pathophysiological mechanism of this insult has marked the last decade. A myriad of molecular and cellular events occurs during ischaemia and reperfusion resulting in endothelial and epithelial cell dysfunction. This knowledge has resulted in new strategies to prevent and to treat IRI although randomised clinical trials to demonstrate an improvement are often lacking. Most publications are limited to personal experience and case series.
After more than 10 yrs of research, extra-cellular type preservation solutions such as low-potassium dextran glucose or Perfadex® and Celsior® have now been introduced, clinically replacing the intra-cellular type solutions such as modified EC and UW. This has resulted in an improved initial graft function and an improved early outcome. The technique of retrograde flush, where the preservation solution is administered *via* the left atrial appendage or *via* the pulmonary veins and drained through the pulmonary artery, is another strategy applied by many transplant teams nowadays. Most surgeons have adopted a technique of controlled reperfusion by slowly releasing the pulmonary artery clamp in order to gradually increase blood flow through the cold graft over a 10-min period. Initial reperfusion with leukocyte-filtered blood, mixed with a crystalloid solution, has also been reported to be beneficial. Controlled ventilation with a low tidal volume or ventilation delayed until the cold graft has re-warmed (32°C) after the onset of reperfusion, may also be important.
Inhaled nitric oxide has been useful, clinically, to treat established IRI because it can improve ventilation/perfusion mismatch and decrease pulmonary artery pressures without affecting systemic pressures. On the basis of experimental evidence, some centres routinely use an infusion of prostaglandin (PG)$E_1$ during the postoperative period after lung transplantation, whereas others reserve $PGE_1$ infusion for the treatment of severe IRI. Experimental studies have found that exogenous surfactant-therapy can improve pulmonary function after lung transplantation, especially when given already in the donor. In cases of life threatening reperfusion oedema, the use of extracorporeal membrane oxygenation (ECMO) has been described as a successful, but ultimate treatment strategy. Weaning of the ECMO support is possible in 60–80% of the patients. In other patients, ECMO may ultimately serve as a bridge to retransplantation. However, this final option for early graft failure is controversial because of the poor results and should,therefore, be very restricted.

**Keywords:** Extra-cellular solutions, extracorporeal membrane oxygenation, ischaemia-reperfusion injury, lung preservation, lung transplantation, surfactant.

*Acknowledgements.* Other co-authors of Working Group 2: W. Coosemans, J.H. Dark, F. Rega, W. De Wever, E. Russi, H.B. Ris, E. Pompeo, W. Weder, P. Evrard, M. Decramer, N. Konietzko, G. Massard, F. Velly.

## References

1. Trulock EP, Edwards LB, Taylor DO, *et al.* The Registry of The International Society for Heart and Lung Transplantation: twentieth official adult lung and heart-lung transplant report-2003. *J Heart Lung Transplant* 2003; 22: 625–635.
2. Trulock EP. Lung Transplantation. *Am J Respir Crit Care Med* 1997; 155: 789–818.
3. Grinyo JM. Reperfusion injury. *Transplant Proc* 1997; 29: 59–62.
4. Kollef MH, Schuster DP. The acute respiratory distress syndrome. *N Eng J Med* 1995; 332: 27–37.
5. Morrison RJ, Bidani A. Acute repiratory distress syndrome epidemiology and pathophysiology. *Chest Surg Clin N Am* 2002; 12: 301–323.

6. Atabai K, Matthay MA. The pulmonary physician in critical care. 5: Acute lung injury and the acute respiratory distress syndrome: definitions and epidemiology. *Thorax* 2002; 57: 452–458.
7. Cooper JD, Vreim CE. Biology of lung preservation for transplantation. *Am Rev Respir Dis* 1992; 146: 803–807.
8. Frost AE, Jammal CT, Cagle PT. Hyperacute rejection following lung transplantation. *Chest* 1996; 110: 559–562.
9. Choi JK, Kearns J, Palevsky HI, *et al.* Hyperacute rejection of a pulmonary allograft; immediate clinical and pathologic findings. *Am J Respir Crit Care Med* 1999; 160: 1015–1018.
10. Paradis IL, Duncan SR, Dauber JH, Yousem S, Hardesty R, Griffith B. Distinguishing between infection, rejection, and the adult respiratory distress syndrome after human lung transplantation. *J Heart Lung Transplant* 1992; 11: S232–S236.
11. Leibowitz D, Michler R, Smith C, *et al.* Complications involving the pulmonary venous anastomoses after lung transplantation: a prospective transesophageal echocardiographic study [abstract]. *J Heart Lung Transplant* 1994; 13: S39.
12. Griffith BP, Magee MJ, Gonzalez IF, *et al.* Anastomotic pitfalls in lung transplantation. *J Thorac Cardiovasc Surg* 1994; 107: 743–753.
13. Birsan T, Kranz A, Mares P, *et al.* Transient left ventricular failure following bilateral lung transplantation for pulmonary hypertension. *J Heart Lung Transplant* 1999; 18: 304–309.
14. Anderson DC, Glazer HS, Semenkovich JW, *et al.* Lung transplant edema: chest radiography after lung transplantation - the first 10 days. *Radiology* 1995; 195: 275–281.
15. Christie JD, Bavaria JE, Palevsky HI, *et al.* Primary graft failure following lung transplantation. *Chest* 1998; 114: 51–60.
16. King RC, Binns OAR, Rodriguez F, *et al.* Reperfusion injury significantly impacts clinical outcome after pulmonary transplantation. *Ann Thorac Surg* 2000; 69: 1681–1685.
17. Khan SU, Salloum J, O'Donovan PB, *et al.* Acute pulmonary edema after lung transplantation; the pulmonary reimplantation response. *Chest* 1999; 116: 187–194.
18. Duarte AG, Lick S. Predicting outcome in primary graft failure. *Chest* 2002; 121: 1736–1738.
19. Lee KH, Martich GD, Boujoukos AJ, Keenan RJ, Griffith BP. Predicting ICU length of stay following single lung transplantation. *Chest* 1996; 110: 1014–1017.
20. Thabut G, Vinatier I, Stern J-B, *et al.* Primary graft failure following lung transplantation; predictive factors of mortality. *Chest* 2002; 121: 1876–1882.
21. Sakka SG, Klein M, Reinhart K, Meier-Hellmann A. Prognostic value of extravascular lung water in critically ill patients. *Chest* 2002; 122: 2080–2086.
22. Matthay MA. Clinical measurement of pulmonary edema. *Chest* 2002; 122: 1877–1879.
23. Ware LB, Golden JA, Finkbeiner WE, Matthay MA. Alveolar epithelial fluid transport capacity in reperfusion lung injury after lung transplantation. *Am J Respir Crit Care Med* 1999; 159: 980–988.
24. Shackleton CR, Ettinger SL, McLoughlin MG, Scoudamore CH, Miller RR, Keown PA. Effect of recovery from ischemic injury on class I and class II MHC antigen expression. *Transplantation* 1990; 49: 641–643.
25. Fiser SM, Tribble CG, Long SM, *et al.* Ischaemia-reperfusion injury after lung transplantation increases risk of late bronchiolitis obliterans syndrome. *Ann Thorac Surg* 2002; 73: 1041–1048.
26. Fisher AJ, Wardle J, Dark JH, Corris PA. Non-immune acute graft injury after lung transplantation and the risk of subsequent bronchiolitis obliterans syndrome (BOS). *J Heart Lung Transplant* 2002; 21: 1206–1212.
27. Novick RJ, Gehman KE, Ali IS, Lee J. Lung preservation: the importance of endothelial and alveolar type II cell integrity. *Ann Thorac Surg* 1996; 62: 302–314.
28. Kelly RF. Current strategies in lung preservation. *J Lab Clin Med* 2000; 136: 427–440.
29. de Perrot M, Liu M, Waddell TK, Keshavjee S. Ischaemia-reperfusion-induced lung injury. *Am J Respir Crit Care Med* 2003; 167: 490–511.
30. Sommers KE, Griffith BP, Hardesty RL, Keenan RJ. Early lung allograft function in twin recipients from the same donor: risk factor analysis. *Ann Thorac Surg* 1996; 62: 784–790.

31. Christie JD, Kotloff RM, Pochettino A, *et al.* Clinical risk factors for primary graft failure following lung transplantation. *Chest* 2003; 124: 1232–1241.
32. Waller DA, Thompson AM, Wrightson N, *et al.* Does the mode of donor death influence early outcome of lung transplantation? A review of lung transplantation from donors involved in major trauma. *J Heart Lung Transplant* 1995; 14: 318–321.
33. Ciccone AM, Stewart KC, Meyers BF, *et al.* Does donor cause of death affect the outcome of lung transplantation? *J Thorac Cardiovasc Surg* 2002; 123: 429–434.
34. Fisher AJ, Donnelly SC, Hirani N, *et al.* Enhanced pulmonary inflammation in organ donors following fatal non-traumatic brain injury. *Lancet* 1999; 353: 1412–1413.
35. Snell GI, Rabinov M, Griffiths A, *et al.* Pulmonary allograft ischemic time: an important predictor of survival after lung transplantation. *J Heart Lung Transplant* 1996; 15: 160–168.
36. Sleiman Ch, Mal H, Fournier M, *et al.* Pulmonary reimplantation response in single-lung transplantation. *Eur Respir J* 1995; 8: 5–9.
37. Kshettry VR, Kroshus TJ, Burdine J, Savik K, Bolman III M. Does donor organ ischaemia over four hours affect long-term survival after lung transplantation? *J Heart Lung Transplant* 1996; 15: 169–174.
38. Ueno T, Snell GI, Williams TJ, *et al.* Impact of graft ischemic time on outcomes after bilateral sequential single-lung transplantation. *Ann Thorac Surg* 1999; 67: 1577–1582.
39. Gammie JS, Stukus DR, Pham SM, *et al.* Effect of ischemic time on survival in clinical lung transplantation. *Ann Thorac Surg* 1999; 68: 2015–2020.
40. Fiser SM, Kron IL, Long SM, *et al.* Influence of graft ischemic time on outcomes following lung transplantation. *J Heart Lung Transplant* 2001; 20: 1291–1296.
41. Novick RJ, Bennet LE, Meyer DM, Hosenpud JD. Influence of graft ischemic time and donor age on survival after lung transplantation. *J Heart Lung Transplant* 1999; 18: 425–431.
42. International Society for Heart and Lung Transplantation. Overall Lung and Adult Lung Transplantation Statistics Slides from the Heart/Lung Transplant Registry. Last accessed 8 June 2004. www.ishlt.org/downloadables /regist_slides_2003/lung_adult.ppt
43. Francalancia NA, Aeba R, Yousem SA, Griffith BP, Marrone GC. Deleterious effects of cardiopulmonary bypass on early graft function after single lung allotransplantation: evaluation of a heparin-coated bypass circuit. *J Heart Lung Transplant* 1994; 13: 498–507.
44. Gammie JS, Cheul LJ, Pham SM, *et al.* Cardiopulmonary bypass is associated with early allograft dysfunction but not death after double-lung transplantation. *J Thorac Cardiovasc Surg* 1998; 115: 990–997.
45. Aeba R, Griffith BP, Kormos RL, *et al.* Effect of cardiopulmonary bypass on early graft dysfunction in clinical lung transplantation. *Ann Thorac Surg* 1994; 57: 715–722.
46. De Santo LS. The effect of cardiopulmonary bypass and extracorporeal membrane oxygenation on early pulmonary allograft function. *Int J Artif Organs* 2000; 23: 727–729.
47. Chatila WM, Furukawa S, Gaughan JP, Criner GJ. Respiratory failure after lung transplantation. *Chest* 2003; 123: 165–173.
48. Bando K, Keenan RJ, Paradis IL, *et al.* Impact of pulmonary hypertension on outcome after single-lung transplantation. *Ann Thorac Surg* 1994; 58: 1336–1342.
49. Boujoukos AJ, Martich GD, Vega JD, Keenan RJ, Griffith BP. Reperfusion injury in single-lung transplant recipients with pulmonary hypertension and emphysema. *J Heart Lung Transplant* 1997; 16: 440–448.
50. Serrick CR, Adoumie A, Giaid A, Shennib H. The early release of interleukin-2, tumor necrosis factor-alpha and interferon gamma after ischaemia reperfusion injury in the lung allograft. *Transplantation* 1994; 58: 1158–1162.
51. Pham SM, Yoshida Y, Aeba R, *et al.* Interleukin-6, a marker of preservation injury in clinical lung transplantation. *J Heart Lung Transplant* 1992; 11: 1017–1024.
52. Fisher AJ, Donnelly SC, Hirani N, *et al.* Elevated levels of interleukin-8 in donor lungs is associated with early graft failure after lung transplantation. *Am J Respir Crit Care Med* 2001; 163: 259–265.

53. de Perrot M, Sekine Y, Fischer S, *et al.* Interleukin-8 release during early reperfusion predicts graft function in human lung transplantation. *Am J Respir Crit Care Med* 2002; 165: 211–215.
54. Eppinger MJ, Ward PA, Bolling SF, Deeb GM. Regulatory effects of Interleukin-10 on lung ischaemia-reperfusion injury. *J Thorac Cardiovasc Surg* 1996; 112: 1301–1306.
55. Fischer S, de Perrot M, Liu M, *et al.* Interleukin 10 gene transfection of donor lungs ameliorates posttransplant cell death by a switch from cellular necrosis to apoptosis. *J Thorac Cardiovasc Surg* 2003; 126: 1174–1180.
56. Keshavjee SH, Davis RD, Zamora MR, *et al.* Inhibition of complement attenuates human lung transplant reperfusion injury: a multicenter clinical trial [abstract]. *J Heart Lung Transplant* 1998; 13: 254.
57. Wittwer T, Grote M, Oppelt P, Franke U, Schaefers HJ, Wahlers T. Impact of PAF antagonist BN 52021 (Ginkolide B) on post-ischemic graft function in clinical lung transplantation. *J Heart Lung Transplant* 2001; 20: 358–363.
58. Hardesty RL, Griffith BP. Autoperfusion of the heart and lungs for preservation during distant procurement. *J Thorac Cardiovasc Surg* 1987; 93: 11–18.
59. Toronto Lung Transplant Group. Unilateral lung transplantation for pulmonary fibrosis. *N Eng J Med* 1986; 314: 1140–1145.
60. Fraser CD, Tamura F, Adachi H, *et al.* Donor core-cooling provides improved static preservation for heart-lung transplantation. *Ann Thorac Surg* 1988; 45: 253–257.
61. Haverich A, Aziz S, Scott WC, Jamieson SW, Shumway NE. Improved lung preservation using Euro-Collins solution for flush-perfusion. *Thorac Cardiovasc Surg* 1986; 34: 368–376.
62. Colquhoun IW, Kirk AJB, Au J, *et al.* Single-flush perfusion with modified Euro-Collins solution: experience in clinical lung preservation. *J Heart Lung Transplant* 1992; 11: S209–S214.
63. Hirt SW, Wahlers T, Jurmann M, Fieguth HG, Dammenhayn L, Haverich A. Improvement of currently used methods for lung preservation with prostacyclin and University of Wisconsin solution. *J Heart Lung Transplant* 1992; 11: 656–664.
64. Hardesty RL, Aeba R, Armitage JM, Kormos RL, Griffith BP. A clinical trial of University of Wisconsin solution for pulmonary preservation. *J Thorac Cardiovasc Surg* 1993; 105: 660–666.
65. Hopkinson DN, Bhabra MS, Hooper TL. Pulmonary graft preservation: a worldwide survey of current clinical practice. *J Heart Lung Transplant* 1998; 17: 525–531.
66. Parry A, Higgins R, Wheeldon D, Bethune D, Wallwork J. The contribution of donor management and modified cold blood lung perfusate to post-transplant lung function. *J Heart Lung Transplant* 1999; 18: 121–126.
67. Keshavjee SH, Yamazaki F, Yokomise H, *et al.* The role of dextran 40 and potassium in extended hypothermic lung preservation for transplantation. *J Thorac Cardiovasc Surg* 1992; 103: 314–325.
68. Steen S, Sjöberg T, Massa G, Ericsson L, Lindberg L. Safe pulmonary preservation for 12 hours with low-potassium-dextran solution. *Ann Thorac Surg* 1993; 55: 434–440.
69. Steen S, Kimblad PO, Sjöberg T, Lindberg L, Ingemansson R, Massa G. Safe lung preservation for twenty-four hours with Perfadex®. *Ann Thorac Surg* 1994; 57: 450–457.
70. Xiong L, Legagneux J, Wassef M, *et al.* Protective effects of Celsior® in lung transplantation. *J Heart Lung Transplant* 1999; 18: 320–327.
71. Kimblad PO, Sjöberg T, Massa G, Solem JO, Steen S. High potassium contents in organ preservation solutions cause strong pulmonary vasocontraction. *Ann Thorac Surg* 1991; 52: 523–528.
72. Strüber M, Ehlers KA, Nielsson FN, Miller VM, McGregor CGA, Haverich A. Effect of lung preservation with Euro-Collins and University of Wisconsin solution on endothelium dependent relaxations. *Ann Thorac Surg* 1997; 63: 1428–1435.
73. Strüber M, McGregor CGA, Locke TJ, Miller VM. Effect of flush perfusion on pulmonary arterial function. *Transplant Proc* 1990; 22: 2206–2211.
74. Chan BBK, Kron IL, Flanagan TL, Kern JA, Hobson CE, Tribble CG. Impairment of vascular endothelial function by high-potassium storage solutions. *Ann Thorac Surg* 1993; 55: 940–945.

75. Ingemansson R, Massa G, Pandita RK, Sjöberg T, Steen S. Perfadex® is superior to Euro-Collins solution regarding 24-hour preservation of vascular function. *Ann Thorac Surg* 1995; 60: 1210–1214.
76. Veldhuizen RAW, Lee J, Sandler D, *et al.* Alterations in pulmonary surfactant composition and function after experimental lung transplantation. *Am Rev Respir Dis* 1993; 148: 208–215.
77. Hohlfeld JM, Tiriyaki E, Hamm H, *et al.* Pulmonary surfactant activity is impaired in lung transplant recipients. *Am J Respir Crit Care Med* 1998; 158: 706–712.
78. Strüber M, Hohlfeld JM, Fraund S, Kim P, Warnecke G, Haverich A. Low potassium dextran solution ameliorates reperfusion injury of the lung and protects surfactant function. *J Thorac Cardiovasc Surg* 2000; 120: 566–572.
79. Maccherini M, Keshavjee SH, Slutsky AS, Patterson GA, Edelson JD. The effect of low-potassium dextran versus Euro-Collins solution for preservation of isolated type II pneumocytes. *Transplantation* 1991; 52: 621–626.
80. Oka T, Puskas JD, Mayer E, *et al.* Low-potassium UW solution for lung preservation. Comparison with regular UW, LPD, and Euro-Collins solutions. *Transplantation* 1991; 52: 984–988.
81. Binns OAR, DeLima NF, Buchanan SA, *et al.* Both blood and crystalloid-based extracellular solutions are superior to intracellular solutions for lung preservation. *J Thorac Cardiovasc Surg* 1996; 112: 1515–1521.
82. Roberts RF, Nishanian GP, Carey JN, Sakamaki Y, Starnes VA, Barr ML. A comparison of the new preservation solution Celsior® to Euro-Collins and University of Wisconsin solutions in lung reperfusion injury. *Transplantation* 1999; 67: 152–155.
83. Chien S, Zhang F, Niu W, Tseng MT, Gray L Jr. Comparison of University of Wisconsin, Euro-Collins, Low-Potassium Dextran and Krebs-Henseleit solutions for hypothermic lung preservation. *J Thorac Cardiovasc Surg* 2000; 119: 921–930.
84. Müller C, Fürst H, Reichenspurner H, Briegel J, Groh J, Reichart B, and the Munich Lung Transplant Group. Lung procurement by low-potassium dextran and the effect on preservation injury. *Transplantation* 1999; 68: 1139–1143.
85. Strüber M, Wilhelmi M, Harringer W, *et al.* Flush perfusion with low potassium dextran solution improves early graft function in clinical lung transplantation. *Eur J Cardiothorac Surg* 2001; 19: 190–194.
86. Fischer S, Matte-Martyn A, de Perrot M, *et al.* Low-potassium dextran preservation solution improves lung function after human lung transplantation. *J Thorac Cardiovasc Surg* 2001; 121: 594–596.
87. Rega F, Dupont L, Verleden G, *et al.* Switch from Euro-Collins to Perfadex® for pulmonary graft preservation resulted in superior outcome in transplant recipients [abstract]. *J Heart Lung Transplant* 2003; 22: S111.
88. Thabut G, Vinatier I, Brugière O, *et al.* Influence of preservation solution on early graft failure in clinical lung transplantation. *Am J Respir Crit Care Med* 2001; 164: 1204–1208.
89. D'Armini AM, Grande AM, Rinaldi M, Goggi C, Vigano M. Prospective randomized clinical study of Celsior® versus University of Wisconsin in double lung transplant [abstract]. *J Heart Lung Transplant* 2001; 20: 183.
90. Baron O, Fabre S, Haloun A, *et al.* Retrospective clinical comparison of Celsior® solution to modified blood Wallwork solution in lung transplantation for cystic fibrosis. *Prog Transplant* 2002; 12: 176–180.
91. Waller DA, Bennett MK, Corris PA, Dark JH. Donor acquired fat embolism causing primary organ failure after lung transplantation. *Ann Thorac Surg* 1995; 59: 1565–1566.
92. Rosendale BE, Keenan RJ, Duncan SR, *et al.* Donor cerebral emboli as a cause of acute graft dysfunction in lung transplantation. *J Heart Lung Transplant* 1992; 11: 72–76.
93. Dawson CA, Jones RL, Hamilton LH. A pulmonary circulation model based on forward and retrograde perfusion of isolated lungs. *J Appl Physiol* 1973; 35: 103–110.
94. Baretti R, Bitu-Moreno J, Friedhelm B, Matheis G, Franchischetti Y, Kreitmayr B. Distribution

of lung preservation solutions in parenchyma and airways: influence of atelectasis and route of delivery. *J Heart Lung Transplant* 1995; 14: 80–91.
95. Chen CZ, Gallagher RC, Ardery P, Dyckman W, Low HBC. Retrograde versus anterograde flush in canine left lung preservation for six hours. *J Heart Lung Transplant* 1996; 15: 395–403.
96. Varela A, Montero CG, Córdoba M, *et al.* Improved distribution of pulmonary flush solution to the tracheobronchial wall in pulmonary transplantation. *Eur Surg Res* 1997; 29: 1–4.
97. Sarsam MA, Yonan NA, Deiraniya AK, Rahman AN. Retrograde pulmonaryplegia for lung preservation in clinical transplantation: a new technique. *J Heart Lung Transplant* 1993; 12: 494–498.
98. Varela A, Montero C, Cordoba M, *et al.* Clinical experience with retrograde lung preservation. *Transplant Int* 1996; 9: Suppl. 1, S296–S298.
99. Varela A, Cordoba M, Serrano-Fiz S, *et al.* Early lung allograft function after retrograde and anterograde preservation. *J Thorac Cardiovasc Surg* 1997; 114: 1119–1120.
100. Alvarez A, Salvatierra A, Lama R, *et al.* Preservation with a retrograde second flushing of Eurocollins in clinical lung transplantation. *Transplant Proc* 1999; 31: 1088–1090.
101. Locicero J III, Massad M, Matano J, Greene R, Dunn M, Michaelis LL. Contribution of the bronchial circulation to lung preservation. *J Thoracic Cardiovasc Surg* 1991; 101: 807–815.
102. Hayama M, Date H, Oto T, Aoe M, Andou A, Shimizu N. Improved lung function by means of retrograde flush in canine lung transplantation with non-heart-beating donors. *J Thorac Cardiovasc Surg* 2003; 125: 901–906.
103. Chen CZ, Gallagher RC, Ardery P, Dyckman W, Donahue S, Low HBC. Retrograde flush and cold storage for twenty-two to twenty-five hours lung preservation with and without Prostaglandin E1. *J Heart Lung Transplant* 1997; 16: 658–666.
104. Wittwer T, Fehrenbach A, Meyer D, *et al.* Retrograde flush perfusion with low-potassium solutions for improvement of experimental pulmonary preservation. *J Heart Lung Transplant* 2000; 19: 976–983.
105. Strüber M, Hohlfeld JM, Kofidis T, *et al.* Surfactant function in lung transplantation after 24 hours of ischaemia: advantage of retrograde flush perfusion for preservation. *J Thorac Cardiovasc Surg* 2002; 123: 98–103.
106. Venuta F, Rendina EA, Bufi M, *et al.* Preimplantation retrograde pneumoplegia in clinical lung transplantation. *J Thorac Cardiovasc Surg* 1999; 118: 107–114.
107. Steen S. Improvement in lung preservation. *In*: Messmer K (ed). Compromised Perfusion. Progress in Applied Microcirculation. Basel, Karger, 1996; vol 22, pp. 50–60.
108. Hopkinson DN, Bhabra MS, Odom NJ, Bridgewater BJM, van Doorn CAM, Hooper TL. Controlled pressure reperfusion of rat pulmonary grafts yields improved function after twenty-four-hours' cold storage in University of Wisconsin solution. *J Heart Lung Transplant* 1996; 15: 283–290.
109. Bhabra MS, Hopkinson DN, Shaw TE, Hooper TL. Critical importance of the first 10 minutes of lung graft reperfusion after hypothermic storage. *Ann Thorac Surg* 1996; 61: 1631–1635.
110. Bhabra MS, Hopkinson DN, Shaw TE, Onwu N, Hooper TL. Controlled reperfusion protects lung grafts during a transient early increase in permeability. *Ann Thorac Surg* 1998; 65: 187–192.
111. Clark SC, Sudarshan C, Khanna R, Roughan J, Flecknell PA, Dark JH. Controlled reperfusion and pentoxifylline modulate reperfusion injury after single lung transplantation. *J Thorac Cardiovasc Surg* 1998; 115: 1335–1341.
112. Halldorsson AO, Kronon M, Allen BS, *et al.* Controlled reperfusion after lung ischaemia: implications for improved function after lung transplantation. *J Thorac Cardiovasc Surg* 1998; 115: 415–425.
113. Halldorsson AO, Kronon M, Allen BS, *et al.* Controlled reperfusion prevents pulmonary injury after 24 hours of lung preservation. *Ann Thorac Surg* 1998; 66: 877–885.
114. Sakamoto T, Yamashita C, Okada M. Efficacy of initial controlled perfusion pressure for ischaemia-reperfusion injury in a 24-hour preserved lung. *Ann Thorac Cardiovasc Surg* 1999; 5: 21–26.

115. Halldorsson AO, Kronon MT, Allen BS, Rahman S, Wang T. Lowering reperfusion pressure reduces the injury after pulmonary ischaemia. *Ann Thorac Surg* 2000; 69: 198–204.
116. Fiser SM, Kron IL, Long SM, *et al.* Controlled perfusion decreases reperfusion injury after high-flow reperfusion. *J Heart Lung Transplant* 2002; 21: 687–691.
117. Ko WJ, Chen YS, Luh SP, Chu SH. Extracorporeal membrane oxygenation support for single-lung transplantation in patients with primary pulmonary hypertension. *Transplant Proc* 1999; 31: 166–168.
118. Chan CY, Chen YS, Ko WJ, *et al.* Extracorporeal membrane oxygenation support for single lung transplantation in a patient with primary pulmonary hypertension. *J Heart Lung Transplant* 1998; 17: 325–327.
119. Pereszlenyi A, Lang G, Steltzer H, *et al.* Bilateral lung transplantation with intra- and postoperatively prolonged ECMO support in patients with pulmonary hypertension. *Eur J Cardiothorac Surg* 2002; 21: 858–863.
120. Ko WJ, Chen YS, Lee YC. Replacing cardiopulmonary bypass with extracorporeal membrane oxygenation in lung transplantation operations. *Artif Organs* 2001; 25: 607–612.
121. Shiraishi Y, Lee JR, Laks H, *et al.* Use of leucocyte depletion to decrease injury after lung preservation and rewarming ischaemia: an experimental model. *J Heart Lung Transplant* 1998; 17: 250–258.
122. Fiser SM, Tribble CG, Long SM, *et al.* Lung transplant reperfusion injury involves pulmonary macrophages and circulating leucocytes in a biphasic response. *J Thorac Cardiovasc Surg* 2001; 121: 1069–1075.
123. Kurusz M, Roach JD Jr, Vertrees RA, Girouard MK, Lick SD. Leucocyte filtration in lung transplantation. *Perfusion* 2002; 17: Suppl, 63–67.
124. Rega FR, Vandezande EJ, Jannis NC, Verleden GM, Lerut TE, Van Raemdonck DEM. The role of leucocyte depletion in *ex vivo* evaluation of pulmonary grafts from non-heart-beating donors. *Perfusion* 2003; 18: 13–21.
125. Lick SD, Brown PS Jr, Kurusz M, Vertrees RA, McQuitty CK, Johnston WE. Technique of controlled reperfusion of the transplanted lung in humans. *Ann Thorac Surg* 2000; 69: 910–912.
126. Allen BS. Controlled pulmonary reperfusion: what is the optimal method of delivery? *Ann Thorac Surg* 2000; 70: 1449–1450.
127. Clark SC, Sudarshan CD, Dark JH. Controlled perfusion of the transplanted lung. *Ann Thorac Surg* 2001; 71: 1755–1756.
128. Alvarado CG, Poston R, Hattler BG, *et al.* Effect of controlled reperfusion techniques in human lung transplantation [abstract]. *J Heart Lung Transplant* 2001; 20: 183–184.
129. Ardehali A, Laks H, Russell H, *et al.* Modified reperfusion and ischaemia-reperfusion injury in human lung transplantation. *J Thorac Cardiovasc Surg* 2003; 126: 1929–1934.
130. Aoe M, Okabayashi K, Cooper JD, Patterson GA. Hyperinflation of canine lung allografts during storage increases reperfusion pulmonary edema. *J Thorac Cardiovasc Surg* 1996; 112: 94–102.
131. Dreyfuss D, Saumon G. Ventilator-induced lung injury. *Am J Respir Crit Care Med* 1998; 157: 294–323.
132. de Perrot M, Imai Y, Volgyesi GA, *et al.* Effect of ventilator-induced lung injury on the development of reperfusion injury in a rat lung transplant model. *J Thorac Cardiovasc Surg* 2002; 124: 1137–1144.
133. Rega FR, Neyrinck AP, Verleden GM, Lerut TE, Van Raemdonck DEM. Controlled ventilation is important during initial reperfusion of the ischemic pulmonary graft. Vienna, Austria, 2nd joint EACTS/ESTS meeting, 2003 (submitted).
134. DeCampos KN, Keshavjee S, Slutsky AS, Liu M. Alveolar recruitment prevents rapid-reperfusion-induced injury of lung transplants. *J Heart Lung Transplant* 1999; 18: 1096–1102.
135. The Acute Respiratory Distress Syndrome Network. Ventilation with lower tidal volumes as compared with traditional tidal volumes for acute lung injury and the acute respiratory distress syndrome. *N Engl J Med* 2000; 342: 1301–1308.
136. Eichacker P, Gerstenberger E, Banks S, Cui X, Natanson C. Meta-analysis of acute lung injury

and acute respiratory distress syndrome trials testing low tidal volumes. *Am J Respir Crit Care Med* 2002; 166: 1510–1514.
137. Van den Berghe G, Wouters P, Weekers F, *et al.* Intensive insulin therapy in critically ill patients. *N Engl J Med* 2001; 345: 1359–1367.
138. Meyer KC, Love RB, Zimmerman JJ. The therapeutic potential of nitric oxide in lung transplantation. *Chest* 1998; 113: 1360–1371.
139. Adatia I, Lillehei C, Arnold JH, *et al.* Inhaled nitric oxide in the treatment of postoperative graft dysfunction after lung transplantation. *Ann Thorac Surg* 1994; 57: 1311–1318.
140. Date H, Triantafillou AN, Trulock EP, Pohl MS, Cooper JD, Patterson GA. Inhaled nitric oxide reduces human lung allograft dysfunction. *J Thorac Cardiovasc Surg* 1996; 111: 913–919.
141. Kemming GI, Merkel MJ, Schallerer A, *et al.* Inhaled nitric oxide (NO) for the treatment of early allograft failure after lung transplantation. *Intensive Care Med* 1998; 24: 1173–1180.
142. Lang JD, Lell W. Pro: Inhaled nitric oxide should be used routinely in patients undergoing lung transplantation. *J Cardiothorac Vasc Anesth* 2001; 15: 785–789.
143. McQuitty CK. Con: Inhaled nitric oxide should not be used routinely in patients undergoing lung transplantation. *J Cardiothorac Vasc Anesth.* 2001; 15: 790–792.
144. Ardehali A, Laks H, Levine M, *et al.* A prospective trial of inhaled nitric oxide in clinical lung transplantation. *Transplantation* 2001; 72: 112–115.
145. Meade MO, Granton JT, Matte-Martyn A, *et al.* A randomized trial of inhaled nitric oxide to prevent ischaemia-reperfusion injury after lung transplantation. *Am J Respir Crit Care Med* 2003; 167: 1483–1489.
146. Thabut G, Brugière O, Lesèche G, *et al.* Preventive effect of inhaled nitric oxide and pentoxyfilline on ischaemia/reperfusion injury after lung transplantation. *Transplantation* 2001; 71: 1295–1300.
147. Aoe M, Trachiotis GD, Okabayashi K, *et al.* Administration of prostaglandin E1 after lung transplantation improves early graft function. *Ann Thorac Surg* 1994; 58: 655–661.
148. de Perrot M, Fischer S, Liu M, *et al.* Prostaglandin E1 protects lung transplants from ischaemia-reperfusion injury: a shift from pro- to anti-inflammatory cytokines. *Transplantation* 2001; 72: 1505–1512.
149. Fiser SM, Cope JT, Kron IL, *et al.* Aerosolized prostacyclin (epoprostenol) as an alternative to inhaled nitric oxide for patients with reperfusion injury after lung transplantation. *J Thorac Cardiovasc Surg* 2001; 121: 981–982.
150. King RJ. Pulmonary surfactant. *J Appl Physiol* 1982; 53: 1–8.
151. Erasmus ME, Petersen AH, Oetomo SB, Prop J. The function of surfactant is impaired during the reimplantation response in rat lung transplants. *J Heart Lung Transplant* 1994; 13: 791–802.
152. Andrade RS, Solien EE, Wangensteen OD, Tsai MY, Kshettry VR, Bolman RM III. Surfactant dysfunction in lung preservation. *Transplantation* 1995; 60: 536–541.
153. Novick RJ, MacDonald J, Veldhuizen RA, *et al.* Evaluation of surfactant treatment strategies after prolonged graft storage in lung transplantation. *Am J Respir Crit Care Med* 1996; 154: 98–104.
154. Erasmus ME, Petersen AH, Hofstede G, Haagsman HP, Bambang OS, Prop J. Surfactant treatment before reperfusion improves the immediate function of lung transplants in rats. *Am J Respir Crit Care Med* 1996; 153: 665–670.
155. Hausen B, Rohde R, Hewitt CW, *et al.* Exogenous surfactant treatment before and after sixteen hours of ischaemia in experimental lung transplantation. *J Thorac Cardiovasc Surg* 1997; 113: 1050–1058.
156. Hohlfeld JM, Strüber M, Ahlf K, *et al.* Exogenous surfactant improves survival and surfactant function in ischaemia-reperfusion injury in minipigs. *Eur Respir J* 1999; 13: 1037–1043.
157. Strüber M, Hirt SW, Cremer J, Harringer W, Haverich A. Surfactant replacement in reperfusion injury after clinical lung transplantation. *Intensive Care Med* 1999; 25: 862–864.
158. Erasmus ME, Hofstede GJ, Petersen AH, Haagsman HP, Oetomo SB, Prop J. Effects of early surfactant treatment persisting for one week after lung transplantation in rats. *Am J Respir Crit Care Med* 1997; 156: 567–572.

159. Novick RJ. Innovative techniques to enhance lung preservation. *J Thorac Cardiovasc Surg* 2002; 123: 3–5.

160. Glassman LR, Keenan RJ, Fabrizio MC, *et al.* Extracorporeal membrane oxygenation as an adjunct treatment for primary graft failure in adult lung transplant recipients. *J Thorac Cardiovasc Surg* 1995; 110: 723–727.

161. Zenati M, Pham SM, Keenan RJ, Griffith BP. Extracorporeal membrane oxygenation for lung transplant recipients with primary severe donor lung dysfunction. *Transpl Int* 1996; 9: 227–230.

162. Ball JW Jr, Noon GP, Short HD, Scheinin SA. Extracorporeal membrane oxygenation for early graft dysfunction in lung transplantation: a case report. *J Heart Lung Transplant* 1997; 16: 468–471.

163. Vlasselaers D, Verleden GM, Meyns B, *et al.* Femoral venoarterial extracorporeal membrane oxygenation for severe reimplantation response after lung transplantation. *Chest* 2000; 118: 559–561.

164. Nguyen DQ, Kulick DM, Bolman RM 3rd, Dunitz JM, Hertz MI, Park SJ. Temporary ECMO support following lung and heart-lung transplantation. *J Heart Lung Transplant* 2000; 19: 313–316.

165. Meyers BF, Sundt TM 3rd, Henry S, *et al.* Selective use of extracorporeal membrane oxygenation is warranted after lung transplantation. *J Thorac Cardiovasc Surg* 2000; 120: 20–26.

166. Fiser SM, Kron IL, McLendon Long S, Kaza AK, Kern JA, Tribble CG. Early intervention after severe oxygenation index elevation improves survival following lung transplantation. *J Heart Lung Transplant* 2001; 20: 631–636.

167. Fiser SM, Kron IL, Long SM, *et al.* Donor lung salvage after neurogenic pulmonary edema with the use of post-transplant extracorporeal membrane oxygenation. *J Thorac Cardiovasc Surg* 2001; 122: 1257–1258.

168. Novick RJ, Kaye MP, Patterson GA, *et al.* Redo lung transplantation: a North American-European experience. *J Heart Lung Transplant* 1993; 12: 5–16.

169. Wekerle T, Klepetko W, Wisser W, *et al.* Lung retransplantation: institutional report on a series of twenty patients. *J Heart Lung Transplant* 1996; 15: 182–189.

170. Haverich A, Hirt SW, Wahlers T, Schäfers H-J, Zink C, Borst H-G. Functional results after lung retransplantation. *J Heart Lung Transplant* 1994; 13: 48–55.

171. Schäfers H-J, Hausen B, Wahlers T, Fieguth H-G, Jurmann M, Borst HG. Retransplantation of the lung. *Eur J Cardiothorac Surg* 1995; 9: 291–296.

*CHAPTER 6*

# Alternatives to lung donor shortage

*D. Van Raemdonck*, W. Coosemans*, W. Klepetko#, J.H. Dark¶, S. Steen+, F. Rega§, and the co-authors of Working Group 2*

**Dept of Thoracic Surgery, University Hospital, Gasthuisberg, §Centre for Experimental Surgery and Anaesthesiology, KUL, Leuven, Belgium, #Dept of Cardiothoracic Surgery, University Hospital, Vienna, Austria, ¶Cardiothoracic Transplant Unit, Freeman Hospital, Newcastle, UK, and +Heart-Lung Division, University Hospital, Lund, Sweden.*

*Correspondence: D. Van Raemdonck, Dept of Thoracic Surgery, University Hospital Gasthuisberg, Herestraat 49, B-3000, Leuven, Belgium.*

Over the last 20 yrs, lung transplantation has become the mainstay of therapy for selected patients suffering from different types of end-stage lung disease refractory to medical management. This form of surgical treatment has enjoyed increasing success with better early and late survival rates [1]. Despite its success, lung transplantation is still hampered by persistent problems such as donor organ shortage, early graft dysfunction (ischaemia reperfusion injury), late graft dysfunction (bronchiolitis obliterans syndrome: BOS), and morbidity related to long-term immunosuppression [2].

As a result of its own success with a proliferation of transplant programmes in every country and an extension of the indications with more patients listed, the main limiting factor to the widespread application of lung transplantation has now become the shortage of suitable donor organs. Strategies to overcome the limited number of organ donors are therefore necessary [3]. All initiatives to increase donation rates should be encouraged including: legislative action; public education and campaigns; and professional training programmes [4–7].

## Lung donor overview

### *Donor management*

It is estimated that only 15–30% of all multi-organ donors have lungs that are suitable for transplantation [8–10]. Out of 1,784 cadaveric donors offered to Eurotransplant in the year 2001, only 489 (27.4%) served as potential lung donors [11]. This percentage is low compared with other solid organs (kidney: 98.3%; liver: 79.6%; heart: 58.9%). This can be explained by the fact that brain death is often associated with lung injury as a result of airway aspiration, infection, neurogenic oedema, atelectasis and contusion [12]. Supportive management strategies to stabilise the donor and to improve the quality of the pulmonary graft prior to retrieval should be considered, these include: antibiotic therapy; fluid and diuretic management [13]; bronchoscopy with pulmonary toilet [14, 15]; inotropic agents [16]; improved ventilatory settings; and steroid administration [17, 18], and may result in a significant increase in suitable organs [3, 15, 19–22].

### *Donor criteria*

Standard criteria for lung donation are listed in table 1. Criteria such as donor age, smoking history, arterial blood gases, chest radiograph findings, bacterial colonisation

Eur Respir Mon, 2004, 29, 89–112. Printed in UK - all rights reserved. Copyright ERS Journals Ltd 2004; European Respiratory Monograph; ISSN 1025-448x. ISBN 1-904097-33-2.

**Table 1. – Standard ideal lung donor criteria**

| Criteria |
|---|
| 1. Age <55 yrs |
| 2. Clear serial chest radiographs |
| 3. Normal gas exchange ($P_{a,O_2}$>300–400 mmHg on $F_{I,O_2}$=1.0, PEEP 5 cm $H_2O$) |
| 4. Absence of chest trauma |
| 5. No evidence of aspiration or sepsis |
| 6. Absence of purulent secretions at bronchoscopy |
| 7. Absence of organisms on sputum Gram stain |
| 8. No history of primary pulmonary disease or active pulmonary infection |
| 9. Tobacco history <20 pack-yrs |
| 10. ABO blood group compatibility |
| 11. Appropriate size match with prospective recipient |

$P_{a,O_2}$: oxygen tension in arterial blood; $F_{I,O_2}$: inspiratory oxygen fraction; PEEP: positive end-expiratory pressure; 1 mmHg=0.133 kPa.

and infection have often been chosen arbitrarily and have not been substantiated in prospective, controlled trials or even large, uncontrolled trials. Most of the currently available data are based on small, centre specific reports from the early days of lung transplantation [23–32]. Therefore, evidence to support these recommendations is often lacking. Acceptability criteria for lung donation were recently reviewed in an extensive consensus report from the Pulmonary Council of the International Society for Heart and Lung Transplantation (ISHLT) [33]. This review concluded that there were no adequate data to provide firm guidelines regarding utilisation of donors with low blood gases, abnormal chest radiographs, purulent secretions, or smoking history of >20 pack-yrs. Extended donor age does not seem to affect early outcome, but may play a role in late functional results as larger registry studies have shown a negative effect on intermediate- and long-term survival, particularly when combined with increased graft-ischaemic-time [34, 35]. Each of the standard lung donor criteria currently in use should be challenged by obtaining, analysing, and using multicentre data from a well designed database [10, 36]. An initiative under the guidance of the Pulmonary Council of the ISHLT is currently under way (personal communication T.K. Waddell, Toronto General Hospital, Toronto, ON, Canada).

## *Donor lung assessment*

Physical examination of the pulmonary graft inside the donor by an experienced transplant surgeon is the best method to assess organ injury and viability. The technique of systematic pulmonary vein gas analysis has been proposed as the ultimate test to assess donor lung function immediately prior to organ retrieval [37]. This method gives an accurate assessment of gas exchange in both individual lungs in comparison with oxygen tension in arterial blood ($P_{a,O_2}$) thereby identifying more potential donor lungs for transplantation. In many circumstances, a single lung could be used from donors with marginal gas exchange who have a unilateral infiltrate with a clear contralateral lung [38]. Even contralateral lung transplantation with an opposite donor lung has been described in cases of an unacceptable ipsilateral graft (*e.g.* left lung implanted in the right thorax) [39].

Studies assessing unsuitable, unused lungs have found that >40% would have been potentially suitable for transplantation [10, 40–42]. It is hoped that new objective indices of donor lung injury at molecular or cellular level may help to rationalise the selection process enabling the transplant physician to accept many of the previously excluded organs [43].

### *Consequences of lung donor shortage*

This critical organ shortage will result in longer waiting times for listed patients with a substantial risk of dying prior to transplantation. According to United Network of Organ Sharing (UNOS) data, mean waiting time to find a suitable organ for a patient with emphysema/chronic obstructive pulmonary disease increased from 480 days in the period 1996–1997 to 667 days in the period 1998–1999 [44]. Waiting list mortality may vary amongst transplant centres and countries. In the year 2001, 3,802 patients were listed for lung transplantation in the USA, of these 1,054 received a suitable organ and 499 patients (13.1%) died awaiting transplantation [44]. In the same year, 414 patients were registered on the lung waiting list in Eurotransplant. A total of 272 patients were transplanted, 19 were delisted and 123 (29.7%) died awaiting a suitable lung offer [11]. Mortality was highest amongst patients with pulmonary fibrosis, cystic fibrosis and pulmonary hypertension and lowest in patients with emphysema [45–47]. It has been postulated that allocation algorithms should, therefore, take into account the type of lung disease and thereby prioritising patients with an increased risk of dying on the waiting list [47, 48].

To overcome this critical organ shortage and to decrease the mortality rate on their waiting list, many transplant programmes have now begun to explore the use of alternative donors. The purpose of this chapter is to describe the worldwide experience with the use of alternative donors for lung transplantation.

## Marginal or extended donors

### *Definition*

A marginal or extended (brain-death) donor does not meet one or more of the strict criteria for lung donation (table 1): age >55 years; smoking >20 pack-yrs; infiltrate on chest radiographs; $P_{a,O_2}$<39 kPa (300 mmHg; inspiratory oxygen fraction: 1.0; positive end-expiratory pressure of 5 cm $H_2O$), purulent bronchoscopic findings; donor ventilator time >5 days; and donor use of inhaled drugs. As a result of the critical donor shortage with increasing waiting times and more patients dying on the waiting list in the nineties, several evolving programmes embarked on using these less-optimal donors; speculating that purulent bacterial secretions could be treated with antibiotics, minor infiltrates due to atelectasis and secretions could be cleared, and abnormalities of gas exchange could be corrected by appropriate fluid and ventilator management [15, 16, 49–53].

### *Reported series*

The percentage of marginal donors in reported series ranges between 33% [49] and 77% (table 2) [16]. The percentage of extended donors failing to satisfy two or more criteria varies between 8% [52] and 38% [15]. Five reports [15, 16, 49, 50, 52] suggested equivalent outcomes with respect to early morbidity and mortality, postoperative time on ventilator and time in intensive care unit (ICU), hospital stay, 30-day survival, pulmonary function and survival at 1 yr post-transplantation (table 2). One study from the Toronto group [53], however, reported a significant increase in early mortality (6.2% in the standard donor group *versus* 17.5% in the extended donor group at 30 days after lung transplant). Mortality was highest (22.2%) in recipients that did not meet the standard guidelines as defined by the ISHLT (older age, colonisation with *Burkholderia cepacia*).

**Table 2. – Published series on marginal donors**

| | First author [Ref.] | | | | | |
|---|---|---|---|---|---|---|
| | Kron [50] | Sundaresan [49] | Gabbay [15] | Bhorade [52] | Straznicka [16] | Pierre [53] |
| Centre | Charlottesville | St Louis | Melbourne | Maywood | Sacramento | Toronto |
| Date | 1993 | 1995 | 1999 | 2000 | 2002 | 2002 |
| Marginal (total) n | 10 (28) | 44 (133) | 64 (112) | 52 (113) | 129 (167) | 63 (123) |
| % marginal | 35 | 33 | 57 | 46 | 77 | 51 |
| Age >55 yrs | N.S. | 2 | 4 | 9 | 10 | 9 |
| Smoking >20 pack-yrs | N.S. | 9 | 5 | 15 | 3 | 26 |
| Abnormal chest radiographs | 6 | 34 | 39 | 5 | 34 | 41 |
| $P_{a,O_2}$ <300 mmHg[#] | 0 | 6 | 20 | 0 | 32 | 0 |
| Purulent secretions | 8 | N.S. | 24 | 0 | 8 | 8 |
| Inhaled drugs | N.S. | N.S. | N.S. | 20 | 13 | N.S. |
| Ventilation >5 days | N.S. | N.S. | N.S. | 7 | N.S. | 27 |
| One criterion | N.S. | 37 | 40 | 48 | 100 | 48 |
| Two criteria | N.S. | 7 | 20 | 4 | 29 | 10 |
| Three criteria | N.S. | 0 | 4 | N.S. | N.S. | 5 |
| Hospital outcome | 9/10 survivors | = | = | = | = | ¶ |
| Early outcome (1 yr) | N.S. | = | = | = | = | N.S. |
| Intermediate outcome | N.S. | = | = | N.S. | = | N.S. |

$P_{a,O_2}$: oxygen tension in arterial blood; N.S.: not stated; #: inspiratory oxygen fraction=1.0, positive end-expiratory pressure of 5 cm $H_2O$; =: identical outcome; ¶: different outcome compared with standard donors.

## *Recipient selection*

Authors have suggested that extended donor lungs, especially with pulmonary infiltrates or contusion, should be used primarily for double-lung replacement in recipients with emphysema. Caution is warranted in patients with pulmonary hypertension, especially in cases of single-lung transplantation, because of the postoperative perfusion imbalance and increased risk of reperfusion-related pulmonary oedema in the graft, aggravating the already existing donor lung dysfunction [49]. Similarly, some degree of reversible donor lung dysfunction is usually tolerable in single-lung transplantation for emphysema, in which the native lung can oxygenate satisfactorily until the graft recovers. One study has found that cardiopulmonary bypass appeared to be necessary to facilitate second graft implantation in bilateral lung transplantation, more often in the marginal donor group than in the ideal donor group [49]. In order to minimise the requirement for cardiopulmonary bypass in bilateral transplants, it is therefore recommended to explant the less functioning of both recipient lungs first and to start with the implantation of the more "normal" donor lung. The Toronto group stated that the increased mortality risk in their patients by using lungs from marginal donors was justified because in their transplant centre waiting times are long and thus mortality on the waiting list is high [53]. Caution, however, is warranted especially in donors with bilateral infiltrates on chest radiographs not related to atelectasis or truly purulent secretions. Finally, the authors pointed out that the experience of the retrieval surgeon is critical to a good outcome when using extended donor lungs [53].

Improved lung preservation techniques [54] and the use of extracellular type flush solutions [55] have resulted in a decrease in the incidence of severe ischaemia-reperfusion injury and a better early outcome. This may also allow the use of more extended donors with less optimal grafts.

## Downsized donor lung

Operative strategies have been developed especially for small and paediatric recipients, *e.g.* cystic fibrosis patients, for downsizing donor lungs in order to allow the use of larger grafts for smaller recipients. This is of special importance for patients with long waiting times or requiring urgent transplantation, where an additional expansion of the potential donor pool can be achieved by the use of initially not size-matched grafts.

### *Peripheral or segmental resection*

Small-to-moderate mismatches between donor organ size and recipient thoracic cavity can be overcome by simple stapler resection of peripheral lung segments [56–59]. On the right side, the middle lobe is resected preferentially, whereas on the left side the lingula can be targeted. This usually allows for a size reduction of ~10–15% and leads to a reduction of the graft not only in its height, but also in its anterior-posterior diameter, since the upper lobe rotates towards the lower lobe. Usually the resection line is completely airtight and only in occasional cases over-sewing with a monofilament suture is warranted.

In 1996, the Vienna group published their first experience with tailoring of the lung in 13 (four single and nine bilateral) of 124 lung transplantations (10.5%) performed between October 1989 and December 1994 [58]. No postoperative complications attributable to the downsizing procedure were observed. In a subsequent report describing their experience up to August 1996, this series was increased to 19 out of 161 transplant patients (11.8%) [59]. In the group's latest experience between 2001 and 2002, tailoring of the lung was carried out in 19 of 98 primary lung transplant patients (19.4%) [60].

### *Cadaveric lobar transplantation*

Extreme size discrepancies can be overcome by transplanting a single lobe instead of a whole lung [61–67]. Usually separation of the donor lobes is performed on the back table. Different combinations of lobar transplantation are applicable. For a bilateral transplantation with an especially small thoracic cavity on one side (*e.g.* after previous lobectomy or in case of a destroyed lung), transplantation of a whole lung together with only one lobe on the opposite side is feasible [65]. For a higher degree of size reduction, bilateral transplantation of lower or upper lobes can be performed as well. On the right side a combination of the lower lobe together with the middle lobe [66] or the upper lobe with the middle lobe can be used as well. The choice of a particular lobe is dependent on its anatomical size and the size of the recipient cavity. If one of the lobes is destroyed due to trauma or otherwise unsuitable for transplantation, the other lobes can still be used. Especially in patients with pulmonary hypertension and enlarged cardiac diameters, the lower part of the left hemithorax is significantly smaller and therefore implantation of a left, upper lobe is preferred.

A meticulous surgical technique is of utmost importance for the success of these challenging operations. Division of parenchymal bridges is performed with commercial stapler devices. As much peribronchial tissue as possible is preserved to guarantee sufficient bronchial blood supply. The bronchial anastomosis is performed in an end-to-end fashion, usually with a 5/0 monofilament suture and size discrepancies are adjusted over the whole circumference. For the vascular anastomoses short stumps are important to avoid any kinking and the venous anastomosis can be either performed with one pulmonary venous stump or with the use of the whole atrial cuff to guarantee a wide lumen. Implantation of the lobes should be performed in general with the use of some cardiopulmonary support to avoid initial overflow of the first implanted lobe, which may result in significant reperfusion pulmonary oedema.

The Vienna group published their experience with lobar transplantation in six out of 161 (3.7%) patients operated upon between November 1989 and August 1996 (left lower lobe plus right middle and lower lobe: n=4; right upper lobe plus left lung: n=1; right middle and lower lobe retransplant 1 yr after first bilateral lung transplant: n=1) [59]. One patient had a prolonged air leak and one other had a pulmonary infection. No bronchial complications were observed. In their latest experience between 2001 and 2002, nine out of 98 (9.2%) primary transplant patients received a lobar transplant [60].

## *Split lung transplantation*

After previous experimental work in dogs [68, 69], the technique of pulmonary bipartitioning in humans was first described by COUETIL *et al.* [70]. With this technique a lung can be split into upper and lower lobe and used for a bilateral transplantation in a recipient with ~50% of total lung capacity (TLC) of the donor. This technique has initially been described for the left lung, whereas the right lung remains for use as a single-lung graft in another patient. Recently, a similar technique for splitting the right lung has also been reported [71].

Some technical details should be mentioned. In case of a left split lung, the oblique fissure is divided with staplers, the pulmonary artery is transected in an oblique way leaving an arterial cuff to the lower lobe including the apical segmental artery (fig. 1). The main stem of the pulmonary artery is shortened and closed with a running suture. The confluence of the pulmonary veins are divided into inferior and superior veins leaving a small cuff of atrial tissue. The orifices of the upper and lower lobe bronchi are transected down to the level of the segmental branches. The donor left, lower lobe is implanted on the left side as in lobar transplantation. The donor left, upper lobe is brought into the right thoracic cavity after 180° rotation in the vertical axis. The left, upper lobe donor bronchus is connected to the intermediate bronchus of the recipient

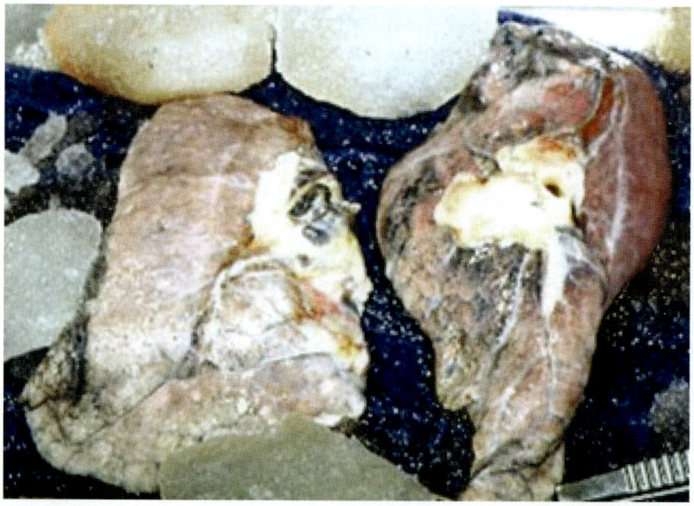

Fig. 1. – The donor left lung is split, on the back table, into upper lobe (right side) and lower lobe (left side) for bilateral lobar implantation. Picture courtesy of W. Klepetko (Dept of Cardiothoracic Surgery, University Hospital, Vienna, Austria).

with the donor's membranous part being sawn to the recipient's cartilaginous part and *vice versa*. The fissural end of the left, upper lobe donor artery is connected to the recipient's right artery. Finally, the left, upper lobe donor vein is connected to the recipients' right superior pulmonary vein.

The initial report by COUETIL *et al.* [70] described the experience with seven patients operated on between May 1993 and November 1994. Indication for transplantation was cystic fibrosis in three patients, primary pulmonary hypertension in two patients and bronchiectasis and idiopathic pulmonary fibrosis in one patient. There were three children aged between 13–17 yrs and four adults aged between 40–53 yrs. One patient died of a systemic Aspergillus infection, the six other patients were alive and well 10–27 months after the procedure. No technical problems were identified and repeated bronchoscopy has demonstrated satisfactory healing of the airways without early stricture formation. Perfect adaptation of the transplanted lobes to the recipient's pleural space was demonstrated on postoperative computed tomography (CT) scan. The Vienna group also reported their initial experience in a 14-yr old female with cystic fibrosis [72]. In the years 2001–2002, two more patients received a split lung transplant in Vienna [60]. Finally, COUETIL *et al.* [71] reported good results in six cystic fibrosis patients using the right split lung technique.

## Living-related donors

The use of living donors is in some ways the most attractive. An elective transplant can be performed with lungs of known quality into a well prepared recipient. Conversely, there is a major ethical dimension to selection of both recipients and donors [73–75]. The donor is exposed to some risk and an obligatory loss of pulmonary function, though the volume of the lung transplanted is small. This approach is based on harvesting lower lobes from healthy donors (usually parents or relatives, of a child or very young adult) to perform bilateral lobar transplantation to patients with cystic fibrosis. Some USA centres have also utilised "unrelated" friends as donors [76].

### *Reported series*

The first living-related donor lung transplant was reported by the Stanford group in 1990 in a 12-yr-old child with bronchopulmonary dysplasia [62, 77]. Most of the experience in this field has been gained by the group based at the University of Southern California (USC) in Los Angeles led by V. Starnes. They now have the experience >120 transplants [78–80]. Recently, other USA transplant centres like St Louis [81, 82], Pittsburgh [83], Chapel Hill [84], and Minneapolis [85] have now embarked on living donor lung transplantations. Up to December 2003, there have been 400 living donor lung transplants reported in the USA [44]. Also in Japan, living donor lobar lung transplantation is now being performed for various lung diseases as the concept of brain-death is not accepted [86]. In contrast, activity in European centres has been small [73, 74, 87].

### *Recipient selection*

Nearly all the recipients in the USC series have had cystic fibrosis [88]. They represent patients of relatively small stature who have a high mortality on the waiting list and usually an excellent history of compliance. A number of other conditions, including pulmonary hypertension, pulmonary fibrosis, bronchiolitis obliterans (BO), and bronchopulmonary dysplasia have been treated in both adults and children [89]. The procedure is not appropriate for very small children, probably those <120 cm, because the volume of an adult lobe will exceed that of the pleural cavity. In this respect the middle lobe and the lingula cannot be regarded as usable units of lung, for transplantation, because of their overlapping venous drainage.

### *Donor selection*

Basic criteria are: that they must be between the ages of 18–55 yrs and have had no thoracic procedure on the side to be used. General health clearly needs to be good and donors are preferred to be significantly taller than the recipients. Investigations include blood typing for compatibility, and chest radiographs and spirometry as a screening procedure. Current smoking is an exclusion criterion. For those who come through the screening process, there is a more rigorous set of investigations including a full cardiopulmonary work up and viral screening. Ventilation and perfusion scanning and high resolution CT are useful adjuncts to ensure that both the lobe to be removed is healthy and the same applies to the rest of the lung. CT will give some clues as to completeness of the fissure and the presence of pleural adhesions and excludes the need for bronchoscopy to detect airway abnormalities [80].

### *Surgical technique*

Transplant centres using this downsized donor lung technique face significant challenges. The surgery involves the use of three surgical teams working simultaneously. The approaches to the donor right and left, lower lobectomies have been well described [63, 78]. The principles are to clearly remove enough of the hilar structures to permit successful anastomosis in the recipient, whilst at the same time preserving the integrity of the remaining lobes in the donor. The tissue available to the implanting surgeon can be considerably reduced compared with the standard transplant. Both airways and vascular structures can be divided at bifurcations. Pericardial patches may be required to ensure continuity, particularly the pulmonary arterial supply and again particularly on the right. Closure of the bronchus on the right can be particularly difficult if there is a high take-off of the orifice of the apical segment of the lower lobe. Bronchoplastic techniques, including detachment and re-implantation of the middle lobe bronchus into the end of the bronchus intermedius may be required.

After the dissection in the donor, but before division of the vessels, 10,000 units of heparin is given and also 500 mg of methylprednisolone. Care is taken to clamp the pulmonary artery before the pulmonary veins so as to avoid engorgement of the removed lobe. It has proved much more straightforward to perfuse the lung retrograde with the standard Perfadex® lung preservation solution on the back table, while using low pressure and a balloon tipped catheter. The lung can be gently ventilated during this phase of the procedure using a sterile airway introduced into the field.

The procedure in the recipient is relatively more standard and straightforward. In the USC group all patients are placed on cardiopulmonary bypass. Bilateral pneumonectomies are performed and then bilateral lobar implants. The bronchus has always been straightforward and bronchial anastomotic problems have not been a source of anxiety, probably because of the closeness of the anastomosis to the lung parenchyma. Adequate lengths of recipient pulmonary artery are left so as to encompass any potential problems on the donor side. The lower lobe pulmonary vein is most conveniently anastomosed directly onto the upper lobe pulmonary vein of the recipient which almost invariably gives a tension free anastomosis. Both lungs are reperfused simultaneously. Inhaled nitric oxide may be used as routine during the implantation and reperfusion. Particular care needs to be taken to avoid ventilator-induced lung injury in view of the small size of the parenchymal bed implanted.

## *Postoperative management*

The major problem is that relatively small lungs are introduced into a large pleural cavity (fig. 2). The problem of over-inflation, resulting in both lung injury and haemodynamic compromise has been described in this setting [90] and is similar to that which has been described after lung transplantation for obstructive airways disease. It may be necessary to leave a pneumothorax in the chest over the first few hours and to avoid the drainage of pleural effusions. Later, the management of the residual pleural space can be particularly difficult. A careful compromise between too much drainage and over-inflation, and lung compression from large osmotically active effusions, has to be reached.

## *Results*

The outcomes in the USC series have been surprisingly disappointing. There is a 1-yr survival rate of only 72% [88] and a 5-yr survival rate of 58% [78]. This may reflect the

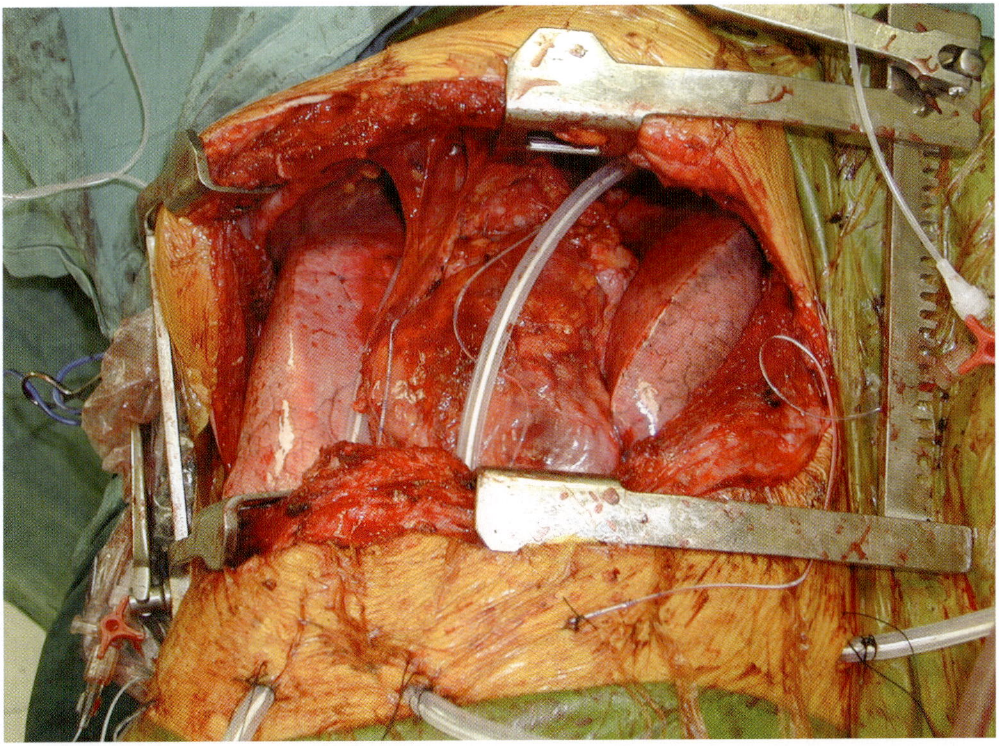

Fig. 2. – Peroperative view taken immediately after reperfusion following living-related bilateral lobar lung transplantation in a young cystic fibrosis patient *via* clam-shell incision. Note the relatively smaller lungs placed into a larger pleural cavity. Picture courtesy of J.H. Dark (Cardiothoracic Transplant Unit, Freeman Hospital, Newcastle UK).

relatively severe nature of the recipients, 76% of whom were in hospital at the time of transplant. A total of 30% were either on invasive ventilation or preoperative noninvasive ventilation. Conversely these risk factors may not be so very different from the general population of cystic fibrosis patients at the time of transplant. Survival was superior in paediatric recipients compared with the adult population (83 and 78 *versus* 65 and 50% for 1 and 5-yr survivals, respectively) [78]. A 1-yr survival was not different between the cystic fibrosis group (72%) *versus* the noncystic fibrosis group (70%) [76].

Early and late rejection remains at least as common as after conventional transplants, but is nearly always asynchronous, affecting one lung at a time [91].

More interesting has been the apparent freedom from BO as a late cause of death. In a paper comparing living donor lobar and cadaveric donors, there was significant preservation of pulmonary function at 2 yrs in the former group [92]. Most of the deaths were a result of infection [88, 93]. It may well be that with appropriate adjustment of immunosuppression and better infection management, long-term outcome from living donor transplant may improve.

No donor deaths have been recorded so far, although donor morbidity may be significant [76, 81, 88]. In the series from the St Louis group, 61.3% of the 62 donors had postoperative complications including pleural effusions necessitating drainage, bronchial stump fistulas, hemorrhage, phrenic nerve injury, and bronchial stricture [81]. There is also regular morbidity as a result of prolonged air leak, postoperative bleeding and atelectasis. There is ~20% fall in forced expiratory volume in one second ($FEV_1$) related to living donor transplant at 6 months follow-up [76, 81].

## Non-heart-beating donors

### *Definition*

Donors who have been declared dead by neurological criteria (brain-death) provide most of the lungs used in transplantation today. Historically, before the introduction of neurological death criteria, the first lung transplantations were realised with organs retrieved from donors after cardiac arrest, so-called non-heart-beating donors (NHBD) [94]. Today, such donors account for only a small percentage of all kidney [95, 96] and less frequent, liver transplantations [97].

### *Categories*

According to the Maastricht classification [98], NHBDs can be classified into four categories (table 3). Categories I and II comprise of the uncontrolled donors. Organ donation in these donors is not discussed until after circulatory arrest. The exact length of the post mortem warm ischaemic period is often not known. Categories III and IV

**Table 3. – Maastricht classification[#] of non-heart-beating donors**

| Category | Definition |
|---|---|
| I | Dead on arrival |
| II | Unsuccessful resuscitation |
| III | Awaiting cardiac arrest |
| IV | Cardiac arrest in a brain-dead donor |

[#]: according to KOOTSTRA [98].

include the controlled donors. The moment of circulatory arrest can be planned in advance and therefore the length of the warm ischaemic interval is precisely known.

### *Controlled non-heart-beating donors*

A category IV NHBD may occur when a heart-beating donor develops cardiac arrest at the time of organ retrieval in the minutes prior to the start of cold flush perfusion. Therefore, the warm ischaemic period will be limited to only a few minutes. Occasional cases of successful lung transplantation with organs from such a donor have been reported [99].

A category III NHBD is a patient with irreversible brain damage (without fulfilling the brain-death criteria) where their next of kin asks for the cessation of life-supporting treatment. In this instance the patient might become an organ donor if they meet the standard criteria for organ, and specifically lung, donation (no gross infection, adequate gas exchange). After informed consent, life support will be withdrawn and the ventilator is switched off in the ICU or in the operating room. Cardiac arrest is awaited. After a period of no touch (5–10 min according to the local protocol), sternotomy is performed and the organs are cooled and flushed *in situ* in the standard way [100]. The first case of successful lung transplantation from such a donor was reported in 1995 by Love *et al.* [101] from the University of Wisconsin. Their 10-yr experience with five such donors was recently presented at the 23rd Annual Meeting of the ISHLT in Vienna [102]. Four single and one double-lung transplantation were performed for various lung diseases. The mean warm ischaemic time prior to cold university of Wisconsin solution (UW) pulmonary flush was 28 min (19–40 min) followed by a cold ischaemic period of 238 min (121–398 min). Transplanted lungs functioned in all cases with no incidence of primary graft failure. The double lung recipient died in hospital from a small bowel perforation and one more patient died from BOS within the first year after transplant. There are three long-term survivors. The current authors are aware of some other case reports of successful lung transplantation from Category III NHBD performed worldwide (personal communication: JH Dark *et al*, Newcastle-upon-Tyne, UK; and GA Patterson *et al*, St Louis, MO, USA;).

### *Uncontrolled non-heart-beating donors*

An uncontrolled NHBD may occur when a person dies unexpectedly inside (category II) or outside (category I) the hospital. In such cases, the deceased person may become a potential donor if his or her organs can be adequately preserved inside the cadaver prior to organ retrieval, and if consent for the retrieval of organs can be obtained from the relatives under such circumstances. As pulmonary graft function can not be assessed in these donors prior to death, lungs should be properly evaluated afterwards prior to organ transplantation in order to reduce the risk of primary nonfunction. The use of lungs from such NHBDs has the potential to eliminate the shortage of donor lungs as it is estimated that approximately one third of all deaths in the Western world are caused by ischaemic heart disease and that 375,000 people in Europe [103] and 275,000 in the USA [104] undergo sudden cardiac arrest yearly.

Steen *et al.* [105] have recently published the first successful case of lung transplantation from such a category II donor . The donor was a 54-yr-old male with an acute myocardial infarction who died in hospital after failed resuscitation of 50 min. After a hands-off period of 65 min and permission from the next of kin, pleural cannulas were inserted and the lungs were cooled to 18°C inside the body with cold Perfadex® for 2 h. The lungs were then harvested and graft function was assessed briefly at 37°C in an *ex vivo* reperfusion circuit and found to be excellent. The lungs were then re-cooled in the circuit to 20°C and further stored at 8°C for >7 h until the recipient was prepared. After a total ischaemic time of >13 h, successful left single-lung transplantation was performed in a 54-yr-old female with emphysema who had previously undergone bilateral thoracoscopic lung volume reduction surgery [105]. No other cases have been reported by Steen's group so far.

VARELA *et al.* [106] very recently reported a series of three patients who underwent bilateral transplantation with lungs retrieved from donors who died unexpectedly outside the hospital (category I NHBD). The immediate and intermediate lung function and quality of life were excellent in all three recipients at 10, 5, and 2 months after surgery. Since this report, a further two patients underwent successful lung transplantation from such donors in Madrid ( personal communication A. Varela, Clinica Puerta de Hierro, Madrid, Spain,).

### *Graft preservation*

The concept of lung transplantation from NHBDs was reintroduced by EGAN and co-workers [107, 108] in 1991. This concept was based on the fact the lung may remain viable for a certain period after death, as a result of the oxygen reserve present in the alveoli [109, 110]. Since then, many groups worldwide have published their experimental work exploring the possibility of transplanting lungs from donors after circulatory arrest [111]. The tolerable period of warm ischaemia after circulatory arrest in the cadaver is limited to between 60–90 min [112], but can be extended if the lungs are continuously ventilated [113], expanded after death [114], or if the lungs are topically cooled *via* chest drains [115]. Post mortem topical cooling was reported to be superior to continued ventilation to protect the lung inside the warm cadaver [116].

### *Ethical issues*

Whether organs from NHBDs can be ethically used for transplantation is still a source of considerable controversy [117–121]. In support of NHBD, it may be acceptable practice if: there is a separation of the rationale to withdraw life support or to withhold cardiopulmonary resuscitation, from the decision to recover organs; if no conflicts of interest exist; if a waiting time precluding spontaneous return of circulation is included; and if NHBD conforms to a standardised protocol. Against NHBD, there are questions regarding the ambiguity and cultural perspectives of death, regarding whether a separation of rationale between withdrawal and donation is sufficient to preclude conflicts of interest, and regarding whether variable protocols arise that subordinate the patient to the goal of donation. Such concerns suggest NHBD may damage the trust in patient–physician relationships and may adversely affect organ donation rates.

## Resuscitated lungs

Approximately 70–80% of lungs from potential multi-organ donors are currently declined for transplantation, the majority as a result of: oedema, contusion, aspiration, atelectasis or pneumonia. If the quality of these organs could be adequately improved outside the donor, some of these lungs may still become suitable for transplantation.

*Ex vivo* reperfusion of human lungs, in an isolated circuit, has previously been reported by STEEN *et al.* [122], as a method to assess the lung from a NHBD prior to transplantation. Such an *ex vivo* assessment enables the transplant surgeon not only to carefully inspect and palpate the organ, but also to assess its functional quality before a potential recipient is called to the hospital. In a porcine model of left, single-lung transplantation with contralateral pneumonectomy, Steen's group recently demonstrated that, after a warm ischaemic interval of 65 min followed by 6 h of intrapleural cooling, all lungs had adequate function during *ex vivo* assessment to serve as donor lungs. Transplanted animals could survive and had normal pulmonary function during a 24-h observation period. Other groups have also reported on functional assessment of NHBD donor lungs in an isolated reperfusion circuit as a method to predict post-transplant function [123–125].

*Ex vivo* reperfusion opens the perspective to re-assess lungs from heart-beating donors, previously rejected by other teams or to condition lungs of inferior quality prior to transplantation. Infected lungs could be treated with high dose antibiotics, administered during isolated reperfusion [126]. Oedematous lungs could be dried out *ex vivo* using a perfusate with a high oncotic pressure [127] or by instillation of drugs with a beneficial effect on the alveolar liquid clearance [128, 129]. Ventilation-perfusion discrepancies could be improved by adding bronchodilating [130] and vasodilating agents [131, 132]. Steen's group previously demonstrated that *ex vivo* reperfusion at normothermia is possible for several hours without the development of oedema, and gas exchange deficiencies (fig. 3) [122]. After the evaluation, the lungs can be cooled to an optimal

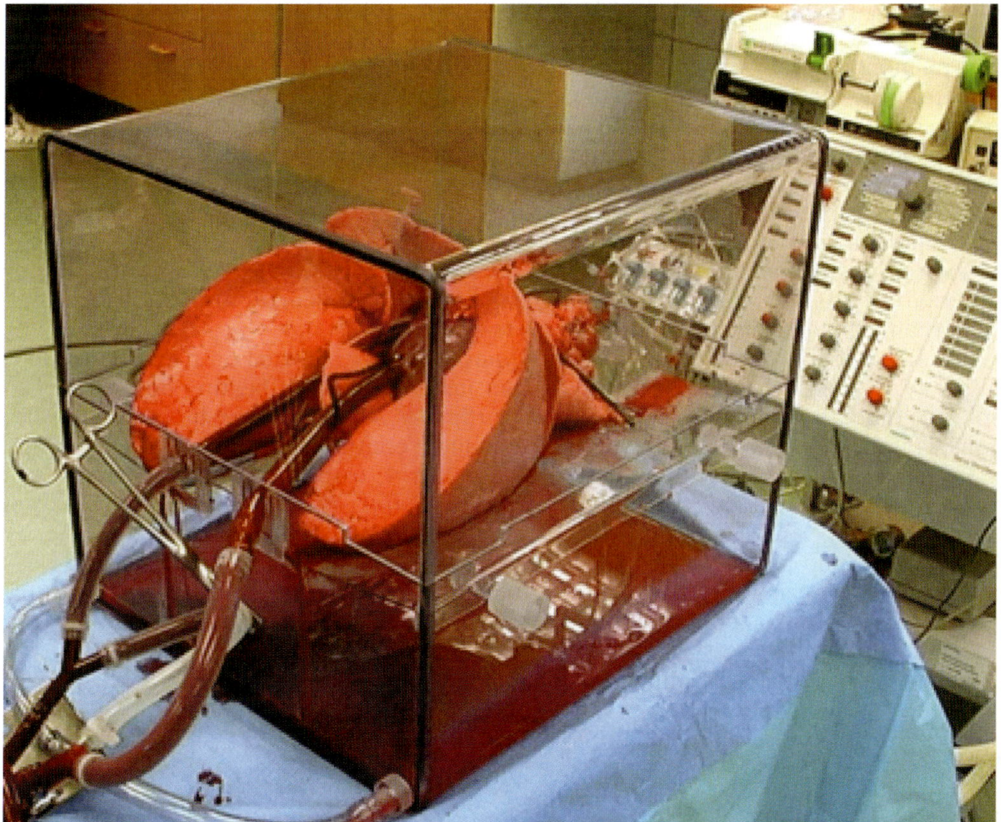

Fig. 3. – Assessment of lung function *ex vivo*. Full perfusion of the lungs are carried out at 37°C with a special medium with a haematocrite of 15±3%. Reproduced with permission [122].

temperature (6–12°C) with a red cell containing oxygenated preservation medium and stored in the same medium (topical extracorporeal membrane oxygenation: ECMO) until the transplantation can be carried out or until repeated reperfusion for further treatment. This method of intermittent *ex vivo* reperfusion has also the potential to preserve lungs for a longer period (> 24h) [133], thereby enabling the transplant surgeon to accept lungs coming from a longer distance or to transform clinical lung transplantation into a daytime practice.

### *Technique*

The basic principle of *ex vivo* evaluation is that lungs can be assessed without additional oedema formation. The prerequisite is that the perfusion is performed at normothermia with an adequate perfusion solution and a perfusion pressure ≤2.66 kPa (20 mmHg). Steen and co-workers (personal communication S. Steen, Heart-Lung Division, University Hospital, Lund, Sweden) performed extensive research to develop the ideal solution for such isolated perfusion that is now marketed under the name Steen Solution® (Vitrolife AB, Gothenburg, Sweden). A pure red blood cell concentrate is added to this solution in order to be able to evaluate gas exchange. STEEN *et al.* [133] found that a haematocrit of ~15% is optimal to obtain an ideal viscosity. After preservation, the heart-lung or lung block is prepared for *ex vivo* evaluation by inserting a cannula in the main pulmonary artery for the inflow and a second cannula in the left atrium for the outflow. In case the heart has already been extracted for heart transplantation, an enlargement of the left atrial patch or stumps of both pulmonary veins can be created with an autologous aortic conduit or pericardial patch to create a neo-atrium in order to facilitate cannulation. The heart-lung or lung block is then mounted in the isolated reperfusion circuit which contains: a blood reservoir, a centrifugal pump, a leukocyte filter, a gas exchanger, and a heater or cooler [124]. The lungs are then reperfused with deoxygenated perfusate, slowly increasing the blood flow by regulating the rate of the pump, thereby controlling the perfusion pressure. Ventilation is not started until the temperature of the pulmonary effluent has reached 32°C and is progressively increased. As soon as lung temperature has reached 37.5°C, functional assessment is performed during a period of 10–20 min with measurements of: gas exchange, haemodynamic and aerodynamic parameters, and indicators of lung oedema.

Van Raemdonck's group in Leuven [134] have recently reported on a feasibility study with *ex vivo* reperfusion of 20 paired human lungs from heart-beating donors in their isolated ventilation and reperfusion model (fig. 4). All lungs had been declined for transplantation for different reasons, these include: contusion, n=3; poor gas exchange, n=3; pneumonia, n=4; high donor age (>55 yrs), n=4; emphysema, n=2; oedema, n=1; donor previous malignancy, n=1; donor Hepatitis C, n=1; and no suitable recipient, n=1. Lungs were reperfused after a mean cold ischaemic interval of 848±58 min (fig. 5). Aerodynamic and haemodynamic parameters in the pulmonary graft remained stable in all experiments during a 2-h period of isolated reperfusion. The authors concluded that *ex vivo* reperfusion of human lungs is technically feasible and can be performed in a stable manner for at least 2 h. This model offers the opportunity to study *ex vivo* conditioning of lungs with inferior quality.

## Future perspectives

### *Xenotransplantation*

High hopes are placed on the research surrounding the use of organs and tissues from animals to man as an alternative source. Lung transplantation, however, has not received

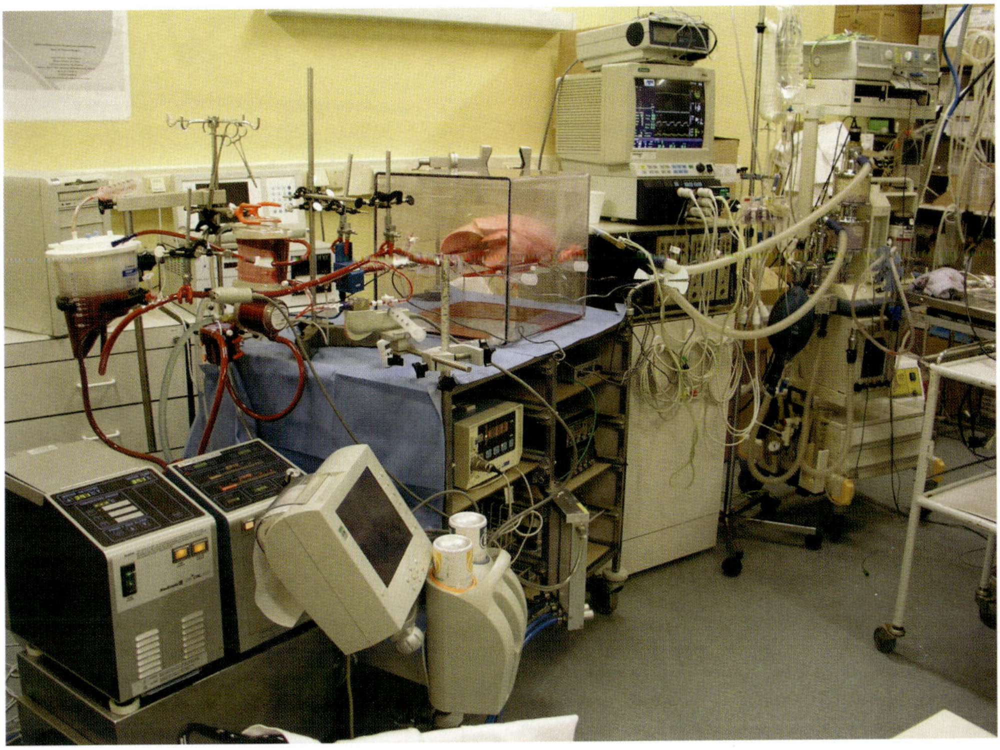

Fig. 4. – Experimental set up for isolated ventilation and reperfusion of human lungs.

nearly as much attention in experimental xenotransplantation as other organs [135]. Historically, few attempts have been made with kidney transplantation from chimpanzees [136], and liver [137] and heart [138] transplantation from baboons.

Many problems still remain unresolved so that xenotransplantation cannot be put forth as a solution for the organ shortage at this time. The main difficulty remains the immunological barrier when transplanting an organ between two largely different species [139]. Complement mediated, hyperacute rejection caused by binding of natural or preformed antibodies will result in endothelial activation and damage, thrombosis with microvascular obstruction and subsequent ischaemic necrosis of the graft. Hopes rest in the research using transgenic animals, placing human complement regulating genes into the organs of pigs [140]. Another problem is the potential transmission of infectious agents from animals to humans (zoonosis), especially endogenous retroviruses [141]. Finally, multiple legal, ethical, and religious aspects will also need extensive review before xenotransplantation becomes a viable reality [142, 143]. Recently, the ISHLT has produced a document with recommendations on the forward progress of cardiac and pulmonary xenotransplantation [144].

## *Artificial Lung*

Organ transplantation, whether living or cadaveric, might be supplemented or replaced by the use of artificial organs. A successful artificial lung could serve as a bridge to transplantation, as a support device immediately post-lung transplantation in case of

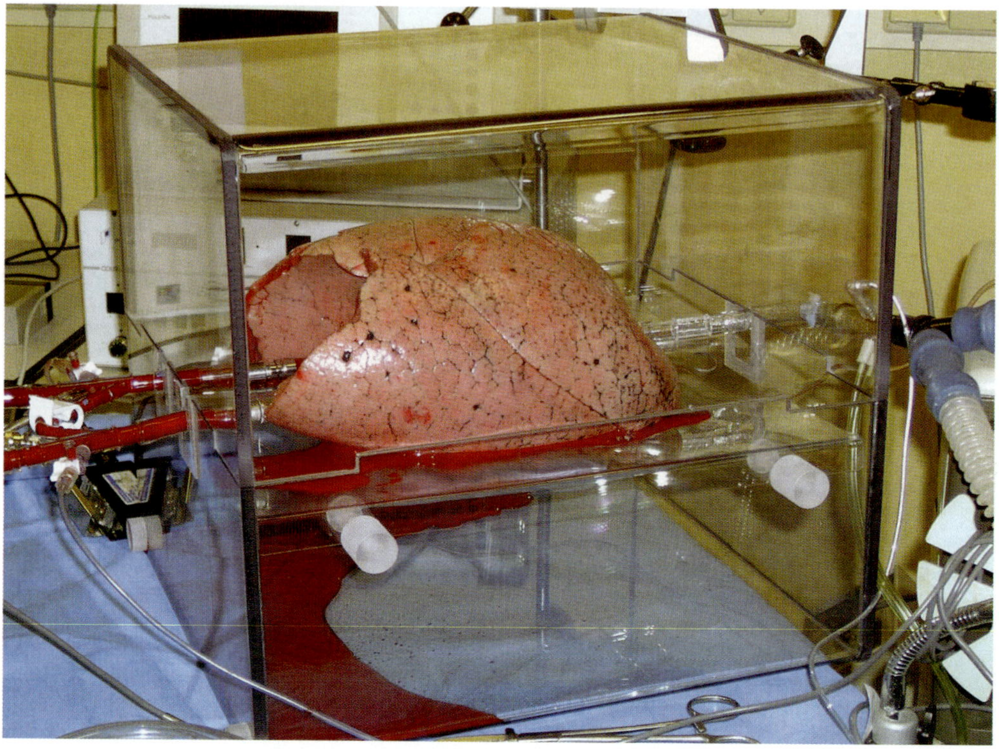

Fig. 5. – Human double-lung block in a plexi-glas box during *ex vivo* assessment. Deoxygenated blood is flowing into the lung *via* a cannula (upper) inserted in the main pulmonary artery and oxygenated blood is draining out of the lung through a cannula (lower) positioned in the left neo-atrium.

primary graft failure or as a temporary support during treatment of severe respiratory failure [145].

Current methods to support patients with lung disease are not efficient enough; although, increasing successes with extracorporeal membrane oxygenation have been reported in adult, paediatric and neonatal respiratory failure [146, 147]. Intravenacaval devices or intravenous membrane oxygenators are still limited by their surface area to provide adequate gas exchange [148]. Research on an implantable artificial lung is ongoing [149, 150] but problems such as power supply, thrombosis, infection, and biocompatibility pose obstacles to long-term function.

A recent survey amongst lung transplant programme directors in the USA revealed that 97% would support a Phase I trial, using an artificial lung as a bridge to lung transplantation. Idiopathic pulmonary fibrosis was the diagnosis thought most appropriate for inclusion in initial clinical trials [151].

## Conclusions

The widespread application of lung transplantation is limited by the shortage of suitable donor organs, resulting in longer waiting times for listed patients with a substantial risk of dying prior to transplantation. Marginal donors not matching the standard donor criteria can be safely used in properly selected recipients. The use of downsized donor lungs, either by peripheral resection of a larger lung or by lobar or split lung transplantation are valuable options for small and paediatric recipients facing long waiting times to find a suitable donor, or requiring urgent transplantation. Living donor lobar transplantation has, as yet, been applied to a relatively small subset of recipients, especially cystic fibrosis patients. There is, however, the promise of improved long-term outcome as the procedure continues to evolve. Transplantation of lungs from controlled, circulation-arrested donors is a valuable option, but the numbers will remain low. The use of lungs from uncontrolled NHBDs is limited by the short tolerable warm ischaemic period and involves methods to adequately preserve the lung inside the cadaver after circulatory arrest. Functional assessment of the graft is mandatory during the cold ischaemic interval in order to safely transplant only quality-approved grafts. The final place of living lobar and NHBD lung transplantation has yet to be established as there are major ethical and technical considerations involved. *Ex vivo* reperfusion has the potential to re-evaluate lungs that have previously been rejected and also to resuscitate lungs of inferior quality by medical treatment outside the body prior to transplantation. Pulmonary xenotransplantation and the implantable artificial lung remain in the future because of currently unsolved immunological and technical problems, respectively.

## Summary

The widespread application of lung transplantation is limited by the shortage of suitable donor organs resulting in longer waiting times for listed patients with a substantial risk of dying prior to transplantation. To overcome this critical organ shortage, many transplant programmes have begun to explore the use of alternative donors.

Several groups have shown that lungs from donors not matching the ideal criteria for lung donation, so called marginal or extended donors, can still be transplanted with no differences in outcome. Nevertheless caution needs to be exercised when transplanting less optimal lungs in recipients with an increased operative risk.

In small or paediatric recipients, successful downsizing techniques by peripheral (segmental) resection, lobar transplantation, and pulmonary bipartitioning have been developed in order to allow the use of larger grafts for smaller recipients facing longer waiting times or requiring urgent transplantation.

The use of lobes from living donors is an option in small recipients, mainly in patients with cystic fibrosis receiving the lower lobes of two family members or even unrelated individuals. Improved long-term outcome with a lower incidence of bronchiolitis obliterans syndrome has been reported.

A few cases of successful transplantation of a lung, retrieved from a donor after cardiac arrest, a so called non-heart-beating donor (NHBD), were recently reported. In the controlled NHBD, the warm ischaemic period of the graft is limited. In the uncontrolled NHBD, topical cooling of the lung with a cold preservation solution inside the cadaver is advocated to minimise the warm ischaemic damage prior to cold flush preservation. Functional evaluation of the graft is mandatory thereafter to assess its viability so that only NHBD lungs of high quality will be transplanted.

Finally, *ex vivo* reperfusion for medical intervention opens the prospect to resuscitate lungs by that have previously been rejected for transplantation because of inferior quality.

Xenotransplantation and the use of an implantable artificial lung are currently still under investigation.

**Keywords:** *Ex vivo* reperfusion, living-related, lobar transplant, marginal donors, non-heart-beating donor, split-lung transplantation.

*Acknowledgements.* Other co-authors of Working Group 2: M. Strüber, F. Venuta, D. Vlasselaers, W. Wisser, M. Erasmus, W. De Wever, E. Russi, H.B. Ris, E. Pompeo, W. Weder, P. Evrard, M. Decramer, N. Konietzko, G. Massard, F. Velly.

# References

1. Trulock EP, Edwards LB, Taylor DO, *et al.* The Registry of The International Society for Heart and Lung Transplantation: twentieth official adult lung and heart-lung transplant report-2003. *J Heart Lung Transplant* 2003; 22: 625–635.
2. Trulock EP. Lung Transplantation. *Am J Respir Crit Care Med* 1997; 155: 789–818.
3. Keller CA. The donor lung: conservation of a precious resource. *Thorax* 1998; 53: 506–513.
4. Roels L, De Meester J. The relative impact of presumed-consent legislation on thoracic organ donation in the Eurotransplant area. *J Transpl Coord* 1996; 6: 174–177.
5. Gäbel H, Roels L. Legislative initiatives to increase organ donation. *Transplant Proc* 1997; 29: 3223.
6. Cohen B, Wight C. A European perspective on organ procurement: breaking down the barriers to organ donation. *Transplantation* 1999; 68: 922–923.
7. Schütt GR. 25 years of organ donation: European initiatives to increase organ donation. *Transplant Proc* 2002; 34: 2005–2006.
8. Egan TM, Boychuk JE, Rosato K, Cooper JD. Whence the lungs? A study to assess suitability of donor lungs for transplantation. *Transplantation* 1992; 53: 420–422.
9. Van Raemdonck D, Roels L, Verleden G, *et al.* Whence the lungs? Assessment of the use of lungs for transplantation from 156 consecutive donors (abstract). Zurich, 3rd International Lung Transplant Symposium, 1993, p. 40.
10. Ware LB, Wang Y, Fang X, *et al.* Assessment of lungs rejected for transplantation and implications for donor selection. *Lancet* 2002; 360: 619–620.
11. Thoracic organs: donation, waiting lists, and transplants. *In*: Persijn GG, Cohen B, eds. Annual Report 2001 of the Eurotransplant International Foundation. Eurotransplant International Foundation, Leiden, 2001; pp. 41–52.
12. Hsieh AH, Bishop MJ, Kubilis PS, *et al.* Pneumonia following closed head injury. *Am Rev Respir Dis* 1992; 146: 290–294.
13. Pennefather SH, Bullock RE, Dark JH. The effect of fluid therapy on alveolar arterial oxygen gradient in brain-dead organs. *Transplantation* 1993; 56: 1418–1422.
14. Riou B, Guesde R, Jacquens Y, *et al.* Fiberoptic bronchoscopy in brain-dead organ donors. *Am J Respir Crit Care Med* 1994; 150: 558–560.
15. Gabbay E, Williams TJ, Griffiths AP, *et al.* Maximizing the utilization of donor organs offered for lung transplantation. *Am J Respir Crit Care Med* 1999; 160: 265–271.
16. Straznicka M, Follette DM, Eisner MD, Roberts PF, Menza RL, Babcock WD. Aggressive management of lung donors classified as unacceptable: excellent recipient survival one year after transplantation. *J Thorac Cardiovasc Surg* 2002; 124: 250–258.
17. Folette DM, Rudich SM, Babcock WD. Improved oxygenation and increased lung donor recovery with high-dose steroid administration after brain death. *J Heart Lung Transplant* 1998; 17: 423–429.
18. McElhinney DB, Khan JH, Babcock WD, Hall TS. Thoracic organ donor characteristics associated with successful lung procurement. *Clin Transpl* 2001; 15: 68–71.
19. Wheeldon DR, Potter CD, Oduro A, Wallwork J, Large SR. Transforming the "unacceptable"

donor: outcomes from the adoption of a standardized donor management technique. *J Heart Lung Transplant* 1995; 14: 734–742.
20. Parry A, Higgins R, Wheeldon D, Bethune D, Wallwork J. The contribution of donor management and modified cold blood lung perfusate to post-transplant lung function. *J Heart Lung Transplant* 1999; 18: 121–126.
21. Lloyd-Jones H, Wheeldon DR, Smith JA, Potter CD, Wallwork J, Large SR. An approach to retrieval of thoracic organs for transplantation. *AORN J* 1996; 63: 416–423.
22. Cummings J, Houck J, Lichtenfield D. Positive effects of agressive resuscitative efforts on cadaver lung procurement. *J Transplant Coord* 1995; 5: 103–106.
23. Harjula A, Baldwin JC, Starnes VA, *et al.* Proper donor selection for heart-lung transplantation. The Stanford experience. *J Thorac Cardiovasc Surg* 1987; 94: 874–880.
24. Calhoon JK, Trinkle JK. Lung transplantation: donor selection and management. *Chest Surg Clin N Am* 1993; 3: 19–28.
25. Cooper JD. The lung donor: special considerations. *Transplant Proc* 1988; 20: 17–18.
26. Zenati M, Dowling RD, Armitage JM, *et al.* Organ procurement for pulmonary transplantation. *Ann Thorac Surg* 1989; 48: 882–886.
27. Griffith BP, Zenati M. The pulmonary donor. *Clin Chest Med* 1990; 11: 217–226.
28. Winton TL, Miller JD, Scavuzzo M, Maurer JR, Patterson GA, and the Toronto Lung Transplant Group. Donor selection for pulmonary transplantation. *Transplant Proc* 1991; 23: 2472–2474.
29. Winton TL. Lung transplantation: donor selection. *Semin Thorac Cardiovasc Surg* 1992; 4: 79–82.
30. Egan T. Selection and management of the lung donor. *In*: Patterson GA, Couraud L, eds. Current topics in general thoracic surgery. Amsterdam, Elsevier, 1995; pp. 103–115.
31. Frost AE. Donor criteria and evaluation. *Clin Chest Med* 1997; 18: 231–237.
32. Aigner C, Seebacher G, Klepetko W. Lung transplantation: donor selection. *Chest Surg Clin N Am* 2003; 13: 429–442.
33. Orens JB, Boehler A, de Perrot M, *et al.* A review of lung transplant donor acceptability criteria. *J Heart Lung Transplant* 2003; 22: 1183–1200.
34. Meyer DM, Bennett LE, Novick RJ, Hosenpud JD. Effect of donor age and ischaemic time on intermediate survival and morbidity after lung transplantation. *Chest* 2000; 118: 1255–1262.
35. Heart/Lung Transplant Registry of the International Society for Heart and Lung Transplantation. Overall lung and adult lung transplantation statistics slides. http://ww accessed: 8 June 2004.
36. Weill D. Donor criteria in lung transplantation. An issue revisited. *Chest* 2002; 121: 2029–2031.
37. Aziz TM, El-Gamel A, Saad RAG, Migliore M, Campbell CS, Yonan NA. Pulmonary vein gas analysis for assessing donor lung function. *Ann Thorac Surg* 2002; 73: 1599–1605.
38. Puskas JD, Winton TL, Miller JD, Scavuzzo M, Patterson GA. Unilateral donor lung dysfunction does not preclude successful contralateral single lung transplantation. *J Thorac Cardiovasc Surg* 1992; 103: 1015–1017.
39. Couetil JP, Argyriadis PG, Tolan MJ, Achkar A, Carpentier AF. Contralateral lung transplantation: a left lung implanted in the right thorax. *Ann Thorac Surg* 2001; 72: 933–935.
40. Stewart S, Ciulli F, Wells FC, Wallwork J. Pathology of unused donor lungs. *Transplant Proc* 1993; 25: 1167–1168.
41. Husain AN, Hinkamp TJ. Donor lung pathology: correlation with outcome of transplanted contralateral lung. *J Heart Lung Transplant* 1993; 12: 932–939.
42. Egan TM. The other lung revisited-again. *J Heart Lung Transplant* 1993; 12: 940.
43. Fisher AJ, Dark JH, Corris PA. Improving donor lung evaluation: a new approach to increase organ supply for lung transplantation. *Thorax* 1998; 53: 818–820.
44. United Network for Organ Sharing scientific registry data. www.unos.org. Date accessed 13 December 2003.
45. De Meester J, Smits JM, Persijn GG, Haverich A. Listing for lung transplantation: life expectancy and transplantation effect, stratified by type of end-stage lung disease, the Eurotransplant experience. *J Heart Lung Transplant* 2001; 20: 518–524.
46. De Meester J, Smits JM, Persijn GG, Haverich A. Lung transplant waiting list: differential

outcome of type of end-stage lung disease, one year after registration. *J Heart Lung Transplant* 1999; 18: 563–571.
47. Egan TM, Bennett LE, Garrity ER, *et al.* Predictors of death on the UNOS lung transplant waiting list: results of a multivariate analysis [Abstract]. *J Heart Lung Transplant* 2001; 20: 242.
48. Dark JH. Priorities for lung transplantation. *Lancet* 1998; 351: 24–27.
49. Sundaresan S, Semenkovich J, Ochoa L, *et al.* Successful outcome of lung transplantation is not compromised by the use of marginal donor lungs. *J Thorac Cardiovasc Surg* 1995; 109: 1075–1080.
50. Kron I, Tribble C, Kern J, *et al.* Successful transplantation of marginally acceptable thoracic organs. *Ann Surg* 1993; 217: 518–524.
51. Shumway S, Hertz M, Petty M, Bolman R. Liberalization of donor criteria in lung and heart-lung transplantation. *Ann Thorac Surg* 1994; 57: 92–95.
52. Bhorade S, Vigneswaran W, McCabe M, Garrity E. Liberalization of donor criteria may expand the donor pool without adverse consequence in lung transplantation. *J Heart Lung Transplant* 2000; 19: 1200–1204.
53. Pierre AF, Sekine Y, Hutcheon MA, Waddell TK, Keshavjee SH. Marginal donor lungs: a reassessment. *J Thorac Cardiovasc Surg* 2002; 123: 421–427.
54. Van Raemdonck D, Strüber M, Venuta F, Vlasselaers D, Wisser W, Erasmus ME. Strategies in the prevention and the treatment of ischaemia-reperfusion injury after lung transplantation. *Eur Respir Mon* 2004; 29: 66–88.
55. Rega F, Dupont L, Verleden G, *et al.* Switch from Euro-Collins to Perfadex for pulmonary graft preservation resulted in superior outcome in transplant recipients [abstract]. *J Heart Lung Transplant* 2003; 22: S111.
56. Lillehei CW, Everts E, Shamberger RC. Reduced size lung transplantation from adult to neonatal sheep. *J Pediatr Surg* 1992; 27: 1153–1156.
57. Cromblehome TM, Adzick NS, Longaker MT. Reduced size lung transplantation in neonatal swine: technique and short-term physiologic response. *Ann Thorac Surg* 1990; 49: 55–60.
58. Wisser W, Klepetko W, Wekerle T, *et al.* Tailoring of the lung to overcome size disparities in lung transplantation. *J Heart Lung Transplant* 1996; 15: 239–242.
59. Artemiou O, Wieselthaler G, Zuckermann A, *et al.* Downsizing of the donor lung: peripheral segmental resections and lobar transplantation. *Transplant Proc* 1997; 29: 2899–2900.
60. Aigner C, Mazhar S, Seebacher G, *et al.* Lobar transplantation, split lung transplantation and peripheral segmental resection: reliable procedures for downsizing donor lungs. *Eur J Cardiothorac Surg* 2004; 25: 179–183.
61. Huggins CE. Reimplantation of lobes of the lung: an experimental technique. *Lancet* 1959; 2: 1059–1062.
62. Starnes VA, Lewiston NJ, Luikart H, Theodore J, Stinson EB, Shumway NE. Current trends in lung transplantation. Lobar transplantation and expanded use of single lungs. *J Thorac Cardiovasc Surg* 1992; 104: 1060–1065.
63. Starnes VA, Barr ML, Cohen RG. Lobar implantation: indications, technique and outcome. *J Thorac Cardiovasc Surg* 1994; 108: 403–411.
64. Spray TL, Mallory GB, Canter CB, Huddleston CB. Pediatric lung transplantation: indications, techniques, and early results. *J Thorac Cardiovasc Surg* 1994; 107: 990–1000.
65. Bisson A, Bonnette P, Perruchou A, *et al.* Left lower lobe transplantation during a bilateral single lung transplantation. *Eur J Cardiothorac Surg* 1992; 6: 568–570.
66. Bisson A, Bonnette P, el Kadi NB, Leroy M, Colchen A. Bilateral pulmonary lobe transplantation: left lower and right middle and lower lobes. *Ann Thorac Surg* 1994; 57: 219–221.
67. Watson TJ, Starnes VA. Pediatric lobar lung transplantation. *Semin Thorac Cardiovasc Surg* 1996; 8: 313–325.
68. Couetil JP, Grousset A, Benaim D, *et al.* Experimental model of pulmonary bipartition with bilateral lobe transplantation in dogs and application to clinical medicine. *Chirurgie* 1994–95; 120: 512–517.

69. Couetil JP, Tolan MJ, Grousset A, *et al.* Experimental bilateral lobar transplantation and its application in humans. *Thorax* 1997; 52: 714–717.
70. Couetil JP, Tolan MJ, Loulmet DF, *et al.* Pulmonary bipartitioning and lobar transplantation: a new approach to donor organ shortage. *J Thorac Cardiovasc Surg* 1997; 113: 529–537.
71. Couetil JP, Argyriadis PG, Amrein C, *et al.* Right split lung technique with bilateral lobar transplantation: an alternative approach to organ shortage [Abstract]. Lisbon, 1st Joint EACTS/ESTS meeting, 2001; 4.
72. Artemiou O, Birsan T, Taghavi S, *et al.* Bilateral lobar transplantation with the split lung technique. *J Thorac Cardiovasc Surg* 1999; 118: 369–370.
73. Dark JH. Lung: living related transplantation. *Br Med Bull* 1997; 53: 892–903.
74. Hodson ME. Transplantation using lobes from living donors. *J Med Ethics* 2000; 26: 419–421.
75. Kramer MR, Sprung CL. Living related donation in lung transplantation. Ethical considerations. *Arch Intern Med* 1995; 155: 1734–1738.
76. Barr ML, Schenkel FA, Cohen RG, *et al.* Recipient and donor outcomes in living related and unrelated lobar transplantation. *Transplant Proc* 1998; 30: 2261–2263.
77. Goldsmith MF. Mother to child: first living donor lung transplant. *JAMA* 1990; 264: 2724.
78. Barr ML, Baker CJ, Schenkel FA, *et al.* Living donor lung transplantation: selection, technique and outcome. *Transplant Proc* 2001; 33: 3527–3532.
79. Cohen RG, Starnes VA. Living donor lung transplantation. *World J Surg* 2001; 25: 244–250.
80. Bowdish ME, Barr ML, Starnes VA. Living lobar transplantation. *Chest Surg Clin N Am* 2003; 13: 505–524.
81. Battafarano RJ, Anderson RC, Meyers BF, *et al.* Perioperative complications after living donor lobectomy. *J Thorac Cardiovasc Surg* 2000; 120: 909–915.
82. Mendeloff EN. Pediatric lung transplantation. *Chest Surg Clin N Am* 2003; 13: 485–504.
83. Gilbert S, Dauber JH, Hattler BG, *et al.* Lung and heart-lung transplantation at the University of Pittsburgh: 1982–2002. *Clin Transpl* 2002; 253–261.
84. Egan TM, Detterbeck FC, Mill MR, *et al.* Long term results of lung transplantation for cystic fibrosis. *Eur J Cardiothorac Surg* 2002; 22: 602–609.
85. Dahlberg PS, Prekker ME, Hertz M, Thompson DJ, Park SJ. Recent trends in lung transplantation: the University of Minnesota experience. *Clin Transpl* 2002: 243–251.
86. Date H, Aoe M, Nagahiro I, *et al.* Living donor lobar lung transplantation for various lung diseases. *J Thorac Cardiovasc Surg* 2003; 126: 476–481.
87. Svendsen UG, Aggestrup S, Heilmann C, *et al.* Transplantation of a lobe of lung from mother to child following previous transplantation with maternal bone marrow. *Eur Respir J* 1995; 8: 334–337.
88. Cohen RG, Barr ML, Schenkel FA, DeMeester TR, Wells WJ, Starnes VA. Living-related donor lobectomy for bilateral lobar transplantation in patients with cystic fibrosis. *Ann Thorac Surg* 1994; 57: 1423–1428.
89. Starnes VA, Barr ML, Schenkel FA, *et al.* Experience with living-donor lobar transplantation for indications other than cystic fibrosis. *J Thorac Cardiovasc Surg* 1997; 114: 917–922.
90. Haddy SM, Bremner RM, Moore-Jefferies EW, *et al.* Hyperinflation resulting in hemodynamic collapse following living donor lobar transplantation. *Anesthesiology* 2002; 97: 1315–1317.
91. Barr ML, Schenkel FA, Cohen RG, *et al.* Living-related lobar transplantation: recipient outcome and early rejection patterns. *Transplant Proc* 1995; 27: 1995–1996.
92. Starnes VA, Woo MS, MacLaughlin EF, *et al.* Comparison of outcomes between living donor and cadaveric lung transplantation in children. *Ann Thorac Surg* 1999; 68: 2279–2284.
93. Woo MS, MacLaughlin EF, Horn MV, Szmuszkovicz JR, Barr ML, Starnes VA. Bronchiolitis obliterans is not the primary cause of death in pediatric living donor lobar lung transplant recipients. *J Heart Lung Transplant* 2001; 20: 491–496.
94. Hardy JD, Webb WR, Dalton ML, *et al.* Homotransplantation in man. *JAMA* 1963; 186: 1065–1074.

95. Kootstra G, Wijnen R, van Hooff JP, van der Linden CJ. Twenty percent more kidneys through a non-heart-beating program. *Transplant Proc* 1991; 23: 910–911.
96. Sanchez-Fructuoso AI, Prats D, Torrente J, *et al.* Renal transplantation from non-heart beating donors: a promising alternative to enlarge the donorpool. *J Am Soc Nephrol* 2000; 11: 350–358.
97. D'Alessandro AM, Hoffman RM, Knechtle SJ, *et al.* Liver transplantation from controlled non-heart-beating donors. *Surgery* 2000; 128: 579–588.
98. Kootstra G, Daemen JH, Oomen AP. Catagories of non-heart-beating donors. *Transplant Proc* 1995; 27: 2893–2894.
99. Shennib H. Discussion on. Egan TM *et al.*. *Ann Thorac Surg* 1991; 52: 1120–1121.
100. D'Alessandro AM, Hoffman RM, Knechtle SJ, *et al.* Controlled non-heart-beating donors: a potential source of extrarenal organs. *Transplant Proc* 1995; 27: 707–709.
101. Love RB, Stringham JC, Chomiak PN, Warner T, Pellett JR, Mentzer RM. Successful lung transplantation using a non-heart-beating donor [Abstract]. *J Heart Lung Transplant* 1995; 14: S88.
102. Love RB, D'Allesandro AM, Cornwell RA, Meyer KM. Ten year experience with human lung transplantation from non-heart beating donors [Abstract]. *J Heart Lung Transplant* 2003; 22: S87.
103. The Hypothermia After Cardiac Arrest Study Group. Mild therapeutic hypothermia to improve the neurologic outcome after cardiac arrest. *N Eng J Med* 2002; 346: 549–556.
104. Curfman GD. Hypothermia to protect the brain: perspective. *N Eng J Med* 2002; 346: 546.
105. Steen S, Sjöberg T, Pierre L, Liao Q, Eriksson L, Algotsson L. Transplantation of lungs from a non-heart-beating donor. *Lancet* 2001; 357: 825–829.
106. Varela A, Nuñez JR, Gamez AP, *et al.* Are out hospital non heart beating donors better than brain death lung donors ? [Abstract]. *J Heart Lung Transplant* 2004; 23: S87.
107. Egan TM, Lambert CJ, Reddick R, Ulicny KS, Keagy BA, Wilcox BR. A strategy to increase the donor pool: use of cadaver lungs for transplantation. *Ann Thorac Surg* 1991; 52: 1113–1120.
108. Egan TM. Non-heart-beating lung donors: yes or no? *Ann Thorac Surg* 2000; 70: 1451–1452.
109. D'Armini AM, Roberts CS, Griffith PK, Lemasters JJ, Egan TM. When does the lung die? I. Histochemical evidence of pulmonary viability after "death". *J Heart Lung Transplant* 1994; 13: 741–747.
110. Alessandrini F, D'Armini AM, Roberts CS, Reddick RL, Egan TM. When does the lung die? II. Ultrastructural evidence of pulmonary viability after "death". *J Heart Lung Transplant* 1994; 13: 748–757.
111. Egan TM. Non-heart-beating donors in thoracic transplantation. *J Heart Lung Transplant* 2004; 23: 3–10.
112. Van Raemdonck DEM, Jannis NCP, De Leyn PRJ, Flameng WJ, Lerut TE. Warm ischaemic tolerance in collapsed pulmonary grafts is limited to 1 hour. *Ann Surg* 1998; 228: 788–796.
113. Roberts CS, Hennington MH, D'Armini AM, Griffith PK, Lemasters JJ, Egan TM. Donor lungs from ventilated cadavers: impact of a free radical scavenger. *J Heart Lung Transplant* 1996; 15: 275–282.
114. Van Raemdonck DEM, Jannis NCP, De Leyn PRJ, Flameng WJ, Lerut TE. Alveolar expansion itself but not continuous oxygen supply enhances postmortem preservation of pulmonary grafts. *Eur J Cardiothorac Surg* 1998; 13: 431–442.
115. Steen S, Ingemansson R, Budrikis A, Bolys R, Roscher R, Sjoberg T. Successful transplantation of lungs topically cooled in the non-heart-beating donor for 6 hours. *Ann Thorac Surg* 1997; 63: 345–351.
116. Rega FR, Jannis NC, Verleden GM, Flameng WJ, Lerut TE, Van Raemdonck DEM. Should we ventilate or cool the pulmonary graft inside the non-heart-beating donor? *J Heart Lung Transplant* 2003; 22: 1226–1233.
117. Whetstine L, Bowman K, Hawryluck L. Pro/con ethics debate: is nonheart-beating organ donation ethically acceptable? *Crit Care* 2002; 6: 192–195.

118. Carlberg A. Transplanting lungs from non-heart-beating donors. *Natl Cath Bioeth Q* 2002; 2: 377–380.
119. Zamperetti N, Bellomo R, Ronco C. Defining death in non-heart beating organ donors. *J Med Ethics* 2003; 29: 127–130.
120. Ethics Committeee, American College of Critical Care Medicine, Society of Critical Care Medicine. Recommendations for nonheartbeating organ donation. *Crit Care Med* 2001; 29: 1826–1831.
121. Van Norman GA. Another matter of life and death. *Anesthesiology* 2003; 98: 763–773.
122. Steen S, Liao Q, Wierup PN, Bolys R, Pierre L, Sjöberg T. Transplantation of lungs from non-heart-beating donors after functional assessment ex vivo. *Ann Thorac Surg* 2003; 76: 244–252.
123. Aitchison JD, Orr HE, Flecknell PA, Kirby JA, Dark JH. Functional assessment of non-heart-beating donor lungs: prediction of post-transplant function. *Eur J Cardiothorac Surg* 2001; 20: 187–194.
124. Rega F, Jannis N, Verleden G, Lerut T, Van Raemdonck D. Long-term preservation with interim evaluation of lungs from a non-heart-beating donor with a warm ischaemic interval of 90 minutes. *Ann Surg* 2003; 238: 782–793.
125. Rega F, Vandezande E, Jannis N, Verleden G, Lerut T, Van Raemdonck D. Role of leucocyte depletion in ex vivo evaluation of pulmonary grafts from non-heart-beating donors. *Perfusion* 2003; 18: Suppl 1, 13–21.
126. Kubo JI, Ohigashi Y, Hamabe M, *et al.* Pharmacokinetic evaluation of high pulmonary disposition of clarithromycin after systemic administration. *Xenobiotica* 2002; 32: 879–893.
127. Lumb PD. A comparison between 25% albumin and 6% hydroxyethyl starch solutions on lung water accumulation during and immediately after cardiopulmonary bypass. *Ann Surg* 1987; 206: 210–213.
128. Ware LB, Fang X, Wang Y, Sakuma T, Hall TS, Matthay MA. Selected contribution: mechanisms that may stimulate the resolution of alveolar edema in the transplanted lung. *J Appl Physiol* 2002; 93: 1869–1874.
129. Berthiaume Y, Folkesson HG, Matthay MA. Lung edema clearance: 20 years of progress: invited review: alveolar edema fluid clearance in the injured lung. *J Appl Physiol* 2002; 93: 2207–2213.
130. Featherstone RL, Kelly FJ, Chambers DJ. Theophylline improves functional recovery of isolated rat lungs after hypothermic preservation. *Ann Thorac Surg* 1999; 67: 798–803.
131. Schutte H, Witzenrath M, Mayer K, *et al.* The PDE inhibitor zaprinast enhances NO-mediated protection against vascular leakage in reperfused lungs. *Am J Physiol Lung Cell Mol Physiol* 2000; 279: L496–502.
132. Murakami S, Bacha EA, Herve P, *et al.* Prevention of reperfusion injury by inhaled nitric oxide in lungs harvested from non-heart-beating donors. Paris-Sud University Lung Transplantation Group. *Ann Thorac Surg* 1996; 62: 1632–1638.
133. Steen S, Kimblad PO, Sjöberg T, Lindberg L, Ingemansson R, Massa G. Safe lung preservation for twenty-four hours with Perfadex. *Ann Thorac Surg* 1994; 57: 450–457.
134. Neyrinck A, Rega F, Jannis N, *et al.* Ex vivo reperfusion of human lungs declined for transplantation: a novel approach to alleviate donor organ shortage? [Abstract 387]. *J. Heart Lung Transplant* 2004; 23: S172–S173.
135. Waddell TK, Peterson MD. Lung transplantation: Xenotransplantation. *Chest Surg Clin N Am* 2003; 13: 559–576.
136. Reemtsma K. Xenotransplantation-a brief history of clinical experiences, 1900–1965. *In*: Cooper DKC, Kemp E, Reemtsma K, *et al*, eds. Xenotransplantation. The transplantation of organs and tissues between species. Berlin, Springer Verlag, 1991; pp. 9–22.
137. Starzl TE, Fung J, Tzakis A, *et al.* Baboon-to-human liver transplantation. *Lancet* 1993; 341: 65–71.
138. Bailey LL, Nehlsen-Cannarella SL, Cencepcion W, Jolley WB. Baboon-to-human cardiac xenotransplantation in a neonate. *JAMA* 1985; 254: 3321–3329.

139. Cooper DK. Clinical xenotransplantation-how close are we? *Lancet* 2003; 362: 557–559.
140. Kemp E. Xenotransplantation. *J Intern Med* 1996; 239: 287–297.
141. Patience C, Takeuchi Y, Weiss RA. Infection of human cells by an endogenous retrovirus of pigs. *Nat Med* 1997; 3: 282–286.
142. Manzetti JD, Ankeny R, Miller D. Psychosocial and ethical issues in surgical approaches to end stage lung disease. *Clin Chest Med* 1997; 18: 383–390.
143. Tibell A, Groth CG. Ethics and public health issues in xenotransplantation. *Current Opinion in Organ Transplantation* 1999; 4: 101–105.
144. Cooper DK, Keogh AM, Brink J, *et al.* Report of the Xenotransplantation Advisory Committee of the International Society for Heart and Lung Transplantation: the present status of xenotransplantation and its potential role in the treatment of end-stage cardiac and pulmonary diseases. *J Heart Lung Transplant* 2000; 19: 1125–1165.
145. Zwischenberger JB, Alpard SK. Artifical lungs: a new inspiration. *Perfusion* 2002; 17: 253–268.
146. Jurmann MJ, Schaefers HJ, Demertzis S, Haverich A, Wahlers T, Borst HG. Emergency lung transplantation after extracorporeal membrane oxygenation. *ASAIO J* 1993; 39: M448–452.
147. Alpard SK, Zwischenberger JB. Extracorporeal membrane oxygenation for severe respiratory failure. *Chest Surg Clin N Am* 2002; 12: 355–378.
148. Jurmann MJ, Demertzis S, Schaefers HJ, Wahlers T, Haverich A. Intravascular oxygenation for advanced respiratory failure. *ASAIO J* 1992; 38: 120–124.
149. Zwischenberger JB, Anderson CM, Cook KE, Lick SD, Mockros LF, Bartlett LH. Development of an implantable artificial lung: challenges and progress. *ASAIO J* 2001; 47: 316–320.
150. Wang D, Lick S, Alpard SK, *et al.* Toward ambulatory arteriovenous $CO_2$ removal: initial studies and prototype development. *ASAIO J* 2003; 49: 564–567.
151. Haft JW, Griffith BP, Hirschl RB, Bartlett RH. Results of an artificial-lung survey to lung transplant program directors. *J Heart Lung Transplant* 2002; 21: 467–473.

*CHAPTER 7*

# Surgery for emphysema: surgical aspects

*T.C. Mineo*, E. Pompeo*, H.B. Ris[#], W. Weder[¶], P. Evrard[+], G. Massard[§], N. Konietzko[f]*

**Division of Thoracic Surgery, Policlinico Tor Vergata, Tor Vergata University, Rome, Italy, [#]Thoracic Surgery Section, CHUV, and [¶]Dept of Thoracic Surgery, University Hospital Zurich, Switzerland. [+]ICU Dept UCL Mont-Godinne University Hospital, Yvoir, Belgium. [§]Dept of Thoracic Surgery, University Hospital of Strasbourg, France. [f]Ruhrlandklinik, Dept of Pneumology, University Duisburg, Essen, Germany.*

*Correspondence: E. Pompeo, Division of Thoracic Surgery, Policlinico Tor Vergata, Tor Vergata University, V.le Oxford 81, 00133 Rome, Italy.*

Emphysema, a form of chronic obstructive pulmonary disease (COPD), is a social problem, which afflicts millions of people in developed countries and causes severe disability and early deaths in up to 45% of the patients [1].

The debilitating symptoms of emphysema and the frustrating results of the medical therapy led surgeons to apply creative solutions. A variety of surgical techniques have been proposed over the past century to improve symptoms and quality of life in patients with severe emphysema [2]. Unfortunately, since all these techniques were based on misconceptions of the underlying pathophysiology, they were inexorably abandoned due to unsatisfactory results.

So far, only three surgical procedures have evolved to survive the test of time and have proven capable of reducing the chronic hyperinflation of the lung caused by the destruction of alveoli, they are: bullectomy, lung volume reduction surgery (LVRS), and lung transplantation. Although similar in their finality, each of the surgical options is unique in its ideal selection criteria and expected outcome.

Bullectomy was first performed in the first half of the last century when external drainage of giant bullae was performed in order to achieve their collapse [3]. This approach has subsequently evolved to include resection of the bulla while sparing the underlying functional lung tissue [4].

Lung transplantation, first attempted by HARDY *et al.* [5] in 1963, after a prolonged period of incremental progress, became clinically feasible in the early 1980s as heart-lung transplantation [6] and isolated lung transplantation [7]. Indications were initially limited to pulmonary fibrosis and pulmonary hypertension, but emphysema was subsequently included [8] and now constitutes the most common diagnosis leading to transplantation.

LVRS, initially proposed by BRANTIGAN *et al.* [9] in 1959, was relaunched into the thoracic surgery scenario by COOPER *et al.* [10] in 1995, and is an effective, palliative surgical option designed to relieve distressing symptoms and improve quality of life in selected patients with advanced emphysema.

The incremental emphysematous destruction of lung tissue decreases the recruitable gas exchange area and leads to a loss of lung elastic recoil. The combined effect of reduced elastic recoil and intrinsic airway disease lead to airflow obstruction, hyperinflation of the lung, overdistention of the chest wall, flattened, disadvantaged diaphragms, and ventilation-perfusion mismatch. When the destruction occurs in a nonuniform manner, the most affected lung tissue can expand to crowd the relatively spared tissue to prevent ventilation of the normal lung.

The relative contributions of lung destruction, lung compression, and small airways

Eur Respir Mon, 2004, 29, 113–128. Printed in UK - all rights reserved. Copyright ERS Journals Ltd 2004; European Respiratory Monograph; ISSN 1025-448x. ISBN 1-904097-33-2.

obstruction to the overall physiological impairment of a given patient, will aid the surgeon in deciding the suitability of that patient for optimal surgical treatment of emphysema.

## Lung volume reduction surgery

LVRS has been shown to improve dyspnoea, respiratory function, exercise capacity and quality of life for up to 4–5 yrs in selected patients with severe emphysema [11–12]. Randomised studies comparing maximal medical therapy, including respiratory rehabilitation, *versus* LVRS have shown a survival advantage and greater improvements in quality of life in the surgical arm, particularly in patients with upper-lobe predominance of disease and low exercise capacity [13]. Conversely, in patients with diffusion capacity for carbon monoxide ($D_{L,CO}$) <20%, forced expiratory volume in one second ($FEV_1$) <20% and homogeneous emphysema, LVRS resulted in an unacceptably high 28% mortality rate.

The operation entails nonanatomical resection of the most diseased lung regions to reduce the overall lung volume by ~25–30% (figs. 1 and 2). It can be performed by different techniques and either in unilateral or bilateral fashion. Cooper *et al.* [10] first preferred to perform LVRS through median sternotomy in order to operate on both lungs during a single anaesthesia, as they considered that incision much less painful than a bilateral thoracotomy. This approach offers good exposure for emphysema located

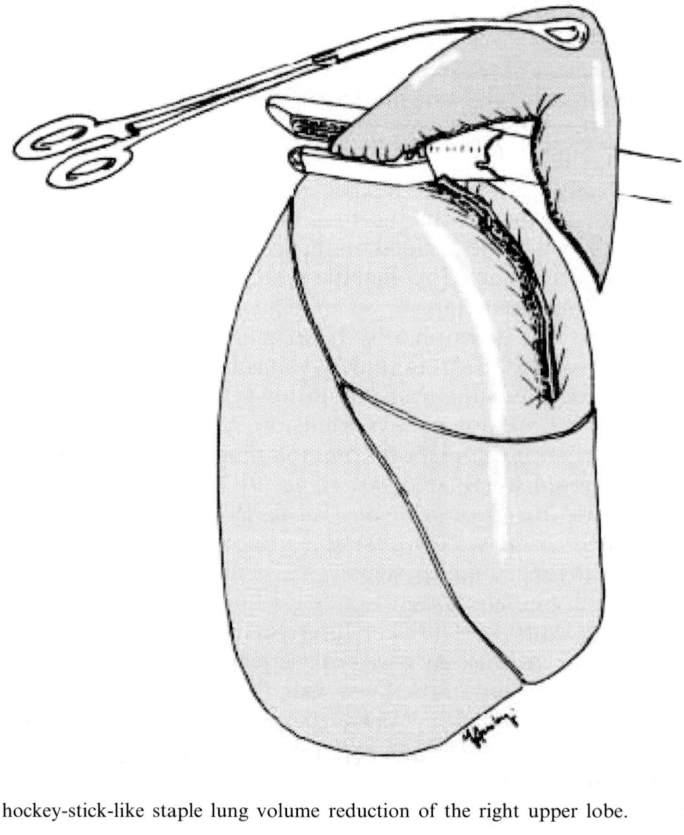

Fig. 1. – Typical hockey-stick-like staple lung volume reduction of the right upper lobe.

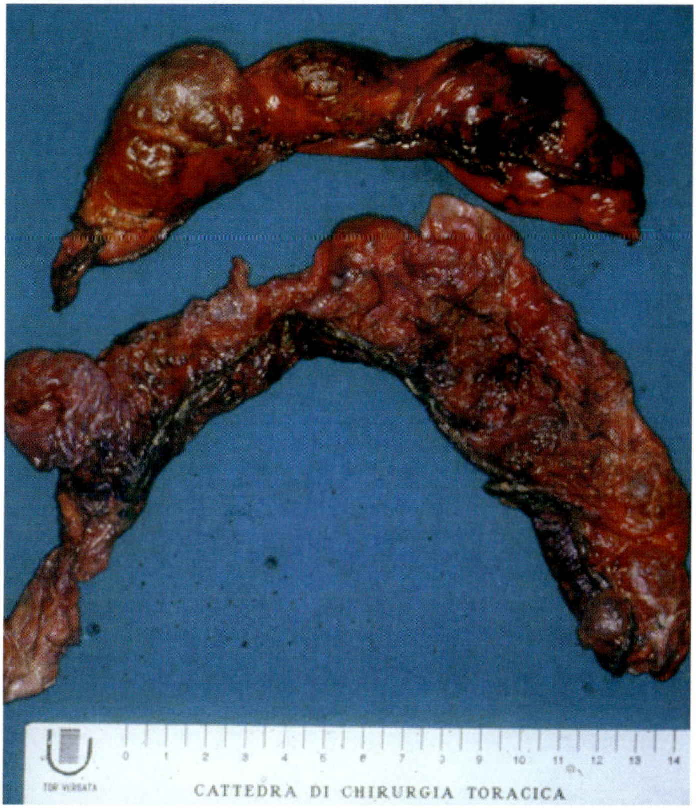


Fig. 2. – Specimens of one-stage bilateral lung volume reduction.

anteriorly and apically whereas posteriorly located areas of emphysema and adhesions are less accessible. Lower lobe resections are more difficult, especially on the left. The procedure can also be performed by video-assisted thoracoscopic surgery (VATS) in the full lateral decubitus position [14]. Through VATS, optimal exposure of all areas of the chest, including the lower lobes is achieved. In a nonrandomised trial comparing VATS with median sternotomy, less morbidity (6.7 *versus* 13.3%) and a trend towards lower mortality (2.5 *versus* 4.2%) was found with the VATS approach [7, 15]. Moreover, in a cost-effectiveness analysis comparing costs and outcome of LVRS performed by sternotomy or VATS, the total inpatient cost was less for patients operated on by VATS [16]. Nonetheless, postoperative improvements after bilateral staple LVRS appears to be comparable, whether the procedure is performed through VATS or median sternotomy. Satisfactory results have also been achieved through bilateral staged thoracotomy [17] or the clamshell incision [18]. VATS-LVRS is also feasible in the presence of pleural adhesions. Whatever the surgical approach, staple resection is now the technique of choice for LVRS although satisfactory results have been reported by the lung plication technique [19]. Conversely, there is no apparent role for current laser technology in the treatment of emphysema.

Operative mortality after LVRS ranges between 0–13.3%, while morbidity is mainly constituted by prolonged air leaks, which occur in 21–53% of patients (tables 1 and 2). Other less frequent complications include: pneumonia, bleeding, respiratory failure, arrhythmias, and gastrointestinal complications. Late complications after LVRS include:

**Table 1. – Operative results after unilateral stapled lung volume reduction surgery**

| First author [Ref.] | Surgical approach | Patients n | Mortality % | Prolonged air leaks % | Hospital stay | $FEV_1$ increase % |
|---|---|---|---|---|---|---|
| KELLER [20] | VATS | 25 | 0 | 32 | 8.8 | 31 |
| KEENAN [21] | VATS | 67 | 5.9 | 46 | 17 | 27 |
| ARGENZIANO [18] | Both | 28 | 3.6 | 46 | | 28 |
| MCKENNA [22] | VATS | 87 | 3.5 | 53 | 11.4 | 31 |
| KOTLOFF [15] | Both | 32 | 0 | | 14.2 | 24 |
| MINEO [23] | VATS | 14 | 0 | 36 | 8.0# | 50 |
| GEISER [24] | VATS | 28 | 0 | 21 | | 18 |

$FEV_1$: forced expiratory volume in one second; VATS: video-asssisted thoracoscopic surgery; Both: sternotomy and VATS; Hospital stay data is expressed as mean or #: median, range.

**Table 2. – Operative results after bilateral stapled lung volume reduction surgery**

| First author [Ref.] | Surgical approach | Patients n | Mortality % | Prolonged air leaks % | Hospital stay | $FEV_1$ increase % |
|---|---|---|---|---|---|---|
| COOPER [25] | Sternotomy | 150 | 4 | 46 | 13.5 | 51 |
| MILLER [26] | Sternotomy | 53 | 5.6 | 40 | 10–59 | 96 |
| BINGISSER (14] | VATS-OS | 20 | 0 | 35 | 15 | 42 |
| BRENNER [27] | VATS-OS | 145 | 4.2 | | 8.8 | 62 |
| WISSER [28] | VATS-OS | 15 | 13.3 | | 12.3 | 60 |
| KOTLOFF [15] | Sternotomy | 80 | 4.2 | | 22 | 40 |
| | VATS-OS | 40 | 2.5 | | 17.3 | 37 |
| MC KENNA [22] | VATS-OS | 79 | 2.5 | 47 | 10.0 | 57 |
| DE PERROT [17] | Thoracotomy-OS | 18 | 0 | 33 | 21 | 54 |
| POMPEO [29] | VATS-ST | 26 | 0 | 52 | 18.4 | 39 |
| | VATS-OS | 33 | 3.0 | 39 | 11.7 | 52 |
| CICCONE [12] | Sternotomy | 250 | 4.8 | 45.2 | 9# | 57 |

$FEV_1$: forced expiratory volume in one second; VATS: video-asssisted thoracoscopic surgery; OS: one-stage; ST: staged; Hospital stay data is expressed as mean, or #: median range.

respiratory failure, pulmonary hypertension [30], secondary pneumothorax; metalloptysis (*i.e.* asymptomatic expectoration of steel staples) [31], and development of giant bullous emphysema [32].

## Unilateral *versus* bilateral lung volume reduction surgery

So far, simultaneous bilateral stapling *via* median sternotomy or VATS is the preferred technique since it produces greater functional improvement than unilateral treatment [22]. The role of unilateral LVRS is controversial but is accepted in patients with markedly asymmetric emphysema or with contraindication to resection on one side, due to previous surgery, previous pleurodesis or radiological evidence of pleural thickening [33]. Conversely, a unilateral approach has the advantage to be less invasive and offers a smoother postoperative course than bilateral LVRS. In addition, unilateral LVRS offers the possibility to operate on the contralateral lung in case of the reappearance of disabling symptoms.

The average $FEV_1$ improves by 52% following a bilateral procedure and 30% after unilateral treatment (tables 1 and 2). However, the magnitude of improvements, following unilateral LVRS, usually exceeds that following bilateral LVRS by >50%. This suggests that unilateral LVRS might also affect the function of the nonoperated lung, possibly due to an interdependence between the hemithoraces [34]. The long-term outcome of unilateral LVRS has been poorly investigated. GEISER *et al.* [24] have found that after unilateral thoracoscopic LVRS, significant improvements of up to 24–36 months for residual volume (RV), dyspnoea index and 6-min walking test (6MWT) measurements while $FEV_1$ remained significantly improved only for 3 months.

In a multi-institutional comparative study, LOWDERMILK *et al.* [35] reported a significantly better improvement of $FEV_1$, forced vital capacity (FVC), RV, quality of life and dyspnoea relief after bilateral than after unilateral LVRS, whereas no difference was found between the procedures with respect to arterial oxygenation, 6MWT and oxygen utilisation.

Surgically oriented visual grading systems have been developed to help identify the best candidates for LVRS, either unilateral or bilateral [36, 37]. In addition, quantitative computed tomography (CT) analysis of emphysema and CT density masks have been used in an attempt to limit interobserver disagreement at visual grading classifications [38].

By applying a visual scoring classification, POMPEO *et al.* [37] reported that in patients with markedly asymmetric emphysema, acute improvement in $FEV_1$ after unilateral LVRS was similar to that achieved in patients undergoing bilateral operation due to heterogeneous but symmetric disease. In a more recent series BLOCH *et al.* [39] reported that at 6 months after bilateral thoracoscopic LVRS, median $FEV_1$ improvement in homogeneous, intermediately heterogeneous, and markedly heterogeneous emphysema was 37, 38 and 63%, respectively. They also noted that the decline in $FEV_1$ was significantly greater in the first postoperative year than in subsequent years and followed an exponential decay over time.

In a retrospective study, SERNA *et al.* [40] reported a 2-yr survival of 86 and 73% after bilateral or unilateral LVRS, respectively. In a recent multi-institutional study [41], 3-yr survival was 69% after unilateral and 74% after bilateral LVRS. BRENNER *et al.* [42] reported a 3-yr survival of 67% after bilateral thoracoscopic LVRS, whereas in a study from YUSEN *et al.* [43], 3–5-yr survival, after one-stage bilateral LVRS *via* median sternotomy, was 82 and 62%, respectively.

The possibility of performing "redo" unilateral procedures in patients who have already undergone a bilateral LVRS is a poorly investigated issue. So far, STAMMBERGER *et al.* [44] reported on one patient with $\alpha_1$-antitrypsin deficiency (AAD) emphysema who underwent redo LVRS with satisfactory results. In addition, POMPEO *et al.* [45] performed completion lobectomy in four patients with a destroyed residual upper lobe.

## The role of staged lung volume reduction surgery

The significant morbidity rates related to one-stage bilateral LVRS and the finding that the annual $FEV_1$ decline following one-stage bilateral LVRS can be steeper than after unilateral treatment [46], renewed the interest for a staged procedure.

Data regarding the outcome of staged LVRS is still scarce. KOTLOFF *et al.* [47] have found that in patients undergoing staged bilateral LVRS, the functional outcome was highly variable. They also found that the maximal improvement of $FEV_1$ was 0.14 L after the first and 0.13 L after the second operation. In 1998, HAZELRIGG *et al.* [48] analysed the results achieved by one-stage or staged bilateral LVRS. Similar complication rates and early functional results were found, although the combination of two hospitalisations for staged procedures was longer than that of one-stage procedures. Incremental improvements in $FEV_1$ were also comparable and almost identical, with those shown in the KOTLOFF *et al.* [47] series. HAZELRIGG *et al.* [48] concluded that staged LVRS do not offer any measurable advantage over a one-stage bilateral procedure.

However, the 3–4-month interval between the two operations, did not allow the advantages of a unilateral approach followed by a contra-lateral operation at the time of reappearance of disabling symptoms, to be explored. This, theoretically, might result in more durable benefit than a simultaneous bilateral treatment.

In a more recent series comparing staged *versus* one-stage LVRS [29], the completion of the bilateral treatment in the staged group was delayed until the clinical benefit of the first operation was lost. This study's results indicated that peak improvements were greater following one-stage bilateral LVR while 4-yr improvements in FEV1, RV and 6MWT were more stable in the staged LVRS group [29]. Yet, long-term survival was 70% in the staged group and 81% in the one-stage group, but the difference was not significant.

In conclusion, the available data indicate that LVRS is an effective surgical tool capable of improving dyspnoea, pulmonary function, exercise capacity and quality of life for up to 5 yrs, in selected patients with severe and heterogeneous nonbullous emphysema. Although one-stage bilateral LVRS remains the most widely applied procedure for patients with severe heterogeneous emphysema, unilateral and staged bilateral LVRS hold promise in offering prolonged benefit in properly selected patients.

## Lung volume reduction surgery *versus* lung transplantation

Lung transplantation and LVRS have both been demonstrated to improve dyspnoea, lung function, exercise capacity, and quality of life. However, selection according to precise criteria is of paramount importance for both procedures. In general, candidates who may be considered for lung transplantation or LVRS are severely disabled with respect to dyspnoea, lung function and exercise capacity. Selection criteria for LVRS and lung transplantation may thus overlap in many aspects.

A working group of transplant physicians and surgeons representing the main scientific societies have formulated guidelines for the selection of lung transplant candidates (table 3). These guidelines should assist physicians throughout the world, who treat patients with pulmonary disease, in identifying potential candidates for lung transplantation.

In the early 1990s, when LVRS was re-introduced by Cooper *et al.* [10], the selection of patient was performed according to criteria that were quite theoretical. Results from a few prospective randomised trials as well as many nonrandomised studies have led to a well accepted selection criteria for LVRS (table 4).

COPD and AAD account for the most common indications for single and bilateral lung transplantations [49]. The average 1-, 3- and 5-yr survival rates of the lung transplantation for COPD is 81.7, 61.9, and 43.4%, respectively as reported in the

**Table 3. – Guidelines for the selection of lung transplant candidates with chronic obstructive pulmonary disease**

| Inclusion criteria | Exclusion criteria |
|---|---|
| FEV1<25% of pred (without reversibility) | Dysfunction of major organs, particularly renal dysfunction, significant untreatable coronary artery disease or left ventricular dysfunction |
| And/or $P_{a,CO_2}$ $\geq$7.3 kPa (55 mmHg) and or elevated pulmonary artery pressures with progressive deterioration, such as cor pulmonale | Active malignancy within past 2–5 yrs |
| Preference should be given to those patients with elevated $P_{a,CO_2}$ with deterioration, who require long-term oxygen therapy | HIV, Hepatitis B antigen positivity, Hepatitis C with histological progressive evidence of liver disease |
| | Psychosocial problems unable to be resolved |

FEV1: forced expiratory volume in one second; $P_{a,CO_2}$: carbon dioxide arterial tension.

**Table 4. – Selection guidelines for lung volume reduction surgery**

| Inclusion criteria | Exclusion criteria |
|---|---|
| Dyspnoea at rest or at minimal physical activity with severe obstructive ventilatory defect ($FEV_1$ <35% predicted) | "Vanishing lung" on CT scan |
| Functional aspects of lung emphysema, *i.e.* irreversible hyperinflation (RV >200% pred; TLC >125% pred) | $FEV_1$ <20% pred, $D_{L,CO}$ <20% pred, hypercapnia with $P_{a,CO_2}$ >7.3 kPa, pulmonary hypertension with mean PAP>35 mmHg or systolic PAP>55 mmHg |
| Heterogeneous emphysema with predominance of upper lobes and low exercise capacity | Coronary artery disease |
| | Recurrent broncho-pulmonary infections, bronchiectasis, chronic sputum production |

$FEV_1$: forced expiratory volume in one second; CT: computed tomography; RV: residual volume; TLC: total lung capacity volume; $D_{L,CO}$: diffusion capacity for carbon monoxide; $P_{a,CO_2}$: carbon dioxide arterial tension; PAP: pulmonary artery pressure; 1mmHg=0.1 kPa.

Registry of the International Society for Heart and Lung Transplantation (ISHLT) [49]. However, several centres report better results with a survival of 88–90% at 1 yr, 75–80% at 3 yrs, and >60% at 5 yrs. In general, older patients have a worse outcome than younger ones. It is therefore recommended that lung transplantations should not be performed above the age of 60–65 yrs. For older patients with advanced emphysema the only surgical option remains LVRS. For younger patients who fulfill the criteria for both treatments, LVRS should be offered first in order to postpone a lung transplantation and avoid the negative side-effects of chronic immunosuppression. This is particularly the case for patients presenting with a heterogeneous emphysema, prevailing in the upper lobes. However, it has been shown that patients with homogeneous emphysema may also profit from LVRS, provided they present a marked hyperinflation, an $FEV_1$ >20% and a $D_{L,CO}$ >20% predicted [36]. The results from the National Emphysema Treatment Trial Research Group (NETT) trial [50] have shown that patients with $FEV_1$ <20% and $D_{L,CO}$ <20% pred have a high risk of perioperative mortality and should be preferably considered for lung transplantation. Patients aged 55–60 yrs are often difficult to manage with respect to LVRS or lung transplantations since symptoms after LVRS may re-appear just at the moment when they reach an age limit for a lung transplantation. All patients with advanced emphysema and a $D_{L,CO}$ <20% pred or vanished lung on the CT scan, should be directed towards a lung transplantation and not to LVRS. In addition, most often, these patients present signs of pulmonary hypertension at the time of evaluation (table 5).

Several groups have demonstrated that LVRS is able to postpone the need for lung transplantation by ~3–4 yrs in selected patients. Furthermore, it has been shown that lung transplantations can be performed safely after LVRS with no additional adverse

**Table 5. – Conditions or facts favoring either lung volume reduction surgery (LVRS) or lung transplantation**

| LVRS | Lung transplantation |
|---|---|
| Age >60–65 yrs | Age <60–65 yrs |
| $FEV_1$ >20–25% predicted | $FEV_1$ <20% pred |
| Heterogeneous emphysema with obvious target areas for resection | Homogenous, diffuse emphysema, vanished lung |
| Marked hyperinflation | $D_{L,CO}$ <20% pred, hypercapnia ($P_{a,CO_2}$>7 kPa) |
| No pulmonary hypertension | Pulmonary hypertension |
| | Pleural scarring, bronchiectasis, recurrent infections |

$FEV_1$: forced expiratory volume in one second; $D_{L,CO}$: diffusion capacity for carbon monoxide; $P_{a,CO_2}$: carbon dioxide arterial tension.

effects in the post-transplant course. However, it has been reported that a relevant number of patients undergoing lung transplantation required blood transfusions due to adhesions, which developed after LVRS [51]. This was particularly true in patients who underwent LVRS with buttressed stapling devices, which also may cause problems in dissecting the lung from the phrenic nerve during lung transplantation. However, the long-term survival was the same when compared with a matched cohort of lung-transplant patients who had not undergone previous LVRS [51].

## Single *versus* double-lung transplantation for emphysema

Lung transplantation has become a widely accepted treatment option for end-stage lung disease. Emphysema, arising from COPD and AAD, account for ~45% of lung transplantations performed worldwide.

The transplantation procedures for emphysema consisted initially of heart-lung transplantation and double-lung transplantation (DLT) [52]. DLT was thought to be necessary to prevent severe ventilation/perfusion mismatch or mediastinal shift compression, which are theoretically linked to single-lung transplantation (SLT). In 1989, MAL *et al.* [8] reported the first clinical series of SLT for emphysema with promising results which were confirmed by other reports. This led to an enthusiasm for SLT as the procedure of choice for emphysema [53].

The bilateral-sequential-lung transplantation procedure (BLT) was developed and excellent results were obtained for emphysema [54]. Since then, whether BLT or SLT represents the optimal procedure for patients with end stage emphysema has been a matter for discussion. This is not simply a medical debate, since ethical and donor organ issues are also considered.

The leading indications for lung transplantations performed between 1995 and 2001 (The Registry of the ISHLT report 2002; n=8,781) were: COPD: 39.4%; idiopathic pulmonary fibrosis (IPF): 16.9%; cystic fibrosis (CF): 16.1%; AAD: 9.3%; and primary pulmonary hypertension: 4.6%. The majority of SLT (n=4,663) were performed for: COPD: 54.4%; IPF: 23.8%: or AAD: 8.7%. Most of the BLTs (n = 4,118) were performed for CF: 33.0%; COPD: 22.5%; or AAD: 9.9% [49].

In some centres, BLT has been performed more often for AAD than for COPD. Perhaps the distribution has been influenced by the younger age of the recipients with AAD or by concerns about SLT for severe emphysema [55, 56]. AAD recipients, despite a younger age, do not achieve significantly superior survival results than those with COPD [55].

The mean age of BLT recipients for AAD and COPD (48 and 54 yrs, respectively) was lower than for SLT recipients in this respect (53 and 57 yrs, respectively). Patients receiving BLT had a longer waiting list time (536±278 days) than patients receiving SLT (382±250 days, $p<0.001$) [55].

The current waiting list algorithm used in the USA is based solely on the waiting time of each listed patient, rather than on the severity of the disease.

Emphysema patients have a 77% diminished risk of dying whilst waiting for a lung transplantation as compared with patients with other diagnoses [57]. The increased longevity of patients with emphysema favours them in terms of obtaining a transplant. Including BLT for patients with emphysema will, therefore, increase the waiting time and mortality rate of recipients who desperately need a BLT such as CF patients.

SLT is simpler, requires a shorter operative time than BLT and may potentially extend the availability of donor organs. In fact, SLT in the early 1990s had a lower perioperative complication rate than BLT [53], which is no longer observed except in recipients >60 yrs of age [58]. SLT offers distinct advantages in older or high-risk candidates for lung transplantation, suffering from emphysema, for patients with a previous thoracic procedure, or for patients with a significant asymmetry in the distribution of the emphysema. If there is no significant disparity between the two native lungs, the choice of the grafted side does not significantly alter the post-transplant lung function [53, 59].

Even if BLT has a longer ischaemic time ($\geq$100 min) [58, 59] and does more frequently require cardiopulmonary bypass [59], many teams have chosen the bilateral operation to prevent hyperinflation of the native lung or ventilation-perfusion mismatch between the native lung and the graft. While such situations still arise, they may be managed with success by double lumen mechanical ventilation, lung volume reduction or even pneumonectomy of the native lung. However, it is usually resolved when the underlying cause has been adequately treated [60].

BLT also provides a greater latitude for donor-recipient size matching than SLT or permits utilisation of marginal lung donor in emphysema recipients [59].

Due to an institutional preference of BLT for emphysema patients, the proportions of BLT may be oversized in some institutions. However, mechanical ventilation duration, intensive care unit or hospital stay and early survival (30 or 90 days) are comparable between SLT and BLT for emphysema [49, 55].

Nevertheless, BLT seems preferable for younger patients with extensive bullae in both lungs, or for patients with chronic sputum production or a bronchiectatic component to their emphysema.

The FVC, FEV1, 6MWT, arterial oxygen tension ($P_{a,O_2}$) and carbon dioxide tension ($P_{a,CO_2}$) showed a benefit up to 5 yrs post-transplant for BLT as compared with SLT, for both AAD and COPD. However, both SLT and BLT showed a statistically significant improvement in all functional measurements when comparing the preoperative measures with those at 1-yr post-transplantation [55, 57, 59]. The improvement in FEV1 and $P_{a,O_2}$ values were reported to be significantly better after BLT than after SLT from 3 months up to 3 yrs after transplantation, respectively [59]. The improvement in exercise tolerance was also better after BLT from 6 months to 3 yrs post-transplantation. However, there was no difference between BLT and SLT with respect to $P_{a,CO_2}$ values [59]. The mean maximal oxygen consumption ($V'_{O_2max}$) after transplantation did not differ between BLT and SLT [56].

Overall hospital mortality after lung transplantation for emphysema has been reported as low as 6.2% [55] with no difference between COPD and AAD recipients. There was no difference in hospital mortality between BLT and SLT.

The current 1-, 3- and 5-yr survival rates after lung transplantation for emphysema are 72, 56 and 43, respectively, as reported by the ISHLT registry [49]. After SLT they were 71, 54 and 40%, respectively; and after BLT, 72, 58 and 48% respectively [49]. Survival seems to be better after BLT than SLT for emphysema recipients, and the survival curves continue to diverge throughout the 7-yr period of follow-up [49, 55, 58].

A subanalysis of data of COPD recipients from USA centres, demonstrate a similar early and long-term survival rate after SLT in patients >60 yrs of age.

The leading cause of mortality behind the first year following transplantation is the development of bronchiolitis obliterans (BOS) with an incidence of 30–50% [49, 55, 61].

BLT has been reported to be associated with a reduced risk for BOS development as compared with SLT.

Post-transplant malignancy occurs in ~9% of lung transplant recipients without differing between COPD and AAD [49, 55]. Lymphoid proliferative disease is the most common malignancy among 1-yr survivors, and skin tumours are the most common neoplasms in 5-yr survivors [49]. Bronchogenic carcinoma develops in the native lung of transplant recipients after SLT for emphysema and IPF with frequencies of 2 and 4%, respectively [62]. This rate is similar to that observed in high-risk patients (*e.g.*, elderly smokers with emphysema or other chronic lung diseases).

In summary, taking into consideration the current shortage of donor lungs, it seems reasonable to recommend: 1) to continue to perform BLT in those patients with an absolute indication for this procedure; 2) to propose BLT also in younger patients with extensive bullae in both lungs and in patients with chronic sputum production; and 3) to suggest SLT in elderly patients with emphysema.

## Surgery for bullous emphysema

A bulla is defined as an enlarged airspace of >1 cm in diameter associated to a variable degree of pulmonary emphysema [63]. The outer surface of a bulla is usually formed by visceral pleura, whereas the inner layer is usually formed of fibrous tissue. The inside of a bulla is crisscrossed by trabeculae of fibrotic interlobular and alveolar septa.

Compression of underlying lung tissue, and the lack of transmission of the respiration mechanics on the lung tissue, as well as ventilation-perfusion mismatch, may explain the impairment of pulmonary function in the presence of a giant bulla.

Bullectomy may be considered in the presence of a large bulla occupying >30–50% of one hemithorax (fig. 3), a decreased $FEV_1$ and radiological signs of compression of nonbullous lung parenchyma [64, 65].

Other less frequent indications for bullectomy include complications arising from bullous disease such as bleeding, infection and malignant degeneration of the bulla [64].

The operation technique is variable. A unilateral lesion may be excised by use of a stapling device through a thoracotomy or VATS. Numerous bullae or bullae that merge indistinctly with the adjacent lung tissue will require a staple wedge resection resembling a typical lung volume reduction. The goal of the operation should be to relieve compression of the underlying lung while preserving the functional lung tissue. A lobectomy is rarely required except if the lobe is destroyed and the fissures are complete. In these cases lobectomy may represent an attractive option and might reduce the risk of postoperative air leaks [65].

Unilateral bullectomy may be performed through lateral thoracotomy or VATS while bilateral bullectomy, by staged thoracotomy, VATS or median sternotomy [66].

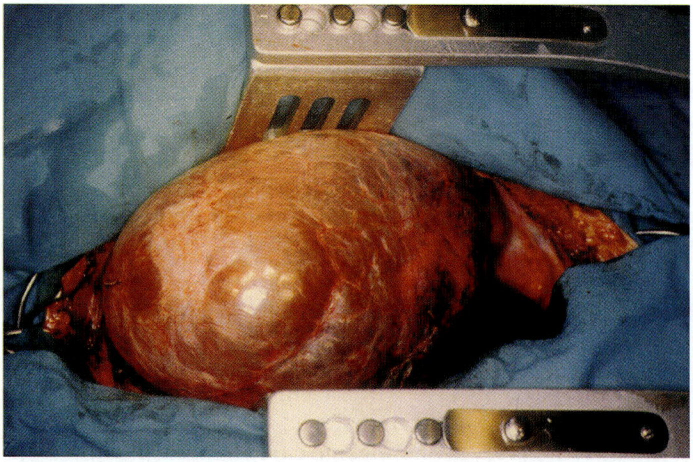

Fig. 3. – Operative view of giant bullous emphysema.

Intracavitary drainage by the Monaldi technique has also been reported to be successful in these situations [67].

Operative mortality in properly selected patients has been low [68]. Prolonged air leaks constitute the most common postoperative complication. Buttressing the staple line or resecting in healthy tissue can help decrease this complication.

As a rule, the functional results of bullectomy depends upon the quality of the underlying lung. Resection of giant bullae occupying at least one third of the hemithorax with relatively well preserved and compressed underlying lung tissue have been followed by the greatest functional improvements [68, 69]. The development of new bullae up to 5 yrs after the operation is a rare event [70].

## Management of prolonged air leaks

Air leaks can occur after pulmonary resection and its incidence and seriousness can vary depending on both the type of resection performed and the characteristics of the underlying lung tissue [71]. Air leaks lasting >7 days are defined as prolonged and may increase costs due to prolonged hospitalisation and the risk for further complications. Due to the fragility of emphysematous lungs, patients undergoing LVRS have a high risk for the development of air leaks, which occur in 21–53% of these patients (table 1 and 2).

Numerous techniques have been described to prevent air leaks, such as pleural tenting [10], staple line buttress with bovine pericardium or use of synthetic material [72], biological glues [73], cyanoacrylate glue [74] and polyethylene glycol-based gel [75]. Air leaks within the fissure have been successfully managed by bovine pericardium patching combined with use of fibrin and cyanoacrylate glues [74]. A randomised two-centre study [76] with 123 patients undergoing unilateral VATS-LVRS showed a decrease in the duration of postoperative air leaks, chest tube drainage time and hospital stay in patients with bovine pericardial strips on the suture lines than those without buttress. The incidence of overall hospital charges was identical, since the costs of the strips offset the saving in hospitalisation length. In a more recent randomised three-centre study, STAMMBERGER *et al.* [77] reported that buttressing the staple line significantly shortened the duration of air leaks and drainage time although the hospital stay did not differ significantly between patients with and without staple lines buttress.

The issue of biocompatibility needs to be carefully considered if a prosthetic material is employed. Currently, little is known regarding host reaction after lung resection procedures. In experimental settings, the intrathoracic use of bovine pericardium was associated with calcification, extensive inflammatory reactions, and formation of fibrosis [78]. In patients undergoing lung transplantation after LVRS, many surgeons have observed that adhesions are more dense if bovine pericardium was previously used [79]. Therefore, bovine pericardium should be used selectively in younger patients who may be transplant candidates in the future.

CERFOLIO *et al.* [80] compared in a randomised trial suction *versus* water seal postoperative drainage and reported that water seal was superior to active suction with respect of prolonged air leaks. However, water seal was not as effective as suction in the case of major expiratory leaks and the development of pneumothorax. To facilitate early discharge of patients with controlled air leaks, the application of a Heimlich valve connected to the chest drainage has been advocated [81].

## Conclusions

Over recent years, surgical management of pulmonary emphysema has evolved. So far, three surgical options namely LVRS, lung transplantation and bullectomy used alone or in the context of more complex surgical strategies are available and can offer a realistic hope of long-lasting improvements to an increasing number of patients. Continuing refinements in patients selection criteria for current surgical options and the development of new, less and less invasive techniques, might increase in the near future the number of patients who will benefit from surgery for emphysema.


## Summary

Surgical treatment of emphysema was designed to improve subjective dyspnoea, respiratory function and quality of life in severely disabled patients. Three surgical options are currently employed, namely bullectomy, lung volume reduction surgery (LVRS) and lung transplantation.

Bullectomy is indicated in presence of giant bullae occupying more than one half of the hemithorax with compression of relatively healthy lung tissue.

LVRS entails nonanatomical resections of severely diseased emphysematous areas of the lungs and is performed in severely disabled patients with hyperinflation, heterogeneous distribution of destruction prevailing in the upper lobes, a forced expiratory volume in one second ($FEV_1$) >20% predicted and a normal carbon dioxide arterial tension. LVRS, can be performed by open or thoracoscopic approaches, in unilateral or bilateral fashion and have been shown to offer prolonged functional benefit with acceptable mortality.

Patients with lower $FEV_1$, hypercapnia, and associated pulmonary hypertension are candidates for lung transplantation. Emphysema, especially in the context of $\alpha_1$-antitrypsin deficiency, is currently one of the most common indications for lung transplantation, accounting for ~45% of cases worldwide. Single-lung transplantation is simpler and shorter than the bilateral transplantation, and there is less frequent need for cardiopulmonary bypass. Yet, it could potentially extend the availability of donor organs. These advantages have to be weighed against bilateral sequential lung transplantation procedure characteristics, which include an improved pulmonary function and the ability to use marginal lung donors as compared with single-lung transplantation.

In conclusion, in properly selected patients, bullectomy, LVRS and lung transplantation can offer prolonged functional benefit and satisfactory long-term survival. Nonetheless, since they are invasive options with a risk of both mortality and morbidity, they are directed only at patients who remain symptomatic despite optimal medical treatment.


**Keywords:** Air leak, bullectomy, emphysema, lung transplantation surgical treatment, lung volume reduction surgery.

## References


1. Anthonisen NR. Prognosis in chronic obstructive pulmonary disease: results from multicenter clinical trials. *Am Rev Resp Dis* 1989; 140: 595–599.
2. Knudson RJ, Gaensler EA. Surgery for emphysema. *Ann Thorac Surg* 1965; 1: 332–362.
3. Head JR, Avery EA. Intracavitary suction (Monaldi) in the treatment of emphysematous bullae and blebs. *J Thorac Cardiovasc Surg* 1948; 18: 761–776.

4. Benfield JR, Cree FM, Pellett JR, *et al.* Current approach to the surgical management of emphysema. *Arch Surg* 1966; 93: 59–70.
5. Hardy JD, Webb WR, Dalton ML, *et al.* Lung homotransplantations in men. *JAMA* 1963; 186: 1065–1074.
6. Retz B, Wallwark J, Hunt S, *et al.* Hearth-lung transplantation: successful therapy for patients with pulmonary vascular diseases. *N Engl J Med* 1982; 306: 557–564.
7. Toronto Lung Transplantation Group. Unilateral lung transplantation for pulmonary fibrosis. *N Engl J Med* 1986; 314: 1140–1145.
8. Mal H, Andreassian B, Pamela F, *et al.* Unilateral lung transplantation in end-stage pulmonary emphysema. *Am Rev Resp Dis* 1989; 140: 797–802.
9. Brantigan OC, Mueller E, Kress MB. A surgical approach to pulmonary emphysema. *Am Rev Respir Dis* 1959; 80: 194–202.
10. Cooper JD, Trulock EP, Triantafillou AN, *et al.* Bilateral pneumectomy (volume reduction) for chronic obstructive pulmonary disease. *J Thorac Cardiovasc Surg* 1995; 109: 106–119.
11. Gelb AF, McKenna RJ Jr, Brenner M, Epstein JD, Zamel N. Lung function 5 yr after lung volume reduction surgery for emphysema. *Am J Respir Crit Care Med* 2001; 163: 1562–1566.
12. Ciccone AM, Meyers BF, Guthrie TJ, *et al.* Long-term outcome of bilateral lung volume reduction in 250 consecutive patients with emphysema. *J Thorac Cardiovasc Surg* 2003; 125: 513–525.
13. National Emphysema Treatment Trial Research Group. A Randomized trial comparing lung-volume-reduction surgery with medical therapy for severe emphysema. *N Engl J Med* 2003; 248: 2059–2073.
14. Bingisser R, Zollinger A, Hauser M, Bloch KE, Russi EW, Weder W. Bilateral volume reduction surgery for diffuse emphysema by video-assisted thoracoscopy. *J Thorac Cardiovasc Surg* 1996; 112: 875–882.
15. Kotloff RM, Tino G, Bavaria JE, *et al.* Bilateral lung volume reduction surgery for advanced emphysema: a comparison of median sternotomy and thoracoscopic approaches. *Chest* 1996; 110: 1399–1406.
16. Ko CY, Waters PF. Lung volume reduction surgery: a cost and outcomes comparison of sternotomy versus thoracoscopy. *Am Surg* 1998; 64: 1010–1013.
17. De Perrot M, Licker M, Spiliopoulos A. Muscle-sparing anterior thoracotomy for one-stage bilateral lung volume reduction surgery. *Ann Thorac Surg* 1998; 66: 582–584.
18. Argenziano M, Thomashow B, Jellen PA, *et al.* Functional comparison of unilateral versus bilateral lung volume reduction surgery. *Ann Thorac Surg* 1997; 64: 321–327.
19. Iwasaki M, Nishiumi N, Kaga K, Kanazawa M, Kuwahira I, Inoue H. Application of the fold application method for unilateral lung volume reduction in pulmonary emphysema. *Ann Thorac Surg* 1999; 67: 815–817.
20. Keller CA, Ruppel G, Hibbett A, Osterloh J, Naunheim KS. Thoracoscopic lung volume reduction surgery reduces dyspnea and improve exercise capacity in patients with emphysema. *Am J Respir Crit Care Med* 1997; 156: 60–67.
21. Keenan RJ, Landreneau RJ, Sciurba FC, *et al.* Unilateral surgical approach for diffuse emphysema. *J Thorac Cardiovasc Surg* 1996; 111: 308–316.
22. Mc Kenna, Brenner M, Fischel RJ, Gelb AF. Should lung volume reduction for emphysema be unilateral or bilateral? *J Thorac Cardiovasc Surg* 1996; 112: 1331–1339.
23. Mineo TC, Pompeo E, Simonetti G, *et al.* Unilateral reduction pneumoplasty for asymmetric emphysema. *Eur J Cardiothorac Surg* 1998; 14: 33–39.
24. Geiser T, Schwizer B, Krueger T, *et al.* Outcome after unilateral lung volume reduction surgery in patients with severe emphysema. *Eur J Cardiothorac Surg* 2001; 20: 674–678.
25. Cooper JD, Patterson GA, Sundaresan RS, *et al.* Results of 150 consecutive bilateral lung volume reduction procedures in patients with severe emphysema. *J Thorac Cardiovasc Surg* 1996; 112: 1319–1330.
26. Miller JI Jr, Lee RB, Mansour KA. Lung volume reduction surgery: lessons learned. *Ann Thorac Surg* 1996; 61: 1464–1469.

27. Brenner M, McKenna RJ, Gelb AF, *et al.* Dyspnea response following bilateral thoracoscopic staple lung volume reduction surgery. *Chest* 1997; 112: 916–923.
28. Wisser W, Tschernko E, Senbaklavaci Ö, *et al.* Functional improvement after volume reduction: sternotomy versus videoendoscopic approach. *Ann Thorac Surg* 1997; 63: 822–828.
29. Pompeo E, Mineo TC. Long-term results of staged versus one-stage bilateral thoracoscopic reduction pneumoplasty. *Eur Cardiothorac Surg* 2002; 21: 627–633.
30. Weg IL, Rossoff L, McKeon K, Graver LM, Scharf SM. Development of pulmonary hypertension after lung volume reduction surgery. *Am J Respir Crit Care Med* 1999; 159: 552–556.
31. Oey I, Waller D. Metalloptysis: a late complication of lung volume reduction surgery. *Ann Thorac Surg* 2001; 71: 1694–1695.
32. Iqbal M, Rossof L, McKeon K, Graver M, Scharf SM. Development of giant bulla after lung volume reduction surgery. *Chest* 1999; 116: 1809–1811.
33. McKenna RJ Jr, Gelb A, Brenner M. Lung volume reduction surgery for chronic obstructive pulmonary disease: Where do we stand? *World J Surg* 2001; 25: 231–237.
34. Becker MD, Berkmen YM, Austin JHM, *et al.* Lung volumes before and after lung volume reduction surgery. *Am J Respir Crit Care Med* 1998; 157: 1593–1599.
35. Lowdermilk GA, Keenan RJ, Landreneau RJ, *et al.* Comparison of clinical results for unilateral and bilateral thoracoscopic lung volume reduction. *Ann Thorac Surg* 2000; 69: 1670–1674.
36. Weder W, Thurnheer R, Stammberger U, Burge M, Russi EW, Bloch KE. Radiologic emphysema morphology is associated with outcome after surgical lung volume reduction. *Ann Thorac Surg* 1997; 64: 313–320.
37. Pompeo E, Sergiacomi GL, Nofroni I, Roscetti W, Simonetti G, Mineo TC. Morphologic grading of emphysema is useful in the selection of candidates for unilateral and bilateral reduction pneumoplasty. *Eur J Cardiothorac Surg* 2000; 17: 680–686.
38. Wisser W, Klepetko W, Kontrus M, *et al.* Morphologic grading of the emphysematous lung and its relation to improvement after lung volume reduction surgery. *Ann Thorac Surg* 1998; 65: 793–799.
39. Bloch KE, Georgescu CL, Russi EW, Weder W. Gain and subsequent loss of function after lung volume reduction surgery in cases of severe emphysema with different morphologic patterns. *J Thorac Cardiovasc Surg* 2002; 123: 845–854.
40. Serna DL, Brenner M, Osann KE, *et al.* Survival after unilateral versus bilateral lung volume reduction surgery for emphysema. *J Thorac cardiovasc Surg* 1999; 118: 1101–1109.
41. Naunheim KS, Kaiser LR, Bavaria JE, *et al.* Long-term survival after thoracoscopic lung volume reduction: a multinstitutional review. *Ann Thorac Surg* 1999; 68: 2026–2032.
42. Brenner M, McKenna RJ, Chen JC, *et al.* Survival following bilateral staple lung volume reduction surgery for emphysema. *Chest* 1999; 115: 390–396.
43. Yusen RD, Pohl MS, Biggar DC, Davis GE, Lefrak SS, Cooper JD. Outcomes through 5 yrs after lung volume reduction surgery. *Chest* 1999; 116: 376s.
44. Stammberger U, Thurnheer R, Schmid RA, Russi EW, Weder W. Redo lung volume reduction surgery in a patient with $\alpha_1$-antitrypsin deficiency. *Ann Thorac Surg* 2000; 69: 632–633.
45. Pompeo E, Mineo D, Bollero P, *et al.* Completion lobectomy after bilateral lung volume reduction for emphysema. Salvage option or fancy? *J Thorac Cardiovasc Surg* 2004; 127: 1212–1214.
46. Brenner M, McKenna RJJ, Gelb AF, Fischel RJ, Wilson AF. Rate of FEV1 change following lung volume reduction surgery. *Chest* 1998; 113: 652–659.
47. Kotloff RM, Tino G, Palevsky HI, *et al.* Comparison of short-term functional outcomes following unilateral and bilateral lung volume reduction surgery. *Chest* 1998; 113: 890–895.
48. Hazelrigg SR, Boley TM, Magee MJ, Lawyer CH, Henkle JQ. Comparison of staged thoracoscopy and median sternotomy for lung volume reduction. *Ann Thorac Surg* 1998; 66: 1134–1139.
49. Hertz MI, Taylor DO, Trulock EP, *et al.* The Registry of the International Society for Heart and Lung Transplantation: Nineteenth Official Report – 2002. *J Heart Lung Transplant* 2002; 21: 950–970.

50. National Emphysema Treatment Trial Research Group. Patients at high risk of death after lung-volume-reduction surgery. *N Engl J Med* 2001; 345: 1075–1083.
51. Burns KEA, Keenan RJ, Grgurich WF, Manzetti JD, Zenati M. Outcomes of lung volume reduction surgery followed by lung transplantation: a matched cohort study. *Ann Thorac Surg* 2002; 73: 1587–1593.
52. Patterson GA. Lung transplantation for chronic obstructive pulmonary disease. *Clin Chest Med* 1990; 11: 547–554.
53. Low DE, Trulock EP, Kaiser LR, *et al.* Morbidity, mortality, and early results of single versus bilateral lung transplantation for emphysema. *J Thorac Cardiovasc Surg* 1992; 103: 1119–1126.
54. Pasque MK, Cooper JD, Kaiser LR, *et al.* Improved technique for bilateral lung transplantation: rationale and initial clinical experience. *Ann Thorac Surg* 1990; 49: 785–791.
55. Cassivi SD, Meyers BF, Battafarano RJ, *et al.* Thirteen-year experience in lung transplantation for emphysema. *Ann Thorac Surg* 2002; 74: 1663–1670.
56. Bavaria JE, Kotloff R, Palevsky H, *et al.* Bilateral versus single lung transplantation for chronic obstructive pulmonary disease. *J Thorac Cardiovasc Surg* 1997; 113: 520–528.
57. De Meester J, Smits JM, Persijn GG, *et al.* Lung transplant waiting list: differential outcome of type of end-stage lung disease, one year after registration. *J Heart Lung Transplant* 1999; 18: 563–571.
58. Meyer DM, Bennett LE, Novick RJ, *et al.* Single vs bilateral, sequential lung transplantation for end-stage emphysema: influence of recipient age on survival and secondary end-points. *J Heart Lung Transplant* 2001; 20: 935–941.
59. Sundaresan RS, Shiraishi Y, Trulock EP, *et al.* Cardiac and pulmonary replacement. Single or bilateral lung transplantation for emphysema? *J Thorac Cardiovasc Surg* 1996; 112: 1485–1495.
60. Weill D, Torres F, Hodges TN, *et al.* Acute native lung hyperinflation is not associated with poor outcomes after single lung transplant for emphysema. *J Heart Lung Transplant* 1999; 18: 1080–1087.
61. Hadjiliadis D, Davis RD, Palmer SM. Is transplant operation important in determining posttransplant risk of bronchiolitis obliterans syndrome in lung transplant recipients? *Chest* 2002; 122: 1168–1175.
62. Collins J, Kazerooni EA, McAdams HP, *et al.* Bronchogenic carcinoma after lung transplantation: frequency, clinical characteristics, and imaging findings. *Radiology* 2002; 224: 131–138.
63. Ciba Guest Symposium Report: terminology, definitions and classifications of chronic pulmonary emphysema and related conditions. *Thorax* 1959; 14: 286.
64. Mehran RJ, Deslauriers J. Indications for surgery and patient work-up for bullectomy. *Chest Surg Clin North Am* 1995; 5: 717–733.
65. Meyers BF, Patterson GA. Chronic obstructive pulmonary disease · 10: Bullectomy, lung volume reduction surgery, and transplantation for patients with chronic obstructive pulmonary disease. *Thorax* 2003; 58: 614–638.
66. Lima O, Ramos L, Di Biasi P, Judice L, Cooper JD. Median sternotomy for bilateral resection of emphysematous bullae. *J Thorac Cardiovasc Surg* 1981; 82: 892–897.
67. Venn GE, Williams PR, Goldstraw P. Intracavitary drainage for bullous, emphysematous lung disease: experience with the Brompton technique. *Thorax* 1988; 43: 998–1002.
68. Connolly JE, Wilson A. The current status of surgery for bullous emphysema. *J Thorac Cardiovasc Surg* 1989; 97: 351–361.
69. Petro W, Hübner Ch, Greschuchna D, Maaßen W, Konietzko N. Bullectomy. *Thorac Cardiovasc Surg* 1983; 31: 342–345.
70. Nickoladze GD. Functional results of surgery for bullous emphysema. *Chest* 1992; 101: 119–122.
71. Cerfolio RJ, Tummala RP, Holman WL, *et al.* A prospective algorithm for the management of air leaks after pulmonary resection. *Ann Thorac Surg* 1998; 66: 1726–1731.
72. Fischel RJ, McKenna RJ Jr. Bovine pericardium versus bovine collagen to buttress staples for lung reduction operations. *Ann Thorac Surg* 1998; 65: 217–219.

73. Thistlethwaite PA, Luketich JD, Ferson PF, Keenan RJ, Jamieson SW. Ablation of persistent air leaks after thoracic procedures with fibrin sealant. *Ann Thorac Surg* 1999; 67: 575–577.
74. Horsley WS, Miller JI. Management of the uncontrollable pulmonary air leak with cyanoacrylate glue. *Ann Thorac Surg* 1997; 63: 1492–1493.
75. Wain JC, Kaiser LR, Johnstone DW, *et al.* Trial of a novel synthetic sealant in preventing air leaks after lung resection. *Ann Thorac Surg* 2001; 71: 1623–1629.
76. Hazelrigg SR, Boley TM, Naunheim KS, *et al.* Effect of bovine pericardial strips on air leak after stapled pulmonary resection. *Ann Thorac Surg* 1997; 63: 1573–1575.
77. Stammberger U, Klepetko W, Stamatis G, *et al.* Butressing the staple line in lung volume reduction surgery: a randomised three-center study. *Ann Thorac Surg* 2000; 70: 1820–1825.
78. Dahm M, Lyman WD, Schwell AB, Factor SM, Frater RW. Immunogenicity of glutaraldehyde-tanned bovine pericardium. *J Thorac Cardiovasc Surg* 1990; 99: 1082–1090.
79. Klepetko W. Surgical aspects and techniques of lung volume reduction surgery for severe emphysema. *Eur Respir J* 1999; 13: 919–925.
80. Cerfolio RJ, Bass C, Katholi CR. Prospective randomised trial compares suction versus water seal for air leaks. *Ann Thorac Surg* 2001; 71: 1613–1617.
81. McKenna RJ, Fischel RJ, Brenner M, Gelb AF. Use of Heimlich valve to shorten hospital stay after lung reduction surgery for emphysema. *Ann Thorac Surg* 1996; 61: 1115–1117.

*CHAPTER 8*

# Surgery for emphysema: medical aspects

*E.W. Russi*, W. De Wever[#], M. Decramer[¶]*

**Pulmonary Division, University Hospital Zurich, Switzerland. [#]Dept of Radiology, and [¶]Respiratory Rehabilitation and Respiratory Division, University Hospital, Catholic University, Leuven, Belgium.*

*Correspondence: E.W. Russi, Pulmonary Division, University Hospital Zurich, Raemistr. 100, CH-8091, Zürich, Switzerland.*

Emphysema with its particular functional consequences, *i.e.* pulmonary hyperinflation and decreased diffusion capacity is usually a major feature in patients suffering from severe chronic obstructive pulmonary disease (COPD). It can be reliably diagnosed and assessed in its severity by computed tomography (CT). Besides smoking cessation and inhalative antiobstructive pharmacotherapy, pulmonary rehabilitation plays a pivotal role in the treatment of these patients, particularly in those who eventually undergo lung volume reduction surgery (LVRS).

Emphysema is defined pathologically as a condition of the lung characterised by abnormal, permanent enlargement of the air spaces distal to the terminal bronchiole, accompanied by destruction of their walls, and without obvious fibrosis [1]. According to the National Heart, Lung, and Blood Institute's committee [2] this air space enlargement corresponds with "an increase in air space size as compared with the air space of normal lungs". This definition is based on lung structure changes, rather than on symptoms or on physiological evidence expressed in impaired ventilation and has been responsible for some controversy in the literature [3]. Being also based on morphological changes, the radiological definition of emphysema has also contributed to this controversy. In addition the radiological diagnosis is often "on/off": a patient has radiological signs of emphysema or not, regardless the presence or absence of symptoms or pulmonary function deterioration. However, as morphological emphysema recognises various grades of disease, the radiological diagnosis should also be quantified. This can be done by evaluating the number of radiological signs that are present when the severity of emphysema increases and by trying to estimate the extent and its distribution [2].

## Radiological diagnosis of emphysema

Conventional chest radiographs and CTs are the most commonly used imaging techniques in the evaluation of lung emphysema.

The roentgenographical signs of emphysema on conventional chest radiographs can be divided in two groups: those related to hyperinflation and those related to the lung destruction and resultant changes in the vascular shadow patterns (table 1). The signs indicating hyperinflation are more objective and more reproducible than the signs that suggest lung destruction. In general, the sensitivity of conventional chest radiographs in detecting emphysema is almost 68% [4].

CT is superior to chest radiography and makes a detailed study of the presence, extent, and severity of emphysema possible because it allows direct visualisation of the lung destruction [5]. Many CT techniques have been used to evaluate lung emphysema: high

Eur Respir Mon, 2004, 29, 129–138. Printed in UK - all rights reserved. Copyright ERS Journals Ltd 2004; European Respiratory Monograph; ISSN 1025-448x. ISBN 1-904097-33-2.

**Table 1. – Roentgenographic signs of emphysema on conventional chest radiography**

| Signs of pulmonary emphysema in the posteroanterior roentgenogram | Signs of pulmonary emphysema in the lateral roentgenogram |
|---|---|
| Depression and flattening of the diaphragm with blunting of costophrenic angles. The actual level of the diaphragm is not as significant as the contour. | Abnormal retrosternal space showing increased radiolucency. |
| Irregular radiolucency of the lung and irregular decrease of vascular markings resulting from irregularity in distribution of the emphysematous tissue destruction. | Flattening or even concavity of diaphragmatic contour. |

resolution computed tomography (HRCT) with 1–2 mm slice thickness at suspended full inspiration and suspended full expiration; spiral CT with 2, 5, 8, 10 mm slice thickness or a combination of spiral and HRCT. CT images can be presented conventionally with a defined window setting, but also as density-masked images [6], where the pixels in a defined interval of Hounsfield Units (HU) representing emphysema are highlighted white [6] or where the pixels are shown in colour depending on their density. Sliding thin slab, minimum intensity projection images with variable slab thickness (*e.g.* 3, 5 and 8 mm) have also been used for evaluating pulmonary emphysema [7].

In general the CT diagnosis of emphysema on CT scans is based on the presence of lung areas with low attenuation and on the visualisation of vascular disruption. A detailed study of these signs allows recognition of the different types of emphysema. In centrilobular emphysema, the abnormalities are usually more severe in the upper parts of the lung and include irregular small round or confluent areas of low attenuation interspersed with normal lung. The localised areas of low attenuation are located near the centre of the secondary pulmonary lobule. Panacinar emphysema involves mainly the lower lung zones and is characterised on CT cans by diffuse areas of low attenuation with little intervening lung. In severe panacinar emphysema, the simplification of lung parenchyma leads to diffuse areas of low attenuation with a paucity of vascular markings that allow distinction between panacinar emphysema and normal lung parenchyma. However, mild or moderately severe panacinar emphysema is often impossible to distinguish from adjacent normal parenchyma on CT scans. Distal acinar or paraseptal emphysema is characterised by areas of low attenuation in the subpleural lung regions and adjacent to vessels and interlobular septa. Because centrilobular and distal acinar emphysema produce localised areas of low attenuation, they are easier to recognise on CT scans than panacinar emphysema [5].

HR CT using the thinnest available collimation, a high spatial-resolution or "sharp" algorithm, the shortest scan time possible, the largest available matrix size, and at least one consistent lung window setting [7] has proven to be the most sensitive CT method for detecting emphysema [8]. Inspiratory HRCT scans are better in the evaluation of pulmonary emphysema than expiratory HRCT scans, as the latter tend to underestimate the degree of emphysema. In several studies it was shown that radiologists subjectively preferred HRCT images to spiral CT images in the evaluation of emphysema. When compared with high spatial-resolution reconstruction images, standard reconstruction images also tend to underestimate the degree of emphysema. However, some studies suggest that spiral CT images are better to study more advanced emphysema and emphysema located in the basal parts of the lung [9]. Vascular pruning, a sign of panacinar emphysema, predominantly located in the basal part of the lungs, is indeed better appreciated in thick slices than in thin slices; while high image detail is necessary to depict small areas of extreme low attenuation seen in early centrilobular emphysema.

Using existing software programs density-mask images can be produced from HRCT or spiral CT images. Each pixel has its own density which is expressed in HU. GEVENOIS *et al.* [10] found that the presence of emphysema correlate with attenuation values lower than -950 HU on inspiratory scans. By highlighting pixels with a density lower than -950 HU a density-masked image showing the regions of emphysema can be produced. In their study CEDERLUND *et al.* [6] showed that visual estimation of emphysema using these density-masked images was better than when emphysema was graded on regular CT images. Pixel density can also be coloured and a coloured-mapped image can be generated. In this way, areas of low attenuation can be demonstrated and the diagnosis of emphysema can be suggested with more certainty.

Sliding thin slab, minimum intensity projection images are images generated from an existing set of contiguous transverse CT scans with a linear interpolation algorithm and a standard reconstruction kernel. The thickness of these slabs can be chosen. Comparing these sliding thin slabs, minimum intensity projection images with thin-section CT scans, detection of emphysema, especially of the smallest lesions, is easier. The superiority of the sliding thin slab, minimum intensity projection technique is directly related to the suppression of hyperattenuating structures such as vessels and fissures, which enables easier depiction of areas of hypo-attenuation against the uniform background of the normal lung. [7].

CT can be used for a quantitative assessment of emphysema. The severity can be evaluated either by a visual grading of the areas of abnormally low attenuation or by an objective quantification based on the measurements of attenuation values [9]. Multiple scoring systems have been used to grade the severity and extent of emphysema. This visual assessment of pulmonary emphysema can be facilitated using density-masked or colour-mapped images. Systemic overestimation and moderate interobserver agreement may compromise subjective visual grading of emphysema. Therefore, objective methods must be preferred to achieve precise, reader-independent quantification of emphysema. Objective quantification of emphysema can be carried out by computer-assisted methods [11]. CT densitometry is a method where measurements are performed with a Pulmo CT software program and where the severity of emphysema can be defined as an emphysema index. This software automatically recognises the lungs, traces lung contours, determines histograms of attenuation values and calculates the lung area occupied by pixels with a predetermined range or attenuation values for a single slice and for the total number of scans. This method can be done for one lung or both lungs [11]. The range of attenuation values indicating emphysema differs in the literature but is mostly between -910 or -950 and -1,024 HU [5, 11]. Measurement of attenuation on CT has, however, several limitations. Scanner types, scan calibration, used kilo voltage and reconstruction algorithms, volume averaging, patient's size and the location of the assessed area are responsible for variation in results.

## Selection of patients with emphysema for surgical lung volume reduction

Several prospective case series [12–14] and, more recently, a few randomised, controlled prospective trials [15–19] have demonstrated that LVRS improves dyspnoea, lung function, exercise tolerance and quality of life in patients suffering from severe forms of emphysema [20]. The amount of improvement is variable and may depend on a variety of factors, including aetiology and morphological type of emphysema, preoperative lung function, and amount of resected emphysematous lung tissue.

The selection of patients for LVRS is based on sound pathophysiological concepts influenced by retrospective analyses of correlations between various preoperative patient characteristics and functional outcome as well as contra-indications, which are known to increase perioperative complication rate and mortality. It is not astonishing that LVRS has a high perioperative complication rate if performed in patients where lung function particularly gas exchange, is extremely impaired due to an almost entirely destroyed lung, *i.e.* in those with so called "vanishing" lung. This has been unambiguously demonstrated by an interims analysis of the National Emphysema Treatment Trial (NETT) [21]. For 69 patients who had a forced expiratory volume in one second ($FEV_1$) that was $\leq$20% of their predicted value, and either a homogeneous distribution of emphysema on CT scan or a carbon monoxide diffusing capacity that was $\leq$20% of their predicted value, the 30-day mortality rate after surgery was 16% (95% CI: 8.2–26.7%), as compared with a rate of 0% among 70 medically treated patients ($p<0.001$). The perioperative mortality is considerably lower (<5%) in centres with experience in selecting and operating suitable patients [22]. In the study by Cooper *et al.* [23] of 150 patients the 30-day mortality was 2%.

Admittedly, many questions concerning LVRS remain unanswered and are difficult to study due to inherent methodological problems that are typical for the scientific investigation of surgical interventions. A fundamental and yet unresolved issue is the lack of accurate information on the amount of tissue removed by the surgeon. This precludes studies, compulsory in pharmacological trials, on the dose effect relationship of LVRS. For theoretical reasons the reduction in hyperinflation is the key issue of LVRS. With respect to the role of emphysema morphology, *i.e.* heterogeneous *versus* homogeneous types of emphysema, as a predictor of outcome, that surgeons will be more courageous to resect larger pieces of severely destroyed lung parts if other areas are better preserved than in cases with evenly affected lungs *i.e.* in homogeneous types of emphysema is considered. Such questions could only be solved by randomised studies, if quantitatively standardised interventions are performed in patients, where not only preoperative lung function but also the quantity and quality of emphysema are characterised in a reproducible and objective manner, *i.e.* by CT-morphometry.

Pivotal in the surgical concept of LVRS are distinctive functional consequences of pulmonary emphysema, *i.e.* the loss of the lung's elasticity accompanied by a reduction in airway calibre and the pulmonary hyperinflation with concomitant impairment of respiratory muscle function. LVRS aims to improve ventilation by restoring the pulmonary elastic recoil and by reducing the size of the hyperinflated lung. Fessler and Permutt [24] emphasised the importance of the decrease in vital capacity resulting of hyperinflation as one of the major mechanisms for impairment in respiratory mechanics and symptoms in severe COPD. Their theoretical model predicts that LVRS improves flow limitation primarily by improving the match between size of the lungs and the rib cage. This is achieved by decreasing residual volume (RV) more than total lung capacity (TLC) and thus achieving a gain in vital capacity. Based on certain theoretical assumptions, Fessler and Permutt [24] anticipated that the effect of LVRS on the direction and magnitude of the change in vital capacity is dominated by RV/TLC. A maximal gain in vital capacity and $FEV_1$ after surgery would be expected in LVRS candidates with the highest RV/TLC ratio. In their view, the measurement of elastic recoil pressure determines neither the best candidates nor the mechanisms of their improvement after LVRS. Supporting these predictions, a major increase in vital capacity after LVRS has been reported by several groups and the gain in $FEV_1$ after LVRS is correlated with the degree of reduction in the RV/TLC ratio [14, 25–30].

The notion that LVRS would be particularly beneficial in patients with heterogeneous distribution of emphysematous destruction, *i.e.* with large bullae and areas that are relatively well preserved, is based on earlier experience with bullectomy [29–31]. Several groups have stressed that patients with distinct regional differences in tissue destruction *i.e*, with markedly heterogeneous emphysema on CT, perfusion scintigram, or both, profit most from LVRS because nonfunctional areas identified by means of imaging techniques are the ideal targets for resection. In previous analyses the present authors corroborated this concept, but more important, they were able to demonstrate that even patients with a uniform pattern of emphysematous destruction (*i.e.* a homogenous type) had significant and clinically relevant improvement after the operation [13]. Therefore, a homogeneous type of emphysema is not a contra-indication for LVRS as long as $FEV_1$ and diffusion capacity are not <20% of their predicted values and if on CT scan, aspects of vanishing lung are absent.

Numerous attempts have been made to find the most reliable radiological method, e.g. visual CT scoring [32–37], semiquantitative CT assessment [28] or CT morphometry [38], to predict functional outcome after LVRS. Since the way patients are assessed differs from group to group, comparability of the results between the centres is limited. For this and other reasons, the question of the most appropriate radiological examination or eventually a combination of examinations, remains open to debate.

## Pre- and postoperative rehabilitation

The benefits of pulmonary rehabilitation programmes were well demonstrated during the last decade [39–46]. Several randomised, controlled trials were conducted. Table 2 provides an overview of the effects obtained in the most significant trials. As can be seen, all trials but one demonstrated an improvement in health related quality of life. The negative trial used the Quality of Well Being Questionnaire (QoWB) [40]. This is a generic instrument that is clearly less sensitive than the disease specific instruments, Chronic Respiratory Disease Questionnaire (CRQ), or St Georges Respiratory Questionnaire (SGRQ), used in the other trials. This effect exceeded the minimal clinically important difference in most trials. Similarly a clear increase in 6-min walking distance or the shuttle walking distance was observed. This increase came close to or exceeded the minimal clinically important difference (table 1). In one trial effects were only obtained in the moderately dyspneic patients and not in the severely dyspnoeic patients [42]. In this study, however, the severely dyspnoeic patients followed a home exercise programme with less supervision than the moderately dyspnoeic patients who exercised in the hospital. This may relate to the smaller effects observed in the latter patients as well.

Besides these improvements in health related quality of life and functional exercise

**Table 2. – Effects of rehabilitation on quality of life and timed walking distance in several large studies**

| First author [Ref.] | Patients n | Duration of programme | QoL | 6-MWD |
|---|---|---|---|---|
| RIES [40] | 119 | 8 weeks | QoWB N.S. | Treadmill endurance +9 min |
| GOLDSTEIN [39] | 89 | 6 months | CRQ=1.04 | 0.74 |
| GRIFFITHS [43] | 200 | 6 weeks | CRQ=0.77<br>SGRQ=1.88 | 0.73# |
| WEDZICHA [42] | Mod. 66 | 8 weeks | Mod<br>CRQ=0.89<br>SGRQ=1.35 | 2.17#<br><br>-0.08# |
| | Sev. 60 | | Sev<br>CRQ=0.02<br>SGRQ=0.23 | |
| TROOSTERS [44, 46] | 100 | 6 months | CRQ=1.4 | 0.96 |

Table shows selected randomised controlled trials on pulmonary rehabilitation, the number of patients, programme duration, and effects on quality of life (QoL) and 6-min walk distance (6-MWD) or shuttle walk are shown (#); Effects are expressed in minimal clinically important difference units; QoWB: Quality of Well Being Questionnaire; CRQ: Chronic Respiratory Disease Questionnaire; SGRQ; St Georges Respiratory Questionnaire; #: Mod: moderately dyspnoeic; Sev: severely dyspnoeic; Reproduced with permission from [47].

capacity, a clear reduction in the utilisation of health care resources was demonstrated. GRIFFITHS *et al.* [43] demonstrated a reduction in the number of hospitalisations (1.9 *versus* 1.4) and the number of days spent in hospital (18.1 *versus* 9.4) in the year following a rehabilitation programme lasting 6 weeks. Interestingly, the number of visits to the pulmonologist decreased, whereas the number of visits to the general practitioner increased. This signals that COPD patients use healthcare resources better after a rehabilitation programme, than before. TROOSTERS *et al.* [44] also found a reduction in the number of hospital days after a rehabilitation programme.

At present, there is no clear demonstration of improved survival after a pulmonary rehabilitation programme. There are three indications that survival might improve after pulmonary rehabilitation. First, RIES *et al.* [40] found greater survival after a rehabilitation programme during 6 yrs follow-up, but the difference did not reach statistical significance. The power, however, of the study to detect a difference in survival was too low. Secondly GRIFFITHS *et al.* [43] found a similar tendency, but the number of patients was too low to reach statistical significance. Thirdly, TROOSTERS *et al.* [46] found a significantly greater survival in patients who were admitted to a training programme after hospitalisation for an acute exacerbation of COPD [46]. These three indications, however, are insufficient to fully demonstrate improved survival after pulmonary rehabilitation. Moreover, it will be difficult to design a large scale trial examining this in the future, as randomisation in a control group would no longer be ethically acceptable now that the benefits of pulmonary rehabilitation are clearly demonstrated [47].

Finally, it was unequivocally demonstrated that the benefits achieved after pulmonary rehabilitation are relatively inexpensive, particularly when the reduction in healthcare resources caused by rehabilitation is taken into account. Indeed, GRIFFITHS *et al.* [48] demonstrated that the cost of the programme outweighed the reduction in healthcare resources, it brought about such that the incremental cost of adding rehabilitation to standard care was negative.

Although it remains difficult to select candidates for rehabilitation on a scientific basis, it is clearly established now that COPD patients with severe airflow obstruction and $FEV_1<30\%$ predicted are good candidates for pulmonary rehabilitation [49–51]. The training effects in these patients are not smaller, but if anything larger, than in patients with less severe airflow obstruction. As a consequence, patients who are candidates for LVRS or transplantation are good candidates for rehabilitation as well. In several departments it is the policy not to admit patients into surgical programmes unless they have followed a rehabilitation programme before. This was also done in several randomised trials published recently [52, 53]. The study by CRINER *et al.* [53] showed that the improvement in health status caused by LVRS is additive to the improvement brought about by rehabilitation. In a recent Canadian study, home rehabilitation was administered in preparation of LVRS, with excellent results [54]. It seems likely that preoperative rehabilitation is useful in the selection of candidates for these procedures, since invalidating complaints of dyspnoea are usually part of the indication for these procedures. These complaints improve substantially with pulmonary rehabilitation. However, at present it is not clear whether preoperative rehabilitation affects the course of the intervention or the results. No randomised controlled study comparing the results of LVRS or transplantation with or without preoperative rehabilitation has ever been performed.

This is also true for postoperative rehabilitation. After these interventions the ventilatory capacity of patients is, without question, improved. There are virtually no data on postoperative rehabilitation after LVRS. More is known on exercise capacity after lung transplantation. Indeed, exercise capacity increases after lung transplantation, but even 1–2 yr after transplantation it often does not exceed 50% of predicted. It is a well known observation that although ventilatory capacity improves, clearly more with double-lung transplantation than with single-lung transplantation, the improvement in exercise capacity is the same after these interventions [55]. The limitation after transplantation remains largely circulatory. This is usually attributed to the muscle alterations that are known to be present after transplantation [56, 57]. Indeed, intramuscular pH is lower in post-transplant patients and it decreases faster than normal with exercise [56]. The proportion of type I fibres and the content in oxidative enzymes are reduced [57]. The mitochondrial function is impaired and more so than expected on the basis of the reduction in the proportion of type I fibres. The mechanism of these changes is unknown. It may be related to disuse, deconditioning, hypertension, heart failure, corticosteroids [58], azathioprine or cyclosporine A. The latter drug is known to affect mitochondrial oxidation in muscle in rats [59, 60]. Rehabilitation may improve this deconditioning and muscle weakness. However, the effects of a structured postoperative rehabilitation programme have never been studied in a critical way [61]. Nevertheless in most departments it is customary to apply a rehabilitation programme after these procedures.

## Summary

Emphysema is usually a major feature in severe Chronic obstructive pulmonary disease. Besides lung function abnormalities, especially pulmonary hyperinflation and decreased diffusion capacity, the imaging patterns on conventional chest radiography and computed tomography are also used to estimate its extent and distribution. The selection of patients for lung volume reduction surgery (LVRS) is based on sound pathophysiological concepts. LVRS is particularly beneficial in heterogeneous distribution of emphysematous destruction. However, many questions concerning LVRS remain unanswered. The benefits of pulmonary rehabilitation programmes have been stressed during the last decade, especially on health related, quality of life and functional exercise capacity, rather than on survival.

**Keywords:** Chronic obstructive pulmonary disease, computed tomography scan, emphysema, high resolution computed tomography, lung function, rehabilitation.

## References

1. Malinen A, Erkinjuntti-Pekkanen R, Partanen K, Rytkönen H, Vanninen R. Reproducibility of scoring emphysema by HRCT. Comparison of visual interpretation methods with pulmonary function tests among farmer's lung patients. *Acta Radiologica* 2002; 43: 54–59.
2. Snider G, Kleinerman JL, Thurlbeck WM, Bengali ZH. The definition of emphysema: report of a National Heart, Lung, and Blood Institute, Division of Lung Disease Workshop. *Am Rev Respir Dis* 1985; 141: 182–183.
3. Philip C, Pratt MD. Role of Conventional Chest Radiography in Diagnosis and Exclusion of Emphysema. *Am J Med* 1987; 82: 998–1006.
4. Sanders C, Nath Ph, Bailey WC. Detection of emphysema with computed tomography. Correlation with pulmonary function tests and chest radiography. *Invest Radiol* 1988; 23: 2626.
5. Thurlbeck WM, Muller NL. Emphysema: Definition, Imaging, and Quantification. *WAJR* 1994; 163: 1017–1025.
6. Cederlund K, Bergstrand L, Högberg S, Rasmussen E, Svane B, Aspelin P. Visual grading of

emphysema severity in candidates for lung volume reduction surgery: comparison between HRCT, spiral CT and "density-masked" images. *Acta Radiologica* 2002; 43: 48–53.
7. Remy-Jardin M, Remy J, Gosselin B, Copin MC, Wurtz A, Duhamel A. Sliding thin slab, minimum intensity projection technique in the diagnosis of emphysema: histopathologic-CT correlation. *Radiology* 1996; 200: 665–671.
8. Klein JS, Gamsu G, Webb WR, Golden JA, Muller NL. High-resolution CT diagnosis of emphysema in symptomatic patients with normal chest radiographs and isolated low diffusing capacity. *Radiology* 1992; 182: 817–821.
9. Cederlund K, Bergstrand L, Högberg S, Rasmussen E, Svane B. Thin-section CT vs spiral CT in candidates for lung volume reduction surgery: a comparison based on radiologists' subjective preferences. *Eur Radiol.* 2001; 11: 402–408.
10. Gevenois PA, De Vuyst P, de Maertelaer V, *et al.* Comparison of computed density and microscopic morphometry in pulmonary emphysema. *Am J Respir Crit Car Med* 1996; 154: 187–192.
11. Bankier AA, De Maertelaer V, Keyzer C, Gevenois PA. Pulmonary emphysema: subjective visual grading versus objective quantification with macroscopic morphometry and thin-section CT densitometry. *Radiology* 1999; 211: 851–858.
12. Cooper JD, Patterson GA, Sundaresan RS, *et al.* Results of 150 consecutive bilateral lung volume reduction procedures in patients with severe emphysema. *J Thorac Cardiovasc Surg* 1996; 112: 1319–1330.
13. Bingisser R, Zollinger A, Hauser M, Bloch KE, Russi EW, Weder W. Bilateral volume reduction surgery for diffuse pulmonary emphysema by video-assisted thoracoscopy. *J Thorac Cardiovasc Surg* 1996; 112: 875–882.
14. Brenner M, McKenna RJJ, Gelb AF, Fischel RJ, Wilson AF. Rate of FEV1 change following lung volume reduction surgery. *Chest* 1998; 113: 652–659.
15. Geddes D, Davies M, Koyama H, *et al.* Effect of lung-volume-reduction surgery in patients with severe emphysema. *N Engl J Med* 2000; 343: 239–245.
16. Pompeo E, Marino M, Nofroni I, Matteucci G, Mineo TC. Reduction pneumoplasty versus respiratory rehabilitation in severe emphysema: a randomized study. Pulmonary Emphysema Research Group. *Ann Thorac Surg* 2000; 70: 948–953.
17. Criner GJ, Cordova FC, Furukawa S, *et al.* Prospective Randomized Trial Comparing Bilateral Lung Volume Reduction Surgery to Pulmonary Rehabilitation in Severe Chronic Obstructive Pulmonary Disease. *Am J Respir Crit Care Med* 1999; 160: 2018–2027.
18. Lödfahl CG, Hillerdal G, Ström K. Preliminary results up to 12 months. *Am J Respir Crit Care Med* 2000; 161: A585.
19. Wilkens H, Demertzis S, Konig J, Leitnaker CK, Schafers HJ, Sybrecht GW. Lung volume reduction surgery versus conservative treatment in severe emphysema. *Eur Respir J* 2000; 16: 1043–1049.
20. Hamacher J, Buchi S, Georgescu CL, *et al.* Improved quality of life after lung volume reduction surgery. *Eur Respir J* 2002; 19: 54–60.
21. National Emphysema Treatment Trial Research Group. Patients at high risk of death after lung-volume-reduction surgery. *N Engl J Med* 2001; 345: 1075–1083.
22. Young J, Fry SA, Hyde C. Lung volume reduction surgery (LVRS) for chronic obstructive pulmonary disease (COPD) with underlying severe emphysema. *Thorax* 1999; 54: 779–789.
23. Tutic M, Bloch K, Weder W, Russi EW. Long term results after bilateral lung volume reduction surgery. *Am J Respir Crit Care Med* 2002; 165: A196.
24. Fessler HE, Permutt S. Lung volume reduction surgery and airflow limitation. *Am J Respir Crit Care Med* 1998; 157: 715–722.
25. Brenner M, McKenna RJ Jr, Gelb AF, *et al.* Objective predictors of response for staple versus laser emphysematous lung reduction. *Am J Respir Crit Care Med* 1997; 155: 1295–1301.
26. Hunsaker AR, Ingenito EP, Reilly JJ, Costello P. Lung volume reduction surgery for emphysema: correlation of CT and V/Q imaging with physiologic mechanisms of improve-ment in lung function. *Radiology* 2002; 222: 491–498.

27. Cederlund K, Berstrand L, Högber S, *et al.* Visual classification of emphysema heterogeneity compared with objective measurements: HRCT vs. spiral CT in candidates for lung volume reduction surgery. *Eur Radiol* 2002; 12: 1045–1051.
28. Cederlund K, Tylen U, Jorfeldt L, Aspelin P. Classification of emphysema in candidates for lung volume reduction surgery. A new objective and surgically oriented model for describing CT severity and heterogeneity. *Chest* 2002; 122: 590–596.
29. Pierce JA, Growdon JH. Physical properties of the lungs in giant cysts: report of a case treated surgically. *N Engl J Med* 1962; 267: 169–173.
30. Gelb AF, Gold WM, Nadel JA. Mechanisms limiting airflow in bullous lung diesase. *Am J Respir Dis* 1973; 107: 571–578.
31. Rogers RM, DuBois AB, Blakemore WS. Effect of removal of bullae on airway conductance and conductance volume rations. *J Clin Invest* 1968; 47: 2569–2579.
32. Slone RM, Pilgram TK, Gierada DS, *et al.* Lung volume recution surgery: comparison of preoperative radiologic features and clinical outcome. *Radiology* 1997; 204: 685–693.
33. Weder W, Thurnheer R, Stammberger U, Burge M, Russi EW, Bloch KE. Radiologic emphysema morphology is associated with outcome after surgical lung volume reduction. *Ann Thorac Surg* 1997; 64: 313–319.
34. Wisser W, Klepetko W, Kontrus M, *et al.* Morphologic grading of the emphysematous lung and its relation to improvement after lung volume reduction surgery. *Ann Thorac Surg* 1998; 65: 793–799.
35. Gierada DS, Yusen RD, Villanueva FS, *et al.* Patient selection for lung volume reduction surgery: an objective model based on prior clinical decisions and quantitative CT analysis. *Chest* 2000; 117: 991–998.
36. Weder W, Thurnheer R, Stammberger U, Burge M, Russi EW, Bloch KE. Radiologic emphysema morphology is associated with outcome after surgical lung volume reduction. *Ann Thorac Surg* 1997; 64: 313–319.
37. Thurnherr R, Engel H, Weder W, *et al.* The role of lung perfusion scintigraphy in relation to chest CT and pulmonary function in the evaluation of candidates for lung volume reduction surgery. *Am J Respir Crit Care Med* 1999; 159: 301–310.
38. Rogers RM, Coxson HO, Sciurba FC, Keenan RJ, Whittall KP, Hogg JC. Preoperative severity of emphysema predictive of improvement after lung volume reduction surgery. Use of CT morphometry. *Chest* 2000; 118: 1240–1247.
39. Goldstein RS, Gort EH, Stubbing D, *et al.* Randomized controlled trial of respiratory rehabilitation. *Lancet* 1994; 344: 1394–1397.
40. Ries AL, Kaplan RM, Limberg TMK, *et al.* Effects of pulmonary rehabilitation on physiological and psychosocial outcomes in patients with chronic obstructive pulmonary disease. *Ann Intern Med* 1995; 122: 823–832.
41. Lacasse Y, Wong E, Guyatt GH, *et al.* Meta-analysis of respiratory rehabilitation in chronic obstructive pulmonary disease. *Lancet* 1996; 348: 1115–1119.
42. Wedzicha JA, Bestall JC, Garrod R, *et al.* Randomized controlled trial of pulmonary rehabilitation in severe chronic obstructive pulmonary disease patients, stratified with the MRC dyspnoea scale. *Eur Respir J* 1998; 12: 363–369.
43. Griffiths TL, Burr ML, Campbell IA, *et al.* Results at 1 year of outpatient multidisciplinary pulmonary rehabilitation: a randomised controlled trial. *Lancet* 2000; 355: 362–368.
44. Troosters T, Gosselink R, Decramer M. Short- and long-term effects of outpatient rehabilitation in patients with chronic obstructive pulmonary disease: a randomised trial. *Am J Med* 2000; 109: 207–212.
45. Lacasse Y, Brosseau L, Milne S, *et al.* Pulmonary rehabilitation for chronic obstructive pulmonary disease. *Cochrane Database Syst Rev* 2002; 3: CD003793.
46. Troosters T, Gosselink R, De Paepe K, *et al.* Pulmonary rehabilitation improves survival in COPD patients with a recent severe acute exacerbation. *Am J Respir Crit Care Med* 2002; 165: A16.

47. Decramer M. Treatment of chronic respiratory failure: lung volume reduction surgery *versus* rehabilitation. *Eur Resp J* 2003; 22; Suppl. 47, 47s–56s.
48. Griffiths TL, Phillips C, Davies S, *et al.* Cost effectiveness of an outpatient multidisciplinary pulmonary rehabilitation programme. *Thorax* 2001; 56: 779–784.
49. ZuWallack RL. Selection criteria and outcome assessment in pulmonary rehabilitation. *Monaldi Arch Chest Dis* 1998; 53: 429–437.
50. Maltais F, LeBlanc P, Jobin J, *et al.* Intensity of training and physiologic adaptation in patients with chronic obstructive pulmonary disease. *Am J Respir Crit Care Med* 1997; 155: 555–561.
51. Casaburi R, Porszasz J, Burns MR, *et al.* Physiologic benefits of exercise training in rehabilitation of patients with severe chronic obstructive pulmonary disease. *Am J Respir Crit Care Med* 1997; 155: 1541–1551.
52. The National Emphysema Treatment Trial Research Group. Rationale and design of the national emphysema treatment trial. *J Cardiopulmonary Rehabil* 2000; 20: 24–36.
53. Criner GJ, Cordova FC, Furukawa S, *et al.* Prospective randomized trial comparing bilateral lung volume reduction surgery to pulmonary rehabilitation in severe chronic obstructive pulmonary disease. *Am J Respir Crit Care Med* 1999; 160: 2018–2027.
54. Debigaré R, Maltais F, Whittom F, Deslauriers J, LeBlanc P. Feasibility and efficacy in home exercise training before lung volume reduction. *J Cardiopulm rehabil* 1999; 19: 235–241.
55. Williams TJ, Patterson GA, McClean PA, Zamel N, Maurer JR. Maximal exercise testing in single and double lung transplant recipients. *Am Rev Respir Dis* 1992; 145: 101–105.
56. Evans AB, Al-Himyary AJ, Hrovat MI, *et al.* Abnormal skeletal muscle oxidative capacity after lung transplantation by 31P-MRS. *Am J Respir Crit Care Med* 1997; 155: 615–621.
57. Wang XN, Williams TJ, McKenn MJ, *et al.* Skeletal muscle oxidative capacity, fiber type, and metabolites after lung transplantation. *Am J Respir Crit Care Med* 1999; 160: 57–63.
58. Decramer M, De Bock V, Dom R. Functional and histologic picture of steroid-induced myopathy in COPD. *Am J Respir Crit Care Med* 1996; 153: 1958–1964.
59. Hokanson JF, Mercier G, Brooks GA. Cyclosporine A decreases rat skeletal muscle mitochondrial respiration in vitro. *Am J Respir Crit Care Med* 1995; 151: 1848–1851.
60. Mercier JG, Hokanson F, Brooks GA. Effects of cyclosporine A on skeletal muscle mitochondrial respiration and endurance time in rats. *Am J Respir Crit Care Med* 1995; 151: 1532–1536.
61. Fournier M, Derenne JPh. Exercise performance in lung transplant candidates and recipients. *Eur Respir Rev* 1995; 25: 38–41.

CHAPTER 9

# Surgery for emphysema and prospects for the future

F. Venuta, A.M. Ciccone, G.F. Coloni

University of Rome, La Sapienza, Dept of Thoracic Surgery, Rome, Italy.

Correspondence: Federico Venuta, University of Rome, La Sapienza, Department of Thoracic Surgery, Policlinico Umberto I, Viale del Policlinico, Rome 00161, Italy.

Chronic obstructive pulmonary disease (COPD) is the third most common cause of death in Europe and the fourth in the UK. Many large longitudinal studies [1–4] on patients with severe COPD demonstrated increased mortality compared with the general population.

The anatomic changes associated with emphysema have been well described by LAENNEC [5], although descriptions of emphysema have previously been reported by BAILLIE [6]. Emphysema is characterised by permanent and anatomically irreversible air-space enlargement, distal to the terminal bronchiole. This definition is probably the only thing that has not been modified in the last 50 yrs. The pathogenesis of emphysema is related to smoking; medical treatment of which primarily consists of drugs such as bronchodilators, steroids, antibiotics, and the administration of supplemental oxygen when required (usually in the most advanced phases of the disease). Most of these drugs will improve symptoms and quality of life, but only oxygen will contribute to improve survival [7–10]. Smoking cessation should always be included in the therapeutic programme, as well as exercise rehabilitation.

A considerable degree of emphysema is suspected when the forced expiratory volume in one second (FEV1) is decreased, the total lung capacity (TLC) is elevated, the residual volume (RV) to RV/TLC is increased and the single-breath carbon monoxide diffusion capacity (DL,CO) is reduced. Major pathophysiological consequences of emphysema can be attributed to a loss of elastic recoil resulting in static and dynamic hyperinflation. The loss of elasticity results in a progressive enlargement of the lung and thoracic diameters; the rib cage expands to an abnormal position and the diaphragm becomes flattened. This results in severely impaired respiratory mechanics with consequent dyspnoea; the work of breathing is markedly increased and the amount of air moved in and out of the chest with each breath is quite limited. The main symptom for patients with severe emphysema is shortness of breath during minimal physical activity.

Over the past 50 yrs, many investigators have attempted to determine which factors influence survival of patients with COPD. Despite all available therapies, the course of the disease is progressively disabling with a significant increase in overall morbidity and mortality: when the FEV1 is <30% of the predicted value, ≤50% of patients will survive for 3 yrs [1, 8]. The biggest challenge today is early diagnosis, *i.e.* before symptoms become disabling.

Various surgical procedures have been promoted in the past to relieve dyspnoea and improve quality of life: costochondrectomy, thoracoplasty, phrenicectomy, pneumoperitoneum, pleural abrasion, denervation of the lung, glomectomy and many others (table 1) [11, 12]. Early results were often encouraging, but poor understanding of the pathophysiology of emphysema was certainly one of the limiting factors for sustained

Eur Respir Mon, 2004, 29, 139–155. Printed in UK - all rights reserved. Copyright ERS Journals Ltd 2004; European Respiratory Monograph; ISSN 1025-448x. ISBN 1-904097-33-2.

**Table 1. – Surgical procedure in patient with emphysema used between 1923–1995**

| Surgical procedure |
|---|
| Costocondrectomy |
| Paravertebral thoracoplasty |
| Phrenicectomy |
| Pneumatic cabinets |
| Abdominal belts |
| Pneumoperitoneum |
| Lung denervation |
| Glomectomy |
| Drainage, plication, excision of bullae |
| Lung transplantation |
| Lung volume reduction |

good results. Controlled trials were almost never carried out to compare the results of standard medical treatment with those of surgery. For these reasons most of them were eventually abandoned due to the lack of documented benefit.

Presently, only resection of the giant bullae and lung transplantation have shown a sustained beneficial effect. Surgical bullectomy has been employed successfully for more than four decades to improve lung function in patients with giant bullous emphysema [13].

Single- and bilateral-lung transplantation are the only therapeutic options for end-stage COPD patients [14] that allowed to achieve prolonged functional improvement with reasonable morbidity and mortality rates.

In 1995, lung volume reduction surgery (LVRS) was proposed, with acceptable results, by COOPER *et al.* [15]; They modified the approach initially described by BRANTIGAN and co-authors [16–18] performing a buttressed staple excision of the more hyperinflated and relatively functionless parts of the lung. This approach would improve the function of the remaining lung, the exercise ability and quality of life and palliate dyspnoea. Lung transplantation and LVRS are currently proposed to a selected group of patients with emphysema, with some limitations that are still debated in the literature.

More recently, other experimental endoscopic procedures have been proposed to improve the quality of life for patients with emphysema; two of these procedures appear to be more promising than others: the airway bypass, and the bronchoscopic lung-volume reduction.

## Surgery for giant bullous emphysema

The only operation that has stood the test of time is bullectomy. This procedure involves the resection of the distended air-spaces, allowing the re-expansion of restricted, but potentially functional, adjacent lung tissue.

Bullous emphysema is histologically referred to as the presence of emphysematous areas with complete destruction of lung tissue producing an air-space >1 cm in diameter. Bullae must be clearly differentiated from other disorders such as lung cysts and blebs. Most of the outer surface of the bullae is made of visceral pleura, while the inner layer consists of fibrous tissue formed mainly by the destroyed adjacent lung. The classification of bullae is useful to evaluate patients with regards their candidacy for surgery and to predict the potential functional outcome [19, 20]. The most frequently used classification is based upon the anatomy of the bulla and the characteristics of the underlying lung, these are: group I, single large bulla with normal underlying lung; group II, multiple bullae with normal underlying lung; group III, multiple bullae with underlying lung diffusely emphysematous; and group IV, multiple bullae with underlying lung affected by other diseases. Patients in groups I and II are ideal candidates for surgery with predicted good results. Patients in groups III and IV must be carefully evaluated and selected; functional results and clinical outcomes are less predictable since the quality and functional impairment of the underlying lung is more difficult to evaluate. Bullous disease may also be associated with a complete destruction of the underlying lung and irreversible respiratory failure; in most of these cases only lung transplantation can be considered if the selection criteria for this procedure are respected.

Surgery is generally indicated to modify the functional status of the underlying lung by relieving restrictive changes, increasing compliance and airway calibre, improving ventilation/perfusion ($V'/Q'$) ratio and decreasing the physiological dead space. These goals are easy to obtain in patients with enlarging bullae and minimal underlying lung disease. These are the best candidates for surgery and optimal results can be expected. Surgery is also indicated to treat complications related to the bullae, *e.g.* pneumothorax, infection, haemoptysis, cancer and pain.

Preventive surgery has been advocated when bullous disease may cause pneumothorax in patients with high risk occupations, independently from the size of the bulla and the state of the underlying lung. The choice of surgery is less unequivocal in asymptomatic patients with one or more bullae of moderate size as their natural history is poorly documented. However, a bulla increasing in size on serial chest radiographs in combination with lesions occupying more than one third of the hemithorax should be resected, even if the patient is asymptomatic.

Another major challenge is represented by dyspnoeic patients with bullae and diffuse emphysema. In this setting it is extremely important to evaluate the actual role of the bulla and the functional status of the underlying nonbullous emphysematous lung. Selection for surgery in this group of patients is extremely difficult. If a bullectomy is considered, it should be interpreted as a lung volume reduction procedure and improvement is mainly due to modifications of pulmonary mechanics [13].

The preoperative work up should always include: a complete clinical and functional evaluation, chest radiographies, computed tomography (CT) scans, $V'/Q'$ scans. Pulmonary angiography has been reported to show some advantages in evaluating the underlying lung; however, it is not routinely performed.

Results can be predicted on the base of the clinical presentation, pulmonary function tests and imaging. Better results are usually anticipated for younger patients with no comorbidity, no weight loss and rapid progression of dyspnoea, normal or slightly decreased forced vital capacity, $FEV_1$ >40% predicted and normal $D_{L,CO}$. Improved results are also expected when radiological work up shows a well localised bulla with evidence of vascular crowding and normal pulmonary density and architecture around the bulla. Angiographs and isotope scans should show preserved distal vascular branching and a well localised matching defect, with normal uptake and washout from the underlying lung.

Surgical treatment of bullous disease is technically not difficult when the correct indications, technique and postoperative management are respected. However, it can lead to serious complications when performed inappropriately.

Surgical bullectomy is usually performed using video-assisted thoracoscopic surgery (VATS) [21]. This approach is ideal both for unilateral and bilateral bullectomy. When a bilateral approach is required, median sternotomy and simultaneous bilateral anterior thoracotomy could also be considered [22]. In this group of patients staged procedures could also be performed. VATS can immediately be converted to open thoracotomy when intraoperative findings require it.

Operative mortality for bullectomy in patients with compression of a relatively normal underlying lung has been low, ranging from 0–8%. Morbidity is primarily related to prolonged air leaks and pulmonary infections. Early results in carefully selected patients have been excellent, with improvement in symptoms occurring within a few weeks after surgery and sustained for a period of years. The best results are seen in patients with large bullae causing the greatest compression of almost normal underlying lung. Symptomatic improvement, including reduction of dyspnoea, is usually observed, which reflects both the lessening of breathing efforts and improvement of diaphragmatic motion. However, clinical and symptomatic improvement is sometimes greater than actual spirometric measurements.

Results in patients with bullae and severe underlying emphysema are more difficult to predict and assess. It has been claimed by some authors [19–21] that bullectomy is not worthwhile in this subset of patients and is associated with a higher morbidity and mortality with a long-term follow-up revealing a more rapid deterioration than in patients with localised disease. The functional decline seems to be similar to that recorded after LVRS in nonbullous emphysema. The present authors postulate that in this subset of patients the effect of bullectomy is related to the reduction of thoracic volumes and the restoration of physiology of the diaphragm and the chest wall mechanics more than to lung re-expansion and recruitment of more functional lung parenchyma. This confirms the impression of other authors who describe bullectomy in patients with severe emphysema as "a special case of lung volume reduction" [19, 21]. In fact, in this subset of patients, bullae can be interpreted as a sign of heterogeneous emphysema, which is usually associated to the most favourable outcome after LVRS.

## Lung transplantation

Lung transplantation has been established as an effective treatment modality for a selected group of patients with end-stage pulmonary disease. On the basis of positive results with single-lung transplantation (SLT) for pulmonary fibrosis [23], this procedure has been considered for other pulmonary diseases and in particular for patients with COPD. However, in the early days of lung transplantation a number of SLTs were performed in patients with emphysema; all of these cases resulted in a fatal outcome [24]. *V'/Q'* imbalance was judged to be a significant problem since the remaining native lung became hyperinflated whereas the transplanted lung received the majority of cardiac output. In the meantime, double-lung transplantation (DLT) was developed and for these reasons it was initially considered the procedure of choice for patients with emphysema [25]. However, the original *en bloc* procedure was associated with a significant incidence of donor-airway ischaemic complications, fatal in most of the cases. The Washington University group subsequently developed the bilateral sequential SLT procedure (BLT), to simplify the operation, reduce the incidence of early complications, and improve results and functional outcome [26]. BLT was performed through a clamshell incision and is currently the procedure of choice in the majority of centres. While these technical innovations were introduced in the clinical practice, Mal *et al.* [27] reported a successful series with single-lung transplantation in COPD patients. Both single- and bilateral-lung transplantation for emphysema [28–32] have subsequently gained popularity.

Emphysema is an attracting disease for transplant surgeons for the following reasons: patients show a rather slow functional deterioration, so that they can tolerate a long wait; patients have enormous chest cavities, adhesions are rare and pulmonary hypertension is not frequent; cardio pulmonary by pass (CPBP) is rarely required; most of the patients do not show a significant parenchimal sepsis; furthermore, results appear to be superior to other disease categories.

According to the International Society for Heart and Lung Transplantation (ISHLT) registry for 2001 [33], ~30% of all lung transplants are performed on emphysema patients (43% of SLT and 37% of DLT). Lung transplantations should be offered only to those ideal candidates who have no other treatment options. The general recipient selection criteria are listed in table 2. The ISHLT has proposed specific criteria crucial for success for each disease category [34]. Reasonable criteria, specific for patients with emphysema, are: postbronchodilator FEV1 <25% pred, with a progressive decline of this parameter; resting hypoxia ($P_{a,O_2}$ <60 mmHg); hypercapnia, significant secondary pulmonary hypertension; deteriorating clinical course; life-threatening exacerbations; and increased frequency of hospitalisations. There are still contraindications to lung transplantation, which have been interpreted differently at each centre (table 3).

The accepted criteria for donor selection have been extensively reported in the literature [35]; it has recently been emphasised that the use of a marginal donor [36] may contribute to increasing the donor pool without a negative impact on outcome.

The choice of the procedure (SLT *versus* DLT) depends upon the experience and the policy of each centre, and on the characteristics of each patient. There remains significant controversy regarding the ideal application of SLT and BLT in patients with obstructive lung disease. Organ sharing and length of waiting time also play a role in the decision making. Younger patients, as well as candidates with giant bullous disease or bronchiectasis, should be considered for a BLT. The worldwide experience suggests an overwhelming international preference for a SLT, which is technically easier and is associated with a lower operative risk; furthermore, this procedure has several advantages in term of organ sharing. However, SLTs for emphysema may pose a number of potential problems, *e.g.* a potentially severe *V'/Q'* mismatch described in an earlier report [24]. Complications occurring in the native lung have also been described [37, 38],

**Table 2. – Lung transplantation: general criteria for patient selection**

| General criteria |
|---|
| Clinically and physiologically severe disease |
| Medical therapy ineffective or unavailable |
| Limitations of activities of daily living |
| Limited life expectancy |
| Adequate cardiac function without significant CAD |
| Ambulatory with rehabilitation potentials |
| Acceptable nutritional status |
| Age <65 yrs |

CAD: coronary artery disease.

**Table 3. – Contraindications for lung transplantation**

| Contraindicator |
|---|
| Active infections |
| Coexisting systemic disease |
| Severe osteoporosis |
| Significant CAD or LV dysfunction |
| Current cigarette smoking |
| High dose steroids |
| Psychosocial problems |
| Drug or alcohol abuse |
| Non compliance with medical management |

CAD: coronary artery disease; LV: left ventricle.

including pneumothorax and severe hyperinflation with compression of the graft as a consequence. Some patients may require native lung lobectomy, bullectomy, pneumonectomy or volume reduction to decompress the allograft [39–41]

BLT is the procedure of choice in younger patients, with functional and survival advantages in the long-term; recipients have more functional reserve in case they develop bronchiolitis obliterans (BO); marginal donors can be used more liberally, potentially increasing the number of transplants. The functional impact of this surgical procedure has been further improved since the old fashioned clamshell incision has been abandoned to perform two anterolateral thoracotomies without sternal division. With this approach early functional outcome is certainly better, with the advantage of avoiding sternal complications [42–44].

During the early postoperative course a number of complications may occur. Despite improved techniques of lung preservation early allograft dysfunction still occurs in 15–20 % of recipients; it can show a wide spectrum of presentations, from reperfusion injury to primary graft failure, and represents a frequent cause of morbidity and potential early postoperative mortality. This condition is characterised by increased pulmonary artery pressures, pulmonary oedema and progressive hypoxaemia. In general, the simple reperfusion injury is self-limited and clears over a period of several days with the administration of diuretics and steroids. Recent laboratory and clinical studies confirm the beneficial effect of inhaled nitric oxide in reducing early allograft dysfunction due to ischaemia-reperfusion injury; it usually causes an immediate fall in pulmonary artery pressure and a significant improvement in oxygenation.

Parenchymal infections represent the most common infectious complication after lung transplantation; most of them are related to nosocomial bacterial pneumonia with Gram-negative organisms predominating. The incidence of these complications is decreasing since appropriate prophylaxis strategies are employed along with judicious use of broad-spectrum antibiotics.

Most patients experience at least one or two acute rejection episodes during the first few postoperative weeks. However, the differential diagnosis between re-implantation response, infection, acute rejection and fluid overload, which represent the most common complications, can be difficult as their clinical presentation and radiographical patterns are similar. The correct diagnosis should be obtained with transbronchial lung biopsy and bronchoalveolar lavage, before starting treatment. The typical histological appearance of acute rejection is that of a perivascular lymphocitic infiltrate. Bolus injection of steroids for the treatment of acute rejection should be started only after parenchymal infections have been excluded; recalcitrant acute rejection requiring more intensive therapy with cytolitic agents is unusual.

Bronchial dehiscence and stenosis formerly represented a frequent cause of morbidity and mortality, they now occur in <10% of patients and are rarely fatal. Conservative strategies *e.g.* mechanical debridement, dilatation, Nd:YAG laser ablation and stent placement proved to be effective in the vast majority of cases. Surgical resection (sleeve resection) and retransplantation are rarely required.

The worst complication during long-term follow-up is represented by chronic rejection. Bronchiolitis obliterans syndrome (BOS) is clinically manifested by a decrease in $FEV_1$ and histologically by fibrotic obliteration of the small airways. This leads to a gradual decline in pulmonary function tests and quality of life, with respiratory insufficiency and recurrent infections with Gram-negative bacteria, and fungi. A lot of effort have been put into the detection of possible risk factors for chronic rejection. This syndrome appears now to be elicited by many donor and recipient factors, including age of the donor, duration of ischaemia, number of acute rejection episodes, and viral infections. Since the histological diagnosis of chronic rejection remains difficult, a clinical grading system has been proposed, enclosing four and, more recently five categories, depending on the severity of airflow obstruction [45]. The only treatment strategy so far is augmented immunosuppression to reduce the speed in which $FEV_1$ declines; however, the results are not encouraging and chronic rejection represents the most common cause of death among lung transplant recipients. Retransplantation may be considered in selected cases [46].

Lung transplantation can produce excellent functional results and satisfactory quality of life in patients without BOS, viral and bacterial infections, and complications related to long-term immunosuppression. Pulmonary function tests demonstrate a dramatic improvement after successful transplantation. The potential functional advantages of DLTs have been extensively described; however, exercise tolerance appears to be improved following both procedures without any significant difference between single and bilateral recipients, unless patients are tested at extremes of exertion or BOS occurs; at this point bilateral recipients present some advantages [47]. Other reports have demonstrated that there is no difference in functional outcome between right or left single-lung allografts in patients with emphysema [48]. It has been documented that emphysema patients have some survival advantages over other disease categories and this is probably related to the differences in early mortality rates. According to the Registry of the ISHLT the 1-yr survival rate for patients with emphysema after lung transplantation is 77% and the 5-yr survival rate is reduced to 50%.

## Lung volume reduction surgery

Emphysematous destruction of the lung is associated with a loss of lung elasticity; as a result the resting volume progressively increases over time, resulting in the expansion of the rib cage and flattening of the diaphragm. This in turn causes the respiratory muscles to be inefficient, contributing to an increase in the amount of work needed to breathe, and to the pervasive sense of breathlessness experienced by these patients. The patient is trapped in a state of permanent hyperinflation and no amount of effort can empty the lungs; the harder the patient strains to empty the lungs, the more the airways collapse and obstruct the outflow of gas.

Brantigan *et al.* [18] in the 1950s noted that patients with severe emphysema had flattened diaphragms and distended chests; in such patients the circumferential pull on the small airways is lost, but it could be restored by downsizing the lungs. From this it was realised that hyperinflation was a consequence, rather than the cause of emphysema, and tested the feasibility of reducing the volume of the lung parenchyma. This would improve elastic recoil and patency of intrathoracic airways. In addition, the reduction in lung size should improve chest wall mechanics. Brantigan and co-workers [16–18] performed an operation through a standard posterolateral thoracotomy with multiple lung resections and plications. A significant clinical and functional improvement in 75% of the patients was reported; however, the procedure was associated with a significant morbidity and a postoperative mortality of 16%.

Cooper *et al.* [15] rediscovered this operation on the base of their observations in emphysema patients undergoing lung transplantation. They noted that the chest cavity size of these patients returned to normal after transplanting lungs of normal sizes. This time, this group performed the procedure of LVRS through median sternotomy, to achieve maximal benefit with the minimum of overall morbidity. The most destroyed areas of the lung, usually located in the upper lobes, were removed with linear staplers buttressed with bovine pericardium. Usually up to one-half of the volume of the most involved lobe is removed. Target areas were carefully selected: these areas should contribute to volume but not to gas exchange. Preoperatively they are identified anatomically and functionally by high resolution CT and $V'/Q'$ scanning respectively. Resection of target areas not only eliminates the nonfunctional space but it also results in the re-expansion and return to function of a significant volume of the restricted adjacent normal lung.

When LVRS was re-introduced it was recognised to be a palliative procedure applicable to a selected group of patients with emphysema. The comparison of patients' outcomes undergoing LVRS with patients receiving medical treatment alone has demonstrated benefits, in the short- and intermediate-terms, for the former group and has confirmed the progressive functional decline in the control group, consistent with the known natural history of emphysema [49–54)

The duration of the benefit following LVRS is uncertain in view of the natural history of the disease; however, several reports have, to date, documented long-term functional results and survival [55–61]. LVRS appears to provide improved pulmonary function and quality of life, increased exercise tolerance, and decreased requirement for supplemental oxygen. However, this surgical procedure is certainly not intended to cure emphysema that continues to progression in the remaining lung parenchima.

Interestingly, LVRS has been shown to be an effective bridge to lung transplantation [62, 63]. LVRS can also be a temporary or permanent alternative to lung transplantation. Whether transplantation or LVRS is the better choice for patients who qualify for either procedure is still an open question and the most appropriate procedure should be selected on a case-by-case base.

Details of the selection process have been extensively reported [64, 65]. Some centres have modified their selection criteria according to personal experience and on the basis of ongoing analysis of the patients outcome [52]. The ideal candidates are those with marked thoracic distention and clear-cut distinction between regions of destruction and regions with preserved pulmonary parenchyma (heterogeneous emphysema); this provides target areas of virtually nonfunctioning lung, accessible to surgical resection (fig. 1). Selection can be performed on the base of morphology on chest radiographs, quantitative $V'/Q'$ lung scanning, and CT scans. Pulmonary function tests are measured with and without bronchodilators, including plethysmography. Eligibility criteria are basically referred to a $FEV_1$ <35% with an increased RV. Predominant small-airways

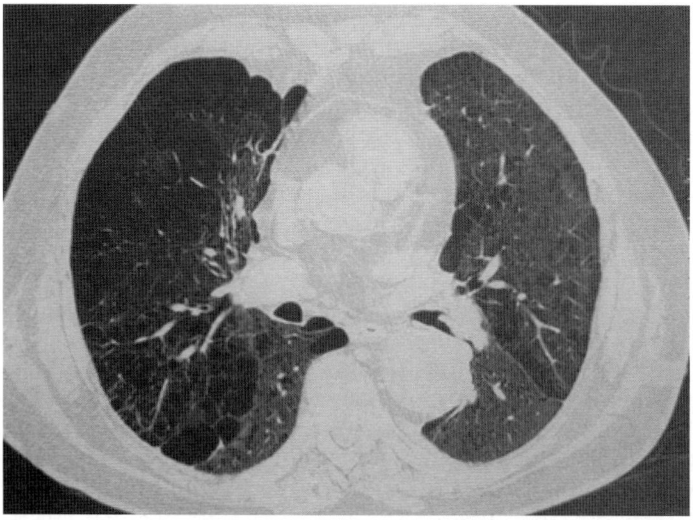

Fig. 1. – Heterogeneous emphysema with target areas accessible to surgical resection for lung volume reduction.

disease, markedly decreased DL,CO, advanced age, hypercapnia, and pulmonary hypertension are considered contraindications for surgery by most centres at the present time.

In addition to the standard initial work-up (medical history, physical examination, serum chemistries, pulmonary function tests with body plethsmography, arterial blood gas analysis, cardiac performance, high resolution CT scans, and $V'/Q'$ scans), evaluation also includes the 6-min walk test and questionnaires assessing quality of life and dyspnoea.

Patients, suitable for surgery, are enrolled in a supervised pulmonary rehabilitation programme based upon graded exercise training, education and bronchial hygiene measures. Before the operation, patients are expected to achieve a goal of 30 min on a treadmill at 1 mile·$h^{-1}$ without stopping. During exercise, the supplemental oxygen is increased as necessary to maintain saturation at >90%. This reconditioning, along with the administration of maximal medical treatment and nutritional counselling, is essential in the preparation of patients for surgery.

There are various surgical approaches to expose the emphysematous lung for volume reduction, but the two most frequently utilised are median sternotomy, as developed by the group at Washington University [15] and VATS, employed at other centres [59, 66, 67].

Median sternotomy provides a good exposure of both lungs, it allows palpation of the parenchyma, it does not interfere with chest wall mechanics and it does not cause excessive pain if the chest tubes are placed below the rib cage. Linear staplers are utilised to excise ~20–30% of the lung. Bovine pericardium continues to be used at many centres to buttress the staple line as proposed by Cooper [68] to prevent air-leaks through the staple holes. In case of total lobar destruction an anatomical lobectomy can be performed rather than wedge excision. If a residual space remains at the apex of the chest a pleural tent can be created [69, 70]

The VATS approach offers better visualisation for posterior and inferior adhesions than that afforded by median sternotomy and it also eliminates the risk of sternal infection or dehiscence. Many patients perceive a VATS procedure to be less invasive, although the postoperative course is comparable with that of a median sternotomy. Several centres have reported their results with a unilateral thoracoscopic resection (fig. 2) [66, 71]. However, bilateral volume reduction not only provides a greater improvement in thoracic mechanics but it also markedly improves alveolar gas exchange [50, 51, 72, 73]. Staged unilateral lung volume reduction can also be performed to prolong palliation of symptoms and functional improvement.

Thoracotomy is used in cases of previous sternotomy, or by groups who prefer open procedures in cases of predominantly unilateral emphysema [74]. VATS can be converted to thoracotomy if extensive adhesions are present.

Various laser techniques have been utilised for LVRS; the analysis of the available data demonstrates that the use of laser is associated with a significant rate of complications and does not produce sufficient benefit to recommend its use [75–77]. Two articles document results by combining the technique of stapled lung resection and laser ablation [78, 79]. Although both reports demonstrate that a combination of these techniques yields significant improvement, it is not clear how much is due either to laser ablation or stapled resection.

Standard postoperative care has been extensively described [49, 55, 69]. Adequate postoperative pain relief is facilitated by the use of continuous analgesia through a thoracic epidural catheter, which also guarantees the use of minimal narcotics. Vigorous chest physiotherapy, early mobilisation and the use of a bedside treadmill are also crucial.

A number of complications may occur after LVRS, but prolonged air leaks are the major source of morbidity reported in the literature [55, 56, 59]. However, the mortality rates are relatively low (2–6%) [55–57].

The improvement of lung function after LVRS is statistically significant in most of the

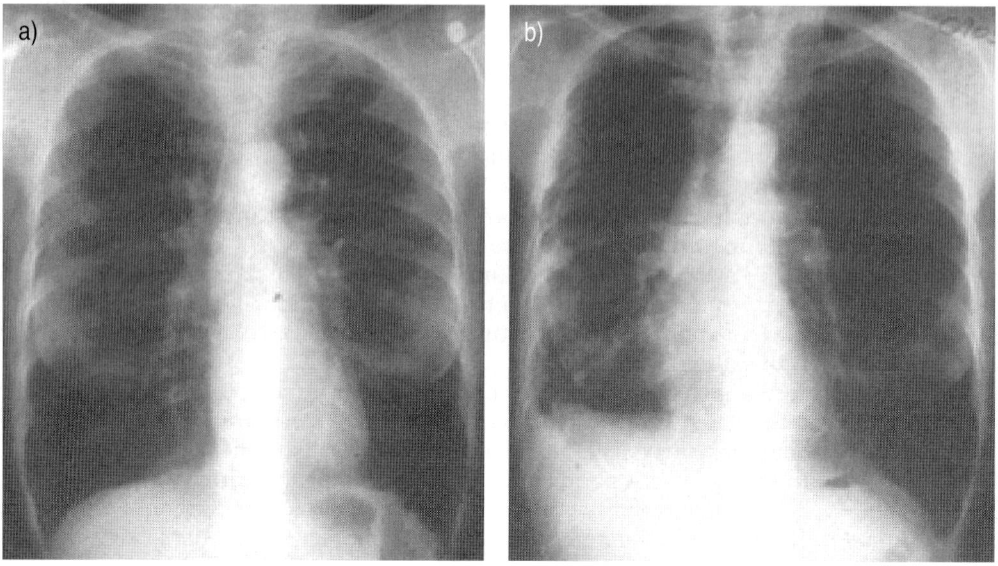

Fig. 2. – Chest radiographs showing the lung before (a) and after (b) right unilateral lung volume reduction surgery.

published reports [55–57]. However, functional deterioration is observed by all authors at different time points after surgery [80] and is probably related to the disease progression in the residual lung. In the majority of patients, despite a decline in $FEV_1$ from the initial peak values, some parameters still remain improved after a considerable interval: dyspnoea score, 6-min walk, supplemental oxygen requirement, overall quality of life, RV and TLC were preserved over 3 yrs following LVRS [55–57, 61, 81). The most recent follow-up data confirms persistent objective benefits at 5 yrs for the majority of patients [55]. Survival rates of patients undergoing LVRS is still under evaluation.

The uncertainty about the risk of LVRS, the magnitude and duration of benefit, and the optimal selection criteria, led to the National Heart, Lung and Blood Institute and the Center for Medicare and Medicaid Services in the USA to sponsor a multicentre, randomised clinical trial: the National Emphysema Treatment Trial (NETT) [82]. A total of 17 centres were enrolled in this trial in North America. The main goal was to compare survival rates and exercise capacity 2 yrs after LVRS with the results obtained after medical treatment alone. An interim report was published in 2001 [83], after randomising 1,033 patients in these two groups. This preliminary report contributed to the identification of high risk patients, with an $FEV_1$ and $D_{L,CO}$ <20% pred and a homogeneous distribution of emphysema at CT scanning. This category of patients is at high risk for death after surgery; they are also unlikely to benefit from surgery. For these reasons caution is warranted in the use of LVRS in case of low preoperative functional parameters, especially when they are associated to an homogeneous distribution of the disease. The final analysis of the results of the NETT will certainly contribute to the improvement of patient selection and predict outcome after surgery.

## Airway bypass

The pathophysiology of emphysema is characterised by a loss of elastic recoil with collapse of the small airways and increased resting-lung volume; this leads to lung hyperinflation and overexpansion of the thoracic cage, with inefficient respiratory muscles, increased work of breathing, and eventually respiratory failure. It has been demonstrated that the resection of nonfunctioning, hyperinflated target areas (LVRS) remodels the residual lung and improves mechanics and function. However, surgical resection may not be required in the future; similar results could be achieved with deflation or atelectasis of the target areas obtained with less invasive procedures.

An experimental endoscopic procedure for the treatment of emphysema is the airway bypass. It is based on the concept of "collateral ventilation", first described by VAN ALLEN *et al.* [84] in 1930. Collateral ventilation is defined as the ability of gas to move from one part of the lung to another through nonanatomical pathways. Collateral ventilation is present in normal lungs but it does not play an important role. In emphysematous lungs, the destruction of alveolar septa create a preferential route for collateral air flow. MACKLEM [85] suggested that creating passageways through the chest wall (spiracles) from the lung surface to the outside, bypassing the small obstructed airways, might alleviate hyperinflation and improve respiratory mechanics, allowing trapped gas to exit from the emphysematous lung.

This concept was recently rescued and simplified by the group at the University of Washington in St. Louis [86]. This group proposed that the creation of artificial communications between lung parenchyma and segmental bronchi would facilitate lung deflation and improve expiratory airflow, and consequently respiratory mechanics; in fact, on expiration, the new bronchial channels could drain the trapped air *via* the collateral pathways bypassing the obstructed small airways. This would be performed by bronchoscopically puncturing the wall of segmental bronchi with a radio-frequency catheter and inserting a stent to create internal bronchopulmonary communications through which air could escape from the lungs on expiration. This would reduce hyperinflation, improve respiratory mechanics and help alleviate dyspnoea. The improvement of $FEV_1$ after creation of new passages has been obtained in an *ex vivo* study on human emphysematous lungs [86]. Flows were experimentally measured in 12 emphysematous lungs resected for lung transplantation; the lungs were closed in a specially designed ventilation chamber and connected to a pneumotacograph to measure expiratory air flow. The baseline $FEV_1$ was measured and then flows were measured after creation of stented passages in the segmental bronchi. As a result of this study, the $FEV_1$ increased from an average of 245 mL at baseline to 447 mL after the creation of three stented passages and 666 ml after six stented passages. The experimental procedure was repeated in normal lungs harvested, but not used, for lung transplantation. After three stented holes, the $FEV_1$ did not differ from baseline, confirming that the modifications in emphysematous lungs, and probably collateral ventilation, are the base of the functional modifications previously described.

Based on these encouraging results, another study was designed and conducted at the University of Rome La Sapienza (Rome, Italy) and at the Washington University in St Louis (USA), to evaluate the feasibility and safety of creation of transbronchial passages in human subjects [87]. A crucial step in the safe perfomance of airway bypass is to create passages while avoiding injury to adjacent blood vessels. The study was conducted creating passages in lobes or lungs to be removed (for cancer or transplantation), after the chest was opened and full control of the pulmonary hilum was obtained. A flexible bronchoscope was introduced into the endotracheal tube. A Doppler probe was introduced through the operating channel of the flexible bronchoscope and used to scan the inner surface of the segmental or subsegmental bronchi to avoid the peribronchial blood vessels. After selection of the target site, the Doppler probe was withdrawn and a radio frequency catheter was advanced to create a passage through the bronchial wall into the lung parenchyma (airway bypass). Twenty-nine passages were performed in the lobectomy patients with two episodes of mild bleeding, and 18 passages in patients with emphysema undergoing transplantation. No major complications were observed.

A clinical study was subsequently designed at the University of Rome, La Sapienza (Rome, Italy) for patients with severe emphysema without other medical or surgical options. Inclusion criteria were homogenous emphysema type, FEV1 <40%, RV >180% and refractivity to medical therapy; all patients required the administration of supplemental oxygen at rest. DL,CO <20%, carbon dioxide arterial tension ($P_{a,CO_2}$ ) >7.3 kPa.(55 mmHg) and mean pulmonary artery pressure >4.0 kPa (30 mmHg) were the main exclusion criteria. In a second phase of the study, after the creation of the passages, a specially designed metallic stent was developed and inserted in the new passageways to maintain the patency. The results observed after the procedure have been controversial: after an initial improvement of symptoms, lung volumes and exercise tolerance, the clinical and functional parameters returned to the pre-treatment values.

The short-term results in these studies demonstrated that the creation of bronchial fenestrations is safe in normal lungs as well as in severely emphysematous patients. However, more studies are required before this procedure can become a real therapeutic option for patients with end-stage emphysema.

## Bronchoscopic volume reduction

The airway bypass is not the only endoscopic procedure proposed to improve symptoms and quality of life in patients with emphysema. Other procedures have been described with the use of occlusive stents and synthetic sealants [88–90]. These procedures were all designed to reduce hyperinflation and obtain atelectasis of the most destroyed, functionless parts of the emphysematous lungs. They have been evaluated to find safer alternatives to LVRS, especially for patients with the most advanced disease. This group of patients showed a higher surgical mortality rate suggesting that LVRS may not be suitable for all of them.

It has been postulated that blocking an airway supplying the over inflaited emphysematous parts of the lung could cause atelectasis of these regions and contribute to alleviate symptoms. The basis of this procedure is the placement of unidirectional valves in the segmental bronchi. Like an Heimlich system the valves favour the expiratory airflow from the emphysematous area with a decrease of lung volumes and an improvement in breathing capacity. The endobronchial valve is a stent supported one-way valve made of silicon and nitilol. This valve prevents air entering the target area of the lung but allows air and mucus to exit. The valves and delivery catheters (Emphasys, Redwood City, CA, USA) are inserted with a flexible bronchoscope and a guidewire; fluoroscopy may or may not be used.

After a series of animal studies, a clinical trial was conducted in eight centres worldwide and >70 patients have been treated so far with the same selection criteria as surgical LVRS. The procedure is safe and may provide benefit for COPD patients, reducing the thoracic volume and improving expiratory flow. The evaluation process includes physiological and radiological criteria: spirometry, DL,CO, exercise tolerance, blood gas analysis, chest radiograph, chest CT scan, and *V'/Q'* scan. The inclusion criteria are: heterogeneous end-stage emphysema visible at CT scan and lung perfusion scan, severe dyspnoea, FEV1 <30% pred and aged between 40–75 yrs. The exclusion criteria are $P_{a,CO_2}$ >6.7 kPa (50 mmHg), DL,CO <30% and evidence of active infection.

This is a day-hospital procedure performed in the operating room under a general anesthetic. The patient is intubated and the flexible bronchoscope is advanced into the endotracheal tube. The target segmental bronchus is chosen and a guidewire is inserted into the operating channel of the bronchoscope to reach the selected segment under direct visualisation. While leaving the guidewire in place, the bronchoscope is withdrawn and the delivery catheter is passed on the guidewire. After the removal of the latter the valve is delivered. Fibreoptic bronchoscopy confirms the correct placement of the valve. It is possible to treat several segments in one set; the valves can be removed easily, if placement is not satisfactory, using rat-tooth graspers through the working channel of the bronchoscope. Unilateral procedures are usually preferred at this initial step.

The current authors performed unilateral bronchoscopic lung volume reduction in six patients and a staged bilateral in two. All patients had heterogeneous emphysema with clear target areas. All patients tolerated the treatment well. Between three and five valves were placed in each target lobe. One homolateral and two contralateral pneumothoraces were observed. One patient had pneumonia in a nontreated lobe; this complication was easily managed with the administration of broad spectrum antibiotics. No other complications were observed. Postoperative hospital stay had been 2 days, as the patients underwent a 24–48 h follow-up after the procedure. It has been slightly longer in patients showing pneumothorax. One of the two patients experienced the contralateral pneumothorax 15 days after the endoscopic procedure.

The functional results were evaluated preoperatively and at intervals during the postoperative period (24–48 h and 1 and 3 months after the procedure). All patients showed an improvement of $FEV_1$ and a decrease of RV. In addition to these results the dyspnoea score, supplemental oxygen requirement and quality of life all significantly improved.

The unilateral approach allows the possibility of a further palliative intervention on the contralateral side when required. With more experience, simultaneous bilateral insertion of the valves could be attempted. One of the advantages of endobronchial lung volume reduction is that the procedure can be reversed and other treatments tried if necessary.

These short-term results are encouraging, but long-term follow-up is necessary to evaluate the therapeutic potential of this procedure.

## Summary

Chronic obstructive pulmonary disease (COPD) is one of the most common causes of death both in Europe and in the USA. At the most advanced phases of the disease, when symptoms become disabling, the quality of life for these patients is extremely compromised. During the last 50 yrs various surgical procedures have been proposed to relieve dyspnoea and improve quality of life: costochondrectomy, pneumoperitoneum, glomectomy and many others. Early results were often encouraging but no sustained good results were obtained. All of these procedures were eventually abandoned.

At the present time, only resection of giant bullae and lung transplantation have shown substantial beneficial effect. Surgical bullectomy has been employed successfully to improve lung function in patients with bullous emphysema for more than four decades; single- and bilateral-lung transplantations are now considered a viable therapeutic option for a selected group of patients with end-stage emphysema. Lung volume reduction has been recently rediscovered; it results in a significant but temporary functional improvement with palliation of dyspnoea and amelioration of quality of life. Also this surgical procedure can now be safely proposed for a selected group of patients with emphysema, with some limitations that are still debated in the literature.

More recently, other experimental endoscopic procedures have been described; two of them seem more promising: the airway bypass and the endoscopic lung-volume reduction.

**Keywords:** Airway bypass, chronic obstructive pulmonary disease, endoscopic-lung volume reduction surgery, lung volume reduction surgery, lung transplantation.

## References

1. Anthonisen NR, Wright EC, Hodgkin JE (IPPB trial group). Prognosis in chronic obstructive pulmonary disease. *Am Rev Respir Dis* 1986; 133: 14–20.
2. Hodgkin J. Prognosis in chronic obstructive pulmonary disease. *Clin Chest Med* 1990; 11: 555–569.
3. Postma DS, Sluiter HJ. Prognosis of chronic obstructive pulmonary disease. *Am Rev Respir Dis* 1989; 140: S95–S99.
4. Traver GA, Cline MG, Burrows B. Predictors of mortality in chronic obstructive pulmonary disease. *Am Rev Respir Dis* 1979; 119: 357–367.
5. Laennec RTH. A treatise on the diseases of the chest and of mediate auscultation. Translated by John Forbes, MD, FRS. 4th Edn. London, Whittaker & Co, 1834.
6. Baillie M. The morbid anatomy of some of the most important pars of the human body. London, printed for J. Jones and G. Nicol, 1793; p.314.
7. Anthonisen N, Connett J, Kiley J, *et al.* Effects of smoking intervention and use of an inhaled anticholinergic bronchodilator on the rate of decline of FEV1. *JAMA* 1994; 272: 1497–1505.
8. Ries AL, Kaplan RM, Limberg TM, Prewitt L. Effects of pulmonary rehabilitation on physiologic and psychosocial outcomes in patients with chronic obstructive pulmonary disease. *Ann Intern Med* 1995; 122: 823–832.
9. Nocturnal Oxygen Therapy Trial Group. Continuous or nocturnal oxygen therapy in hypoxemic chronic obstructive lung disease. *Ann Intern Med* 1980; 93: 391–398.
10. Report of the Medical Research Council Working Party. Long-term domiciliary oxygen therapy in chronic hypoxic cor pulmonale complicating chronic bronchitis and emphysema. *Lancet* 1981; 1: 681–685.
11. Cooper JD. The history of surgical procedures for emphysema. *Ann Thorac Surg* 1997; 63: 312–319.
12. Deslauriers J. History of surgery for emphysema. *Semin Thorac Cardiovasc Surg* 1996; 8: 43–51.
13. Snider GL. Reduction pneumoplasty for giant bullous emphysema: implications for surgical treatment of non-bullous emphysema. *Chest* 1996; 109: 540–548.
14. Kaiser LR, Cooper JD, Trulock EP, *et al.* The evolution of single lung transplantation for emphysema. *J Thorac Cardiovasc Surg* 1991; 102: 333–341.
15. Cooper JD, Trulock EP, Triantafillou AN, *et al.* Bilateral pneumonectomy (volume reduction) for chronic obstructive pulmonary disease. *J Thorac Cardiovasc Surg* 1995; 109: 106–119.
16. Brantigan OC, Mueller E. Surgical treatment of pulmonary emphysema. *Am Surg* 1957; 23: 789–804.
17. Brantigan OC, Mueller E, Kress MB. A surgical approach to pulmonary emphysema. *Am Rev Respir Dis* 1959; 80: 194–202.
18. Brantigan OC, Kress MC, Mueller EA. The surgical approach to pulmonary emphysema. *Dis Chest* 1961; 39: 485–501.
19. Shamji FM. Classification of cystic and bullous lung disease. *Chest Surg. Clin. N. Am.* 1995; 5: 705–716.
20. Mehran RJ, Deslauriers J. Indications for surgery and patient work up for giant bullous emphysema. *Chest Surg. Clin. North Am.* 1995; 5: 717–734.

21. De Giacomo T, Venuta F, Rendina EA, *et al.* Video – assisted thoracoscopic treatment of giant bullae associated with emphysema. *Eur. J. Cardiothorac. Surg.* 1999; 15: 753–757.
22. Lima O, Ramos L, Di Biasi PD, *et al.* Median sternotomy for bilateral resection of emphysematous bullae. *J. Thorac. Cardiovasc. Surg.* 1981; 82: 892–897.
23. Grossman RF, Frost A, Zamel N, *et al.* Results of single lung transplantation for bilateral pulmonary fibrosis. *N Engl J Med* 1990; 727: 33–37.
24. Wildevuur CRH, Benfield JR. A review of 23 human lung transplantations by 20 surgeons. *Ann. Thorac. Surg.* 1970; 9: 489–515.
25. Cooper JD, Patterson GA, Grossman R, Maurer J. Double lung transplant for advanced chronic obstructive lung disease. *Am Rev Respir Dis* 1989; 139: 303–307.
26. Pasque MK, Cooper JD, Kaiser LR, Haydock DA, Triantafillou A, Trulock EP. Improved technique for bilateral lung transplantation: rationale and initial clinical experience. *Ann Thorac Surg* 1990; 49: 785–791.
27. Mal H, Andreassian B, Pamela F, *et al.* Unilateral lung transplantation in end-stage pulmonary emphysema. *Am Rev Respir Dis* 1989; 140: 797–802.
28. Kaiser LR, Cooper JD, Trulock EP, *et al.* The evolution of single lung transplantation for emphysema. *J Thorac Cardiovasc Surg* 1991; 102: 333–341.
29. Low DE, Trulock EP, Kaiser LR, *et al.* Morbidity, mortality and early results of single versus bilateral lung transplantation for emphysema. *J Thorac Cardiovasc Surg* 1992; 103: 1119–1126.
30. McGregor CGA, Daly RC, Peters SG, *et al.* Evolving strategies in lung transplantation for emphysema. *Ann Thorac Surg* 1994; 57: 1513–1521.
31. Patterson GA, Maurer JR, Williams TJ, *et al.* Comparison of outcomes of double and single lung transplantation for obstructive lung disease. *J Thorac Cardiovasc Surg* 1991; 101: 623–632.
32. Levine SM, Anzueto A, Peters JL, *et al.* Medium term functional results of single lung transplantation for end stage obstructive lung disease. *Am J Respir Dis Crit Care Med* 1994; 150: 398–402.
33. Hosenpud, JD, Bennett LE, Keck BM, Boucek MM, Novick RJ. The Registry of the International Society for Heart and Lung Transplantation: eighteenth Official Report – 2001. *J Heart Lung Transplant* 2001; 20: 805–815.
34. Maurer JR, Frost AE, Estenne LF, *et al.* International guidelines for the selection of lung transplant candidates. *J Heart Lung Transplant* 1998; 17: 703–709.
35. Sundaresan S, Trachiotis GD, Aloc M, *et al.* Donor lung procurement: assessment and operative technique. *Ann Thorac Surg* 1993; 56: 1409–1413.
36. Sundaresan S, Semenkovich J, Ochoa L, *et al.* Successful outcome of lung transplantation is not compromised by the use of marginal donor lungs. *J Thorac Cardiovasc Surg* 1995; 109: 1075–1080.
37. Mal H, Brugiere O, Sleiman C, *et al.* Morbidity and mortality related to the native lung in single lung transplantation for emphysema. *J Heart Lung Transplant* 2000; 19: 220–223.
38. Venuta F, Boehler A, Rendina EA, *et al.* Complications in the native lung after single lung transplantation. *Eur J Cardiothorac Surg* 1999; 16: 54–58.
39. Venuta F, De Giacomo T, Rendina EA, *et al.* Thoracoscopic volume reduction of the native lung after single lung transplantation for emphysema. *Am J Respir Crit Care Med* 1997; 156: 292–293.
40. Yonan NA, El-Gamel A, Egan J, Kakadellis J, Rahman A, Deiraniya AK. Single lung transplantation for emphysema: predictors for native lung hyperinflation. *J Heart Lung Transpl* 1998; 17: 192–201.
41. Negri JC, Dunning J, Sharples LD, Mcneil K. Native lung volume reduction surgery following single lung transplantation (SLTX) for emphysema. *J Heart Lung Transplant* 2001; 20: 177.
42. Meyers BF, Sundaresan RS, Guthrie T, Cooper JD, Patterson GA. Bilateral sequential lung transplantation without sternal division eliminates post transplantation sternal complications. *J. Thorac Cardiovasc Surg* 1999; 117: 358–364.
43. Taghavi S, Birsan T, Setelberger R, *et al.* Initial experience with two sequential anterolateral thoracotomies for bilateral lung transplantation. *Ann Thorac Surg* 1999; 67: 1440–1443.

44. Venuta F, Rendina EA, De Giacomo T, *et al.* Bilateral sequential lung transplantation without sternal division. *Eur. J Cardiothorac. Surg.* 2003; 26: 895–898.
45. Estenne M, Maurer JR, Bohler A, *et al.* Bronchiolitis obliterans syndrome 2001: an update of the diagnostic criteria. *J. Heart Lung Transplant* 2002; 21: 297–310.
46. Novick RJ, Stitt L. Pulmonary retransplantation. *Semin Thorac Cardiovasc Surg* 1998; 10: 227–236.
47. Williams TJ, Patterson GA, McClean PA, *et al.* Maximal exercise testing in single and double lung transplant recipients. *Am Rev Respir Dis* 1992; 145: 101–105.
48. Levine SM, Anzueto A, Gibbons WJ. Graft position and pulmonary function after single lung transplantation for obstructive lung disease. *Chest* 1993; 103: 444–448.
49. Cooper JD, Patterson GA, Sundaresan S, *et al.* Results of 150 consecutive bilateral lung volume reduction procedures in patients with severe emphysema. *J Thorac Cardiovasc Surg* 1996; 112: 1319–1330.
50. McKenna RJ, Brenner M, Fischel RJ, Gelb AF. Should lung volume reduction for emphysema be unilateral or bilateral? *J Thorac Cardiovasc Surg* 1996; 112: 1331–1339.
51. Kotloff RM, Tino G, Palevsky HI, *et al.* Comparison of short-term functional outcomes following unilateral and bilateral lung volume reduction surgery. *Chest* 1998; 113: 890–895.
52. Russi EW, Stammberger U, Weder W. Lung volume reduction surgery for emphysema. *Eur Respir J* 1997; 10: 208–218.
53. Criner G, Cordova F, Furukowa S, *et al.* Prospective randomized trial comparing bilateral lung volume reduction surgery to pulmonary rehabilitation in severe chronic obstructive pulmonary disease. *Chest* 1999; 160: 2018–2027.
54. Meyers BF, Yusen RD, Lefrak SS, *et al.* Outcome of Medicare patients with emphysema, selected for, but denied, a lung reduction operation. *Ann Thorac Surg* 1998; 66: 331–336.
55. Ciccone AM, Meyers BF, Guthrie TJ, *et al.* Long-term outcome of bilateral lung volume reduction in 250 consecutive emphysema patients. *J Thorac Cardiovasc Surg* 2003; 125: 513–525.
56. Fujimoto T, Teschler H, Hillejan L, Zaboura G, Stamatis G. Long-term results of lung volume reduction surgery. *Eur J Cardiothorac Surg* 2002; 21: 483–488.
57. Flaherty KR, Kazerooni EA, Curtis JL, *et al.* Short-term and long-term outcomes after bilateral lung volume reduction surgery: prediction by quantitative CT. *Chest* 2001; 119: 1337–1346.
58. Geddes D, Davies M, Koyama H, *et al.* Effect of lung volume reduction surgery in patients with severe emphysema. *N Engl J Med* 2000; 343: 329–345.
59. Naunheim KS, Kaiser LR, Bavaria JE, *et al.* Long-term survival after thoracoscopic lung volume reduction: a multiinstitutional review. *Ann Thorac Surg* 1999; 68: 2026–2032.
60. Brenner M, McKenna RJ Jr, Chen JC, *et al.* Survival following bilateral staple lung volume reduction surgery for emphysema. *Chest* 1999; 115: 390–396.
61. Gelb AF, McKenna RJ, Brenner M, Schein MJ, Zamel N, Fischel R. Lung function 4 years after lung volume reduction surgery for emphysema. *Chest* 1999; 116: 1608–1615.
62. Gaissert HA, Trulock EP, Cooper JD, Sundaresan RS, Patterson GA. Comparison of early functional results after volume reduction or lung transplantation for chronic obstructive pulmonary disease. *J Thorac Cardiovasc Surg* 1996; 111: 296–307.
63. Wisser W, Deviatko E, Simon-Kupilik N, *et al.* Lung transplantation following lung volume reduction surgery. *J Heart Lung Transplant* 2000; 19: 480–487.
64. Yusen RD, Lefrak SS, and the Washington University Emphysema Surgery Group. Evaluation of patients with emphysema for lung volume reduction surgery. *Semin Thorac Cardiovasc Surg* 1996; 8: 83–93.
65. Slone R, Gierada D. Radiology of pulmonary emphysema and lung reduction surgery. *Semin Thorac Cardiovasc Surg* 1996; 8: 61–82.
66. Keenan R, Landreneau R, Sciurba F, *et al.* Unilateral thoracoscopic surgical approach for diffuse emphysema. *J Thorac Cardiovasc Surg* 1996; 111: 308–316.
67. McKenna RJ, Brenner M, Gelb AF, *et al.* A randomized, prospective trial of stapled lung

reduction versus laser bullectomy for diffuse emphysema. *J Thorac Cardiovasc Surg* 1996; 111: 317–322.
68. Cooper JD. Technique to reduce air leaks after resection of emphysematous lung. *Ann Thorac Surg* 1994; 57: 1038–1039.
69. Cooper JD, Patterson GA. Lung volume reduction surgery for severe emphysema. *Semin Thorac Cardiovasc Surg* 1996; 8: 52–60.
70. Venuta F, De Giacomo T, Rendina EA, Ricci C, Coloni GF. Thoracoscopic pleural tent. *Ann. Thorac. Surg.* 1998; 66: 1833–1834.
71. Naunheim KS, Keller CA, Krucylak PE, Singh A, Ruppel G, Osterloh J. Unilateral video-assisted thoracic surgical lung reduction. *Ann Thorac Surg* 1996; 61: 1092–1098.
72. Tino G, Kotloff R, Palevsky H, *et al.* Lung volume reduction surgery by median sternotomy vs. video thoracoscopy: functional outcomes. *Am J Respir Crit Care Med* 1996; 153: A449.
73. Keenan R, Sciurba F, Landreneau R, *et al.* Superiority of bilateral versus unilateral thoracoscopic approaches to lung reduction surgery. *Am J Respir Crit Care Med* 1996; 153: A268.
74. Miller JI Jr, Lee RB, Mansour KA. Lung volume reduction surgery: lessons learned. *Ann Thorac Surg* 1996; 61: 1464–1469.
75. Mc Kenna RJ, Brenner M, Mullin MJ, *et al.* A randomized, prospective trial of stapled lung reduction versus laser bullectomy for diffuse emphysema. *J Thorac Cardiovasc Surg* 1996; 111: 317–321; discussion 322.
76. Little AG, Swain JA, Nino JJ, Prabhu RD, Schlachter MD, Barcia TC. Reduction pneumonoplasty for emphysema. Early results. *Ann Surg* 1995; 222: 365–371; discussion 371–374.
77. Hazelrigg S, Boley T, Henkle J, *et al.* Thoracoscopic laser bullectomy: a prospective study with three-month results. *J Thorac Cardiovasc Surg.* 1996; 112: 319–326; discussion 326–327.
78. Eugene J, Ott RA, Gogia HS, Dos Santos C, Zeit R, Kayaleh RA. Video-thoracic surgery for treatment of end-stage bullous emphysema and chronic obstructive pulmonary disease. *Am Surg* 1995; 61: 934–936.
79. Wakabayshi A. Thoracoscopic laser pneumoplasty in the treatment of diffuse bullous emphysema. *Ann Thorac Surg* 1995; 60: 936–942.
80. Brenner M, McKenna RJ, Gelb AF, Fischel RJ, Wilson AF. Rate of FEV1 change following lung volume reduction surgery. *Chest* 1998; 113: 652–659.
81. Cooper JD, Lefrak SS. Lung-reduction surgery: 5 years on. *Lancet* 1999; 353: Suppl. I, 26–27.
82. National Emphysema Treatment Trial Research Group: Rationale and design of the National Emphysema Treatment Trial (NETT): a prospective randomised trial of lung volume reduction surgery. *J. Thorac. Cardiovasc. Surg.* 1999; 118: 518–528.
83. National Emphysema Treatment Trial Research Group. Patients at high risk of death after lung volume reduction surgery. *N. Engl. J. Med.* 2001; 15: 1075–1083.
84. Van Allen CM, Lindskog GE, Richter HT. Gaseous interchange between adjacent lung lobules. *Yale J Biol Med* 1930; 2: 297–300.
85. Macklem PT: Collateral ventilation. *New Engl J Med* 1978; 298: 49–50.
86. Lausberg HF, Chino K, Patterson GA, Meyers BF, Toeniskoetter PD, Cooper JD. Bronchial fenestration improves expiratory flow in emphysematous human lungs. *Ann Thorac Surg* 2003; 75: 393–397.
87. Rendina EA, De Giacomo T, Venuta F, *et al.* Feasibility and safety of the airway bypass procedure for emphysema. *J Thorac Cardiovasc Surg* 2003; 125: 1294–1299.
88. Snell GI, Smith GA, Silòvers AJ, *et al.* Broncoscopic volume reduction: a pilot study. ACCP Meeting 2001; Paper 25.
89. Ingenito EP, Berger RJ, Henderson AC, Reilly JJ, Tsai L, Hoffman A. Bronchoscopic volume reduction using tissue engineering principles. *Am J Respir Crit Care Med* 2003; 167: 771–778.
90. Toma TP, Hopkinson NS, Hansell DM, *et al.* Bronchoscopic volume reduction with valve implants in patients with severe emphysema. *Lancet* 2003; 15: 931–933.

*CHAPTER 10*

# Extrapulmonary function-improving surgery

N. Konietzko*, R. Meister#

*Ruhrlandklinik, Essen and #Karl-Hansen-Klinik, Bad Lippspringe, Germany.

Correspondence: N. Konietzko, Ruhrlandklinik, Tueschener Weg 40, 45239, Essen, Germany.

## Diseases of the ribs

Most congenital rib abnormalities as well as diseases of the ribs, *e.g.* osteomyelitis or tumours, cause little interference with the respiratory function. However, in contrast with this severe chest wall injuries, *e.g.* in traffic road accidents or in elderly patients with household trauma, may lead to significant morbidity and, especially in flail chests, to mortality rates up to 12%.

Flail chest occurs when there is a fracture of at least four ribs in at least two places. The flail segment moves paradoxically and may severely disturb the mechanics of breathing often leading, together with pain and lung contusion, to respiratory insufficiency. There are various techniques for operative stabilisation of the flail chest and several reports demonstrating advantages of surgical intervention, but all reports are retrospective, nonrandomised and small in number. Currently, it seems appropriate to stabilise a flail rib segment only operatively if surgical intervention is performed for other reasons. Otherwise internal stabilisation by prolonged mechanical ventilation should be applied for several days.

Thoracoplasty was used as part of lung-collapse therapy for cavernous lung tuberculosis between 1930–1955, before effective drug treatment was available, and leads to restrictive defects of the lung function. The degree of restriction is directly correlated with the extent of the thoracoplasty, leading to a reduction in predicted vital capacity (VC) of ~45% in a thoracoplasty with a resection of 9–11 ribs. Respiratory insufficiency and cor pulmonale develop usually 4–5 decades after the operative procedure [1]. The reduction in lung volume can be more pronounced if the contralateral lung has been affected by the tuberculous process and additional scarring occurs in both the parenchyma of the lung and in the pleural space. There are no surgical options for the improvement of the respiratory function in thoracoplasty. Long-term oxygen therapy in severe hypoxaemic patients and noninvasive ventilation in hypercapnic patients are highly effective with most patients experiencing a better quality of life and up to 80% of patients surviving for up to 5 yrs [2].

## Diseases of the sternum

### *Instability of the sternum*

Congenital aplasia of the sternum is easily clinically recognised and can be confirmed on using computer tomography (CT) of the thorax. It leads to extreme mobility of the shoulders, but has no impact on respiratory function. In traumatic fractures of the sternum, and following sternotomy, the sternum can become unstable and lead to

Eur Respir Mon, 2004, 29, 156–167. Printed in UK - all rights reserved. Copyright ERS Journals Ltd 2004; European Respiratory Monograph; ISSN 1025-448x. ISBN 1-904097-33-2.

paradoxical inward movement during inspiration. Surgical fixation in the case of respiratory embarrassment poses many problems, the management is usually conservative with prolonged ventilation.

## *Pigeon breast:* pectus carinatum

In congenital pigeon breast, the sternum protrudes anteriorely and mostly asymmetrically. The respiratory sequelae in patients with *pectus carinatum* are of no functional relevance, operative correction may be indicated for cosmetic reasons.

## *Funnel chest:* pectus excavatum

***Definition.*** *Pectus excavatum* is characterised by an inward displacement of the lower part of the sternum, decreasing the anterio-posterior diameter of the chest wall. It can displace and in severe instances can even compress the heart and reduce the lung volume. The incidences of *pectus excavatum* vary in the literature between 0.031–2.3%. It is more often seen in male children; the ratio male to female is 4:1. Funnel chest is often present soon after birth and may be associated with straight back syndrome, thoracic scoliosis and mitral valve prolapse. *Pectus excavatum* of later onset may be a manifestation of Marfańs disease, but is usually idiopathic. Funnel chest is often seen in families with an increased frequency of up to 39% [1].

***Pathophysiology.*** The majority of children have no complaints; usually the first problems arise during adolescence. Half of the young patients, usually aged between 16–20 yrs, complain of shortness of breath during exercise, palpitation of the heart, a feeling of pressure behind the sternum and precordial pain. On auscultation, a systolic click or a late systolic murmur is typically recorded. The chest radiograph shows a displacement of the heart to the left (fig. 1) and the electrocardiogram shows a rotation of the electrical axis [3, 4].

In rare instances the right heart can be compressed between the spine and the dorsally displaced sternum. The cardiac filling can thus become impaired. This reduced filling of the right ventricle is especially pronounced during exercise in the upright sitting position [5–7]. The heart lies more caudally in the upright position and the compression between the spine and the sternum is more pronounced. In the right heart catheterisation, an early diastolic pressure dip and a late diastolic plateau are typically demonstrated (fig. 2). Another typical finding is the inadequate increase of the stroke volume and the cardiac output during exercise in the sitting position, while the haemodynamic reaction for the

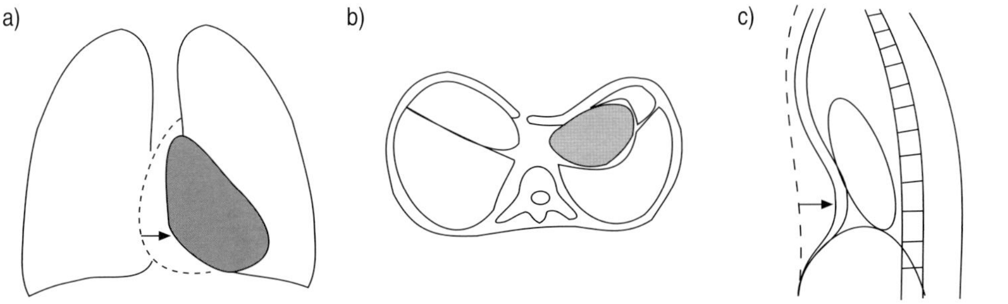


Fig. 1. – Funnel chest: effect of thoracic deformity on the position of the heart and effect on the lung volume. a) Heart displacement, b) decreased antero-posterior diameter, c) decreased lung volume.

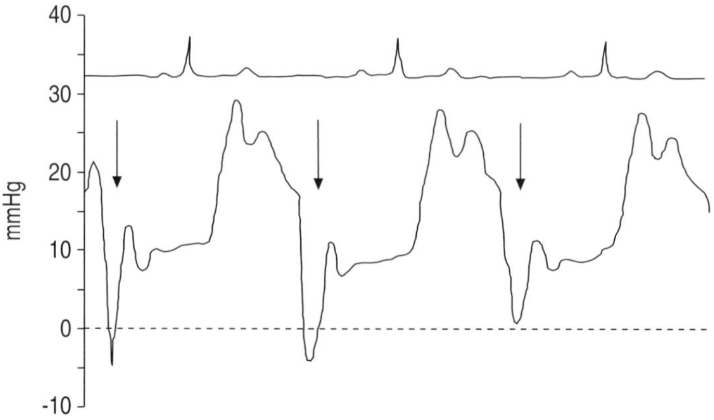


Fig. 2. – Funnel chest: early diastolic deep (arrow) and late diastolic plateau of the right ventricular pressure. ECG-tracing (upper line) and right ventricular pressure tracing (lower line) showing three cardiac actions.

same workload may be normal in the supine position [4, 5, 7, 8]. This phenomenon can also be demonstrated by noninvasive exercise testing *e.g.* the working capacitiy (physical work capacity: 170) in patients with substantial funnel chest is >20–25% higher in the supine position compared with the sitting position [4]. By surgical correction the compression can be completely relieved [4, 9].

Lung function is usually either not or only slightly reduced. In accordance with the small volume, which is lost by the deformity of the chest wall (fig. 2), the static lung volumes are slightly smaller than in a normal population (fig. 3). Dynamic lung volumes (forced expiratory volume in one second: FEV1, and FEV1/VC), mechanics of breathing including lung compliance, airway resistance, and gas exchange at rest and during exercise, are essentially normal [4, 10, 11].

***Indications for surgery.*** The indications for surgical correction of the deformity, usually accomplished by reconstruction of the chest wall and by internal fixation, are: severe degree of the funnel chest; and proven functional abnormalities, usually due to cardiac

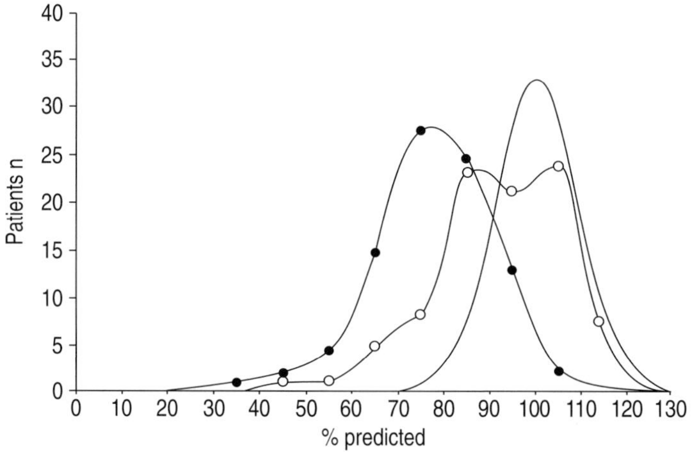


Fig. 3. – Funnel chest: frequency distribution of vital capacity (VC; ●) and total lung capacity (TLC; ○) in 96 patients with funnel chest compared with the normal distribution for VC and TLC (—).

compression. The operation should be performed in late childhood, usually at 12–14 yrs of age, in younger children the relapse rate is higher. Patients with Marfan's syndrome should be excluded from corrective surgery of the sternum.

Reduction in lung volume in the pattern of restrictive lung function is *per se* not an indication for the operation, although there is often a strong desire for surgical intervention from all sides; the affected children, the parents and the surgeons, generally for cosmetic reasons [12, 13]. However, in most instances, the desire to get the funnel chest surgically corrected disappears when the patient reaches adulthood [14–16].

***Surgical approach.*** There are various surgical techniques used to correct a funnel chest. All the approaches follow two principles (fig. 4) which include: the reconstruction of the normal rib cage and chest wall; and the internal fixation of the rib cage, to prevent a relapse of the funnel chest, which is usually accomplished with metallic clasps [4, 17, 18].

***Complications.*** Common, minor complications, as observed in up to 30% of cases, are haematoma, wound infection and haemato-pneumothorax. Rare and more severe complications, observed in up to 10% of cases, include: pneumonia, mediastinitis, dislocation and fracture of the implanted material. The mortality rates reported in the literature range from 0.33–0.96% [4, 18].

***Outcome.*** The surgical correction of the deformity usually normalises the haemodynamic abnormalities, if the compression of the heart was substantial prior to surgery. Improvement in pulmonary function, *e.g.* an increase in VC, is only observed if surgery was done during adolescence. The increase in lung volume is due to growth of the body and the lung. Cosmetic results are satisfying in up to 96% of cases in the early phase, but

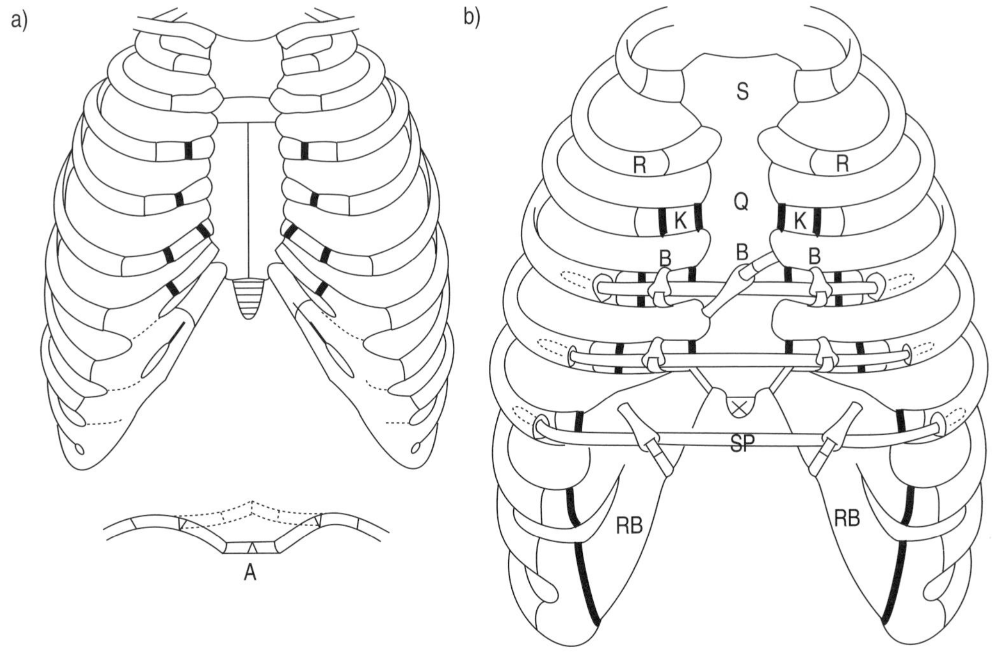


Fig. 4. – Funnel chest: surgical approach with techniques for reconstruction and internal fixation. S: sternum; Q: transverse osteotomy; R: rib; K: costal cartilage; B: metal band; SP: funnel chest metal splint; RB: costal arch.

8–10 yrs after surgery results are judged acceptable only in half of the patients [4, 9, 12, 13, 16, 17, 19, 20].

***Summary.*** In the presence of substantial compression of the heart, surgery can improve haemodynamics. In severe cases, pulmonary function shows restriction and can become a limiting factor during strong physical exertion. If performed during adolescence, surgery can improve lung volumes, which is due to the growth of the body and the lung. Surgical correction of the deformity should not be performed for psychological or cosmetic reasons only, because most patients accept their problem later in adulthood. There is no progress in the deformity of the sternum anymore after adolescence.

# Diseases of the spine

Deformities of the spine can have profound implications upon the respiratory system. Hippocrates observed, over 2,000 yrs ago, an abnormal breathing pattern in a humpbacked female child, and concluded that the breathing pattern would be normalised if the spine could be stretched, an erroneous assumption as present science shows.

## *Scoliosis of the spine*

***Definition.*** Scoliosis is characterised by a lateral outward bending and rotation of the spine, more or less fixed, and is usually combined with a curvature in the sagittal front (kyphoskoliosis; fig. 5). The aetiology is, in most cases, unknown. Idiopathic scoliosis is predomonantly seen in female children and is progressive during childhood and adolescence (fig. 6). Rarely are babies born with scoliosis (inborn scoliosis). Myopathic scoliosis, due to poliomyelitis, was very common during the last century, but nowadays it is rarely found as poliomyelitis has virtually disappeared. However, it can still occur in other neuromuscular diseases like Morbus Duchenne or Syringomyelia.

***Pathophysiology.*** The torsion of the spine has major pathophysiological consequences [21–39] which include: antagonisms of the ribcage and malfunction of the respiratory muscles (fig. 5); overinflation of the lung on the side of scoliosis (fig. 5); an overall decrease in VC (fig. 7) and asymmetry of the system with ventilation-perfusion

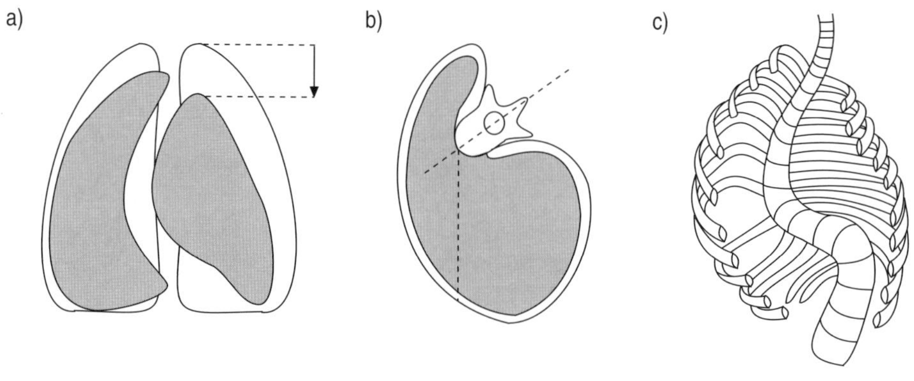


Fig. 5. – Scoliosis of the spine: leading reasons for restriction due to the chest deformity. a) The amount of loss in thoracic height (-----), b) the deviation of the thoracic medline (-----) and c) antagonism of the ribcage.

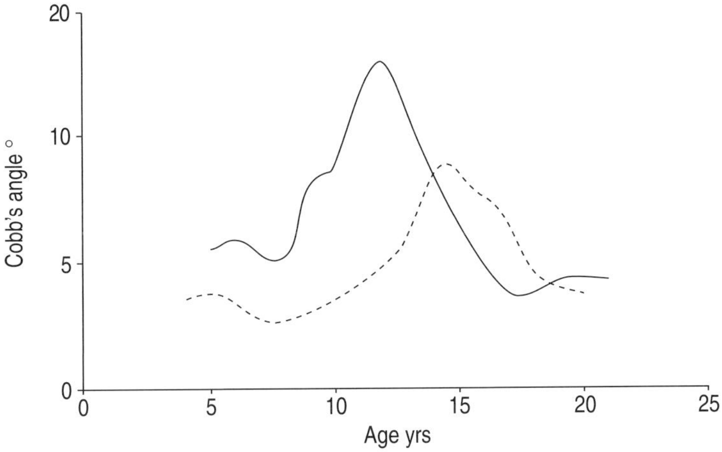


Fig. 6. – Scoliosis of the spine: mean annual progression of Cobb's angle in children and adolescents depending upon age and sex (——: female, n=62; -----: male, n=21) of patients with idiopathic scoliosis.

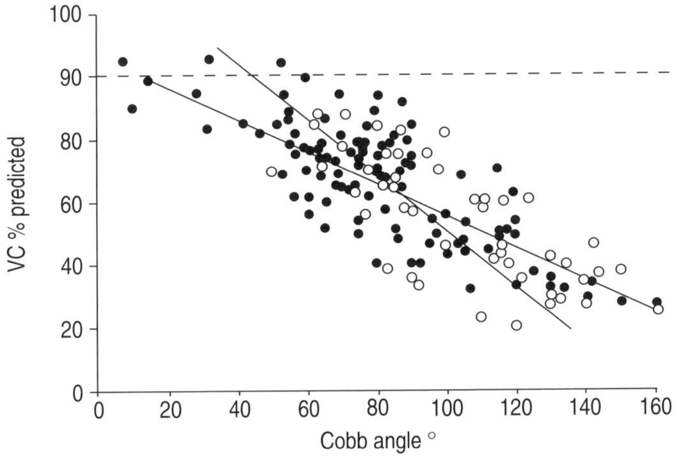


Fig. 7. – Scoliosis of the spine: correlation between Cobb's angle and vital capacity (VC) in adolescents (●) and adults (○). ——: represents the regression lines for the total collective (adolescents plus adults); ··········: represents 100% predicted value.

inequalities, leading to arterial hypoxia (fig. 8). Ineffective function of the respiratory muscles can lead, in severe cases, to: alveolar hypoventilation and arterial hypercapnia (fig. 8), pulmonary hypertension and cor pulmonale due to alveolar hypoventilation, and alveolar hypoxia (fig. 9).

Before hypercapnia can be detected at rest, it is observed during exercise and in rapid eye movement (REM) phase during sleep. The functional disturbances are closely correlated with the degree of spine distortion, reflected by the bending angle (Cobb), which can be easily measured on radiographs of the spine [1, 22, 23, 32, 37].

***Indications for surgery.*** Patients with severe scoliosis (Cobb $\geq 50°$) may undergo surgery: for functional reason, to improve pulmonary function; for orthopaedic reasons, to relieve

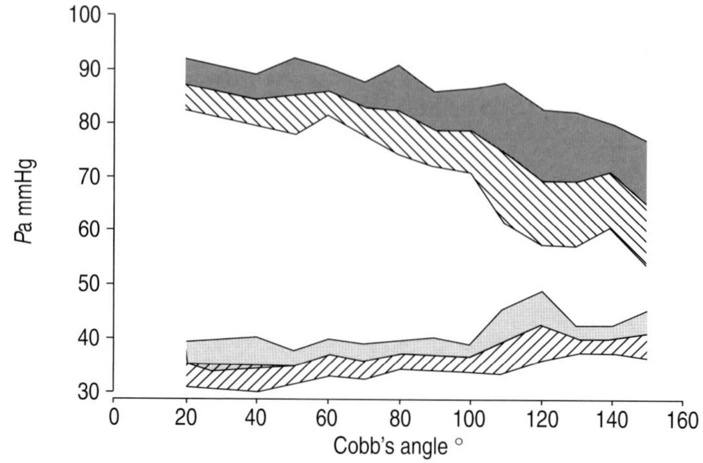


Fig. 8. – Scoliosis of the spine: relationship between Cobb's angle and arterial tension (*P*a) blood gases (oxygen tension in arterial blood: $P_{a,O_2}$; and carbon dioxide tension in arterial blood: $P_{a,CO_2}$). The different shaded areas represent for both the $P_{a,O_2}$ (●, ▧) and $P_{a,CO_2}$ (▒, ▨) the range above and below the mean values (n=150).

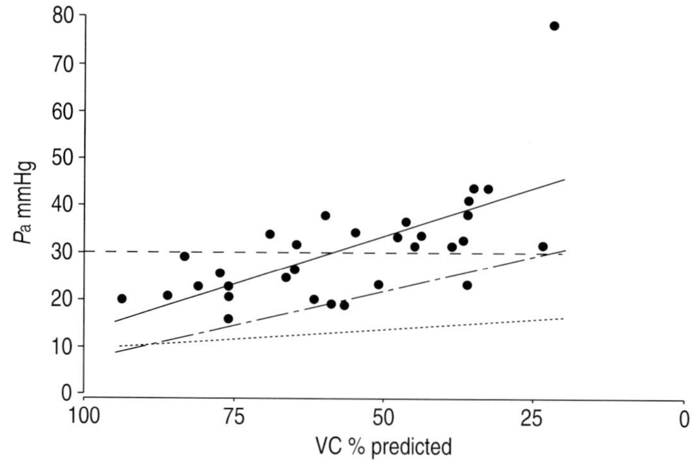


Fig. 9. – Scoliosis of the spine: pulmonary arterial mean pressure (——), pulmonary arterial diastolic pressure (*P*pad; — - — -) and wedge pressure (*P*pev) during exercise in relation to lung volume (vital capacity: VC in % predicted; ·········). The four different stages of restriction in terms of VC are: I: 100–75; II 74–50; III 49–25; and IV: <25% pred. The dashed line represents the two-fold standard deviation for the mean *P*pap under exercise (normal collective). The shaded area represents the pressure gradient between *P*pad and *P*pev. The pressure gradient correlates with the pulmonary vascular resistance.

compression and pain; for cosmetic reasons, to reduce the deformity of the spine and to increase the size of the body. Usually the latter two reasons prevail, when the discussion about surgical correction arises, and it is largely expected that lung function and dyspnoea also improve. But improvement of pulmonary function is accomplished only in rare instances [32, 40–42]. The timing of surgery is important, since the best orthopaedic results are obtained if the surgical procedure is performed during adolescence (fig. 6).

***Contraindication for surgery.*** The main cardiopulmonary contraindications are: clinically decompensated cor pulmonale; respiratory failure, measured by arterial blood gas analysis (partial arterial carbon dioxide $\geq$6.65 kPa: 50 mmHg); concomiting chronic airway disease with obstructive pattern proven by pulmonary function testing.

***Surgical approach.*** The most widely used method, to correct the scoloiosis of the spine, goes back to Harrington, who in 1962 described an operative procedure, using implanted steel bars for stabilisation of the scoliotic segment of the spine. There are numerous modifications of this method, but all follow the same principle [42–44].

***Complications.*** The main complications include: neurological defects, infection, and postoperative respiratory insufficiency. The morbidity is generally high and the mortality little less than 1% [32, 45].

***Outcome.*** In the first year following surgical correction, only the over inflation of the lung decreases (functional residual capacity decreases), all other parameters remained constant. Although there is an increase in body size due to the erection of the spine, the VC does not increase simultaneously (table 1 and fig. 10).

In the following 4–5 yrs, the gas exchange improves at rest and during exercise. The static lung volumes improve by up to 25%, but only if surgery was performed during adolescence. This improvement in lung function is mainly explained by the growth of the lung during adolescence (fig. 11) [4, 42, 46, 47].

***Summary.*** Surgical erection of a scoliotic spine has positive orthopaedic and cosmetic effects, but operative intervention does not improve pulmonary function. In advanced disease, long term oxygen therapy or noninvasive ventilation is indicated, when severe hypoxia, hypercarbia and/or cor pulmonale become manifest [1, 48–50].

## *Kyphosis*

Respiratory function is nearly never disturbed in kyphosis to a substantial degree; over inflation of the lung is observed when testing the pulmonary function, but overt lung emphysema is not seen in nonsmoking subjects with kyphosis. Only if the spine deformity develops early in childhood, as seen in spondylitis tuberculosa (Pott's disease), does respiratory impairment due to insufficient lung growth develop. In Morbus Bechterew,

**Table 1. – Lung function results before and 1 yr after an operation for scolisosis**

| | Preoperative | Postoperative | p-value |
|---|---|---|---|
| Patients n | 50 | 50 | |
| TLC | 3.73±1.06 | 3.84±0.92 | NS |
| TLC % pred | 79.4±17.9 | 78.8±14.0 | NS |
| VC | 2.43±0.75 | 2.44±0.70 | NS |
| VC % pred | 67.0±16.6 | 64.8±14.7 | NS |
| RV | 1.30±0.44 | 1.40±0.36 | 0.05 |
| FRCBP | 2.08±0.65 | 2.35±0.60 | 0.001 |
| RV/TLC % | 34.5±7.3 | 36.6±6.6 | 0.05 |
| FRC/TLC % | 55.4±6.2 | 60.9±6.8 | 0.001 |

Data are shown in L unless otherwise stated; TLC: total lung capacity; % pred: percentage predicted; VC: vital capacity; RV: Residual volume; FRCBP: functional residual capacity measured by bodyplethxsmography; FRC: functional residual capacity.

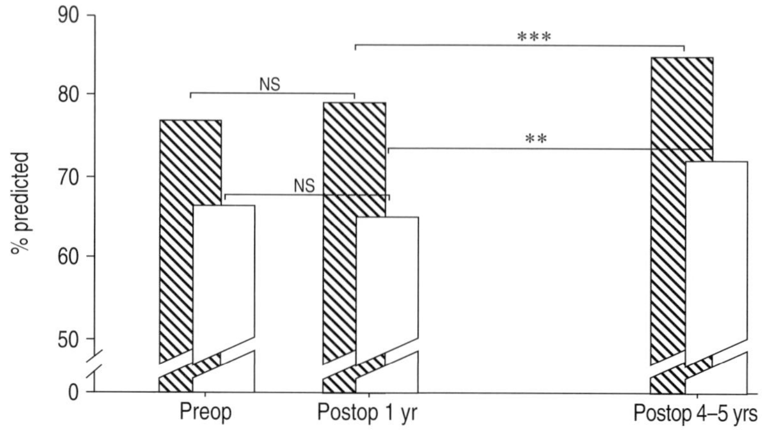


Fig. 10. – Scoliosis of the spine: change in lung volume (▧: total lung capacity; □: vital capacity) in 24 adolescent scoliosis patients before and after orthopaedic correction (dorsal spondylodesis and internal fixation by Harrington's spine instrumentation). **: p<0.01; ***: p<0.001.

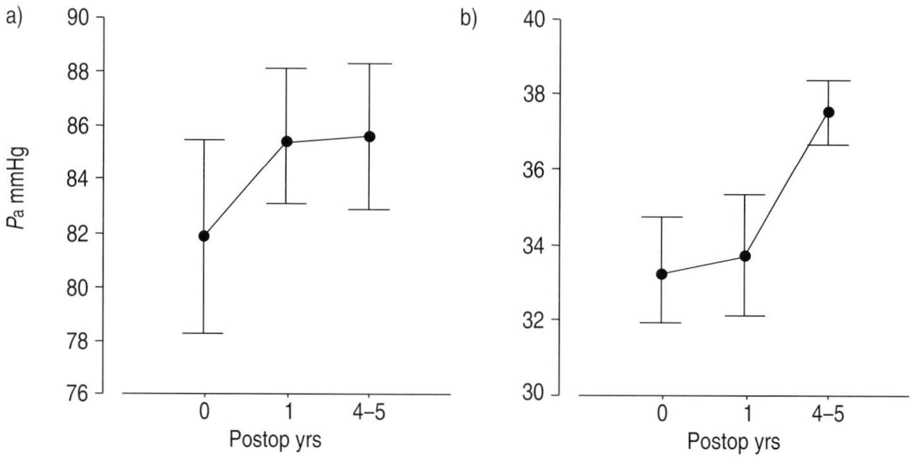


Fig. 11. – Scoliosis of the spine: blood gases (oxygen and carbon dioxide tension in arterial blood: $P_a$) during exercise in 23 adolescents with idiopathic thoracic scoliosis before and after orthopaedic correction.

respiratory function may become disturbed to a substantial degree, but there are no surgical options for the improvement of the lung function [1, 51].

# Diseases of the diaphragm

Unilateral paralysis of the diaphragm is associated with a decrease in static lung volumes, *e.g.* in VC by ~30%, hypoxaemia due to ventilation/perfusion (inequalities and REM), and sleep associated alveolar hypoventilation [48, 52].

Bilateral paralysis of the diaphragm is always associated with severe respiratory insufficiency, leading to hypercapnia, cor pulmonale and death if not treated. The treatment of choice is usually noninvasive mechanical ventilation. Stimulation of the diaphragm by implanted pacemakers poses many problems in the long run, although it works transiently.

Following traumatic rupture of the diaphragm or in tumour surgery, it may become necessary to replace the diaphragmatic muscle by dacron or other materials. This procedure obviously does not change pulmonary function, but merely separates the abdominal and thoracic cavity.

## Summary

Most extrapulmonary function-improving surgical techniques were developed some 25–60 yrs ago and the indications, results and complications are well known. They comprise of the correction for funnel chest and severe scoliosis of the spine. However, for some abnormalities such as diaphragm paralysis or thoracoplasty, surgery cannot offer clear extrapulmonary function improving solutions.

**Keywords:** Diaphragm, flail chest, funnel chest, kyphosis, scoliosis thoracoplasty.

## References

1. Meister R. $0_2$-Langzeittherapie bei Thoraxdeformitäten: Pathophysiologische Grundlagen. *Prax Klin Pneumol* 1981; 35: 523–527.
2. Jackson M, Smith l, King M, Shneerson J. Long term non invasive domiciliary assisted ventilation for respiratory failure following thoracoplasty. *Thorax* 1994; 49: 915–919.
3. Hecker WCh, Pöschl U, Billinger W. Trichterbrust und Kielbrust. *Münch Med Wschr* 1977; 119: 559.
4. Meister R. Trichterbrust und Trichterbrustoperation: Auswirkungen auf Herz, Hämodynamik und Lunge. *Prax Klin Pneumol* 1982; 36: 223–243.
5. Bevegard S. Postural circulatory changes at rest and during exercise in patients with funnel chest, with special reference to factors affecting the stroke volume. *Acta Med Scand* 1962; 171: 695–713.
6. De Leon AC Jr, Perloff JK, Twigg H, Majd M. The straight back syndrome. Clinical cardiovascular manifestations. *Circulation* 1965; 32: 193–203.
7. Gattiker H, Bühlrnann A. Cardiopulmonary function and exercise tolerance in supine and sitting position in patients with pectus excavatum. *Helv Med Acta* 1966; 33: 122–138.
8. Nolan SP, Epstein SE, Levitsky S, Geiser GD, Goldstein RE, Stampfer M. Does pectus excavatum cause functional disability? *J Thorac Cardiovasc Surg* 1976; 71: 148.
9. Haller JA, Peters GN, Mazur D, White JJ. Pectus excavatum. A 20 year surgical experience. *J Thorac Cardiovasc Surg* 1970; 60: 375–383.
10. Aigner A, Baumgartl P, Bolzano K, Raas E. Zur klinischen Differentialdiagnose und deren sportrnedizinische Bedeutung bei Trichterbrust. *Med Welt* 1970; 39: 1703–1706.
11. Kleine P, Fabel H, Ringe B. Ruhe. Lungenfunktion und Belastungsverhalten bei Patienten mit Trichterbrustdeformität. *Atemwegs- u. Lungenkh* 1980; 6: 1143.
12. Hegemann G. Kosmetische und funktionelle Ergebnisse operativer Maßnahmen bei Trichterbrust. Langenbecks. *Arch Chir* 1967; 319: 5–26.
13. Jensen NX, Schmidt WR, Garamella JJ, Lvnch MF. Pectus excavatum and carinatum: the how, when, and why of surgical correction. *J Ped Surg* 1970; 5: 4–13.

14. Meissner F, Bennek J, Gottschalk M. Die Altersabhängigkeit der Trichterbrust. Operation. *Zentralbl Chir* 1977; 102: 1432–1440.
15. Randolph JG, Tunel WP, Morton D Jr. Repair of pectus excavatum in children under 3 years of age: a twelve year experience. *Ann thorac Surg* 1977; 23: 364–366.
16. Stauffer UG. Spätresultate nach Trichterbrustoperationen im Kindesalter. Zur Problematik der Operationsindikation. *Helv Paediatr Acta* 1975; 30: 459.
17. Geroulanos S, Hahnloser P, Senning A. Trichterbrustkorrektur. Indikation, operatives Vorgehen und Resultate nach einer vereinfachten und modifizierten Methode. *Helv Chir Acta* 1974; 41: 101–108.
18. Sbokos CG, McMillan LK, Akins CW. Surgical correction of pectus excavatum using a retrosternal bar. *Thorax* 1975; 30: 40–45.
19. Haller JA, Shermeta DW, Tepas JJ, Bittner HR, Golladay ES. Correction of pectus excavatum without prostheses or splints: objective measurement of severity and management of asymmetrical deformities. *Ann Thorac Surg* 1978; 16: 73–79.
20. Liese W, Bühlmann AA. Arbeitskapazität und Lungenvolumina vor und nach chirurgischer Korrektur einer Trichterbrust. Spätresultate bei Erwachsenen. *Schweiz Med Wsch* 1974; 104: 83–86.
21. Baydur A, Milic-Emili J. Respiratory mechanics in kyphoscoliosis. *Monaldi Arch Chest Dis* 1993; 48: 69–79.
22. Bergofsky EH, Turino GM, Fishman AP. Cardiorespiratory failure in kyphoscoliosis. *Medicine* 1959; 38: 263–317.
23. Bergofsky EH. Respiratory failure in disorders of the thoracic cage. *Amer Rev Resp Dis* 1979; 119: 643–669.
24. Branthwaite MA. Cardiorespiratory consequences of unfused idiopathic scoliosis. *Br J Dis Chest* 1986; 80: 360–369.
25. Cooper DM, Rojas JV, Mellins RB, *et al.* Respiratory mechanics in adolescents with idiopathic scoliosis. *Am Rev Respir Dis* 1984; 130: 16–22.
26. Dollery CT, Gillam PMS, Hugh-Jones P, Zorah PA. Regional lung function in kyphoscoliosis. *Thorax* 1965; 20: 175–181.
27. Jones RS, Kennedy JD, Haslam F, *et al.* Mechanical inefficiency of the thoracic cage in scoliosis. *Thorax* 1981; 36: 456–461.
28. Kafer ER. Idiopathic scoliosis. Mechanical properties of the respiratory system and the ventilatory response to carbon dioxide. *J Clin Invest* 1975; 55: 153–163.
29. Kafer ER. Idiopathic scoliosis. Gas exchange and the age dependence of arterial blood gases. *J Clin Invest* 1976; 58: 825–833.
30. Kesten S, Garfinkel FK, Wright T, Rebuck AS. Impaired exercise ability in adults with moderate scoliosis. *Chest* 1991; 99: 663–666.
31. Klempt HW, Meister R, Most E, Heine J. Die Hämodynamik des Lungenkreislaufs bei Thoraxdeformitäten. Kongr Ber Wiss Tag. *Norddtsch Ges Lungen u Bronchialhk* 1975; 14: 47.
32. Meister R. Atemfunktion und Lungenkreislauf bei thorakaler Skoliose. [Respiratory function and pulmonary circulation in thoracic scoliosis.] Bücherei des Pneumologen, Bd. 5, Stuttgart, Thieme, 1980.
33. Midgren B, Petersson K, Hansson I, *et al.* Impairment exercise ability in adults with moderate scoliosis. *Chest* 1991; 99: 663–666.
34. Muirhead A, Conner AN. The assessment of lung function in children with scoliosis. *J Bone Joint Surg Br* 1985; 67B: 699–702.
35. Sawicka EH, Branthwaite MA. Respiration during sleep in kyphoscoliosis. *Thorax* 1987; 42: 801–808.
36. Shneerson JM, Sutton GC, Zorah PA. Causes of death, right ventriculary hypertrophy, and congenital heart disease in scoliosis. *Clin Orthop Rel Res* 1978; 135: 52–57.
37. Shneerson JM. The cardiorespiratory response to exercise in thoracic scoliosis. *Thorax* 1978; 33: 457–463.

38. Swank SM, Winter RB, Moe JH. Scoliosis and cor pulmonale. *Spine* 1982; 7: 343–354.
39. Sakic K, Pecina M, Pavicie F. Pulmonary function in adolescents with idiopathic scoliosis. *Int Orthop* 1992; 16: 207–212.
40. Beiser GL, Epstein SE, Stampfer M, Goldstein RE, Nolan SP, Levitisky S. Impairement of cardiac function in patients with pectus excavatum, with improvement after operative correction. *N Engl J Med* 1972; 287: 267–272.
41. Rom WN, Miller A. Unexpected longevity in patients with severe kyphoscoliosis. *Thorax* 1978; 33: 106–110.
42. Savini R, Parisini P, Vicenzi G. Respiratory function in severe scolosis before and after treatment (a review of 76 cases). *Ital J Orthop Traumatol* 1976; 2: 247–259.
43. Kinnear WJ, Johnston ID. Does Harrington instrumentation improve pulmonary function in adolescents with idiopathie scoliosis? A metaanalysis. *Spine* 1993; 18: 1556–1559.
44. Kumano K, Tsuyama N. Pulmonary function before and after surgical correction of scoliosis. *J Bone Joint Surg Am* 1982; 64: 242–248.
45. Kinnear WJ, Kinnear GC, Watson I, *et al.* Pulmonary function after spinal surgery for idiopathic scoliosis. *Spine* 1992; 17: 708–713.
46. Vedantam R, Lenke LG, Bridwell KH, Haas J, Linville DA. A prospective evaluation of pulmonary function in patients with adolescent idiopathic scoliosis relative to the surgical approach used for spinal arthrodesis. *Spine* 2000; 25: 82–90.
47. Wong CA, Cole AA, Watson L, Webb JK, Johnston ID, Kinnear Wj. Pulmonary function before and after anterior spinal surgery in adult idiopathic scoliosis. *Thorax* 1996; 51: 534–536.
48. Ferris G, Pieras E, Vergara P, *et al.* Kyphoscoliosis ventilation insufficiency: noninvasive management outcome. *Am J Phys Med Rehabil* 2000; 79: 24–29.
49. Hill NS, Eveloff SE, Carlisle CC, Goff SG. Efficacy of nocturnal nasal ventilation in patients with restrictive thoracic disease. *Am Rev Respir Dis* 1992; 145: 305–371.
50. Simonds AK, Elliott MW. Outcome of domiciliary nasal intermittent positive pressure ventilation in restrictive and obstructive disorders. *Thorax* 1995; 50: 604–609.
51. Meister R, Merkel Th. Beziehungen zwischen Wirbelsäulenfunktion und Atmung bei ankylosierender Spondylitis (M. Bechterew). *Prax Klin Pneumol* 1983; 37: 691–694.
52. Nava S, Zanotti E, Ambrosino N, *et al.* Evidence of acute diaphragmatic fatigue in a 'natural' condition. *Am Rev Resp Dis* 1992; 140: 1226–1230.

# CHAPTER 11

# Treatment of suppurative lung disease

G. Massard

Correspondence: G. Massard, Cardio-thoracic Surgery/Université Louis Pasteur, Service de Chirurgie Thoracique, Hôpitaux Universitaires de Strasbourg, F-67091, Strasbourg, France.

The conjunction of a well working social system, together with the major advances in the treatment of infectious diseases over recent decades, might explain why surgery for suppurative lung diseases has become rare in Western Europe. As a consequence, surgeons with extensive experience in this field have also become greatly outnumbered. The presented chapter summarises the experience drawn from the author's own centre and from recently published series. For the sake of clarity, the chapter is divided into four sections: aspergillus-related diseases, bronchiectasis, multi-drug resistant tuberculosis, and pneumonectomy for destroyed lung.

## Thoracic aspergillosis

Thoracic aspergillosis is by far the most common fungal disease of the lung and the pleura requiring surgical treatment in Western Europe. Traditionnally, thoracic aspergillosis has been classified into three categories: the saprophytic infection, leading to fungus balls within parenchymal or pleural cavities; the invasive aspergillosis observed in neutropenic or immunocompromised patients; and the allergic broncho-pulmonary aspergillosis. In classic textbooks, only the saprophytic aspergilloma has received surgical interest.

During the past decade, an increasing amount of publications have underlined that surgical management may improve the outcome of selected patients with invasive aspergillosis. Futhermore, at least three distinct new clinical entities have been described: semi-invasive aspergillosis; ulcerative tracheo-bronchitis in transplant recipients; and anecdotal cutaneous aspergillosis or osteomyelitis.

### *Classic saprophytic pulmonary aspergilloma*

Despite being considered an old-fashioned disease, at least six articles dealing with aspergilloma have been published in major medical journals during the past four years, illustrating the renewed interest in this disorder.

Surgical resection in such patients is known to be technically challenging and to convey a huge mortality and morbidity. Therefore, many authors have restricted surgical indications to heavily symptomatic patients, and advocate simple surveillance in asymptomatic patients. The main aim of this chapter is to defend an aggressive surgical management whenever possible: symptomatic patients need to be alleviated, and asymptomatic patients should be operated on to prevent further progression of their disease.

The authors of all recent publications validate the radiological classification of Belcher and Plummer [1], distinguishing simple and complex aspergilloma. Complex

Eur Respir Mon, 2004, 29, 168–180. Printed in UK - all rights reserved. Copyright ERS Journals Ltd 2004; European Respiratory Monograph; ISSN 1025-448x. ISBN 1-904097-33-2.

aspergilloma is characterised by thick-walled cavities and associated parenchymal or pleural fibrosis; this presentation is characteristic for aspergilloma growing in former tuberculous caverns. Simple aspergilloma is characterised by a thin-walled cavity surrounded by normal lung and pleura, and is observed together with the so-called bronchial aspergilloma.

The clinical presentation closely follows this radiological classification: many data show that patients with simple aspergilloma are usually asymptomatic; patients with complex aspergilloma have marked symptoms such as haemoptysis or bronchorrhea, and often have a poor nutritional and/or functional status [2, 3] (table 1).

The postoperative outcome is also related to this classification. Surgical morbidity such as intraoperative bleeding, postoperative bleeding, prolonged air-leak, need for thoracoplasty, and respiratory failure are significantly lower in patients with simple aspergilloma. In previous work, excessive bleeding was seen in 20% of simple aspergillomas, and in 60% of complex aspergillomas, the rates for pleural space disease were 20 and 36% respectively [2]. Except in one series [3], there were virtually no postoperative deaths following resection for simple aspergilloma (table 2).

A further observation is an obvious shift from a majority of complex aspergillomas towards a current predominance of simple aspergillomas [8]. All these data arguments confirm the recommendation for the liberal use of surgery in patients with aspergilloma, since there is no alternative in very symptomatic patients, whilst in asymptomatic patients the operation carries a low risk and may prevent further complications (table 3).

The choice of the adequate procedure is of paramount importance. The ideal treatment consists of resection of both the mycetoma and the underlying cavity. Lobectomy is therefore the option of choice [2, 3, 7]. Segmentectomy is subjected to a higher incidence of prolonged air-leak, and might favour intraoperative seeding. Pneumonectomy carries a prohibitive risk for empyema and/or bronchial fistula and should be avoided whenever possible [9]. In patients with seriously disabled lung function, parenchymal resection is contraindicated. In such patients, cavernostomy and removal of the fungal material, followed by thoracoplasty, may yield excellent medium term results; however, operative risk is substantial, as shown by a mortality rate in excesss of 10% [2].

**Table 1. – Comparative demographic data of patients with various forms of aspergilloma**

| | Pulmonary aspergilloma | Bronchial aspergilloma | Pleural aspergilloma |
|---|---|---|---|
| Subject n | 55 | 6 | 16 |
| Mean age yrs | 48.2 | 40.2 | 54.6 |
| Mean weight % of ideal | 86.2 | 111.8 | 83.8 |
| Mean VC % of predicted | 77.5 | 97.5 | 65.5 |

VC: vital capacity. Table adapted from [2].

**Table 2. – Comparative operative mortality following resection of simple and complex aspergilloma**

| First author [Ref.] | Patients n | Mortality | |
|---|---|---|---|
| | | Simple aspergilloma | Complex aspergilloma |
| BATTAGLINI [4] | 15 | 0 | 18.1 |
| DALY [3] | 53 | 4.7 | 34.3 |
| STAMATIS [5] | 29 | 0 | 11.7 |
| SHIRAKUSA [6] | 24 | 0 | 0 |
| MASSARD [2] | 63 | 0 | 10 |
| REGNARD [7] | 87 | 0 | 6.2 |

Data presented as % unless otherwise stated.

**Table 3. – Demographic and postoperative data comparing two chronological subsets of patients**

| Postoperative data | Years | |
|---|---|---|
| | 1974–1991 | 1992–1997 |
| Mean age yrs | 49 | 46 |
| Tuberculosis | 57.4 | 16.6 |
| Complex aspergilloma | 80 | 41.6 |
| Excessive bleeding | 44.1 | 8.3 |
| Prolonged air-leak | 47 | 16.6 |
| Hospital stay >30 days | 32.3 | 8.3 |

Data shown as % unless otherwise stated; Table adapted from [8].

## *Pleural aspergilloma*

Pleural aspergilloma is a rare disease, which has seldom been addressed in the literature [2]. There are two possible presentations. Early pleural aspergilloma presents as a postoperative empyema, during the first 4–6 weeks in patients who have undergone surgery for aspergilloma and who have prolonged air-leak. The most probable mechanism is intraoperative seeding. Late postoperative pleural aspergilloma occurs months or years following parenchymal resection and usually develops in a residual pleural space. Presence of a small bronchopleural fistula is required to carry aerosolised fungal spores towards the cavity. Treatment of such patients is tedious as they are usually in a poor general condition, and present with invalidating symptoms. Decortication is only feasible in patients who did not undergo parenchymal resection, as previous partial lung resection precludes complete obliteration of the pleural cavity by re-expansion of the residual lung. When loss of parenchymal volume is obvious, thoracoplasty remains the only surgical option. Muscle transfers are likely to fail because of previous thoracotomy and poor nutritional status. Due to the poor nutritional and functional status of these patients, there is a high rate of complications. In a series of 13 patients, two died postoperatively; nine experienced excessive bleeding; and eight required prolonged drainage. Hospital stay was in excess of 30 days for nine patients [2].

## *Semi-invasive aspergillosis*

Semi-invasive aspergillosis is rarely reported in the literature, although many centres have anecdotal experience with such patients [10]. This disease occurs preferentially in patients who underwent previous irradiation therapy; the onset mimicks an acute lobar pneumonia with high fever, which does not respond to antibiotics. After 2–3 weeks, a cavitation appears in the fibrosed lung, suggesting a complex aspergilloma. In such patients, completion pneumonectomy following previous lobectomy and irradiation therapy would have a tremendous risk owing to pleural adhesions and hilar fibrosis; operative mortality may reach 25% [11]. Thoracoplasty with removal of fungal material is a valuable option.

## *Invasive aspergillosis*

Invasive aspergillosis accounts for 30% of all fungal infections in patients with leukaemia; at least 5% of patients treated with leukaemia will develop invasive aspergillosis. Prevalence increases to 70% if neutropenia exceeds 34 days. Mortality is high despite early antifungal treatment; the overall mortality rates are 50% during neutropenia, and in excess of 90% after bone marrow graft. Approximately 15% of all patients with invasive aspergillosis could be subjected to surgical care [12].

The onset of invasive aspergillosis occurs usually during neutropenia. Fungal hyphae invade pulmonary vessels and produce peripheral infarctions; at this stage, a computed tomography (CT) scan reveals a rounded opacity surrounded by a low density halo [12, 13]. While bone marrow recovers, neutrophiles colonise the infarcted areas and cause further tissue necrosis; which presents radiologically as the air-crescent sign. Necrosis may lead to haemoptysis, especially when the lesions are close to major branches of the pulmonary artery.

In a patient receiving chemotherapy, any three of the following items may be suggestive of invasive aspergillosis: neutropenia; pneumonia; haemoptysis; persistent fever despite antibiotics; chest pain; halo sign; or air crescent sign [12].

Noninvasive diagnosis may rely on detection of aspergillus antigen and culture of aspergillus on bronchoalveolar lavage fluid (BALF). Although identification of antigen is correlated with a strong positive predictive value >90%, BALF is negative for aspergillus in >50% of patients [14].

Surgical management may be indicated to serve two main purposes. Firstly, to prevent massive haemoptysis [13], in this situation, radiology demonstrates a necrotic lesion close to a major vessel. Operations are performed on an emergency basis in patients who may not have a completely recovered bone marrow. In a series including eight patients, who were operated on during aplasia, there was no operative death; however, aspergillosis recurred and caused death in two patients [13]. Secondly, to prevent reinfection during subsequent chemotherapy [12], in this situation, an elective operation is scheduled to remove mycotic sequestra, which could be a source for reinfection during subsequent neutropenia. Such operations are planned once the patients' bone marrow has fully recovered. Several reports describe successful bone marrow transplantation after such procedures. Operative risk is acceptable with a mortality rate of >10%. Medium term results are acceptable with a recurrence rate of <10% (table 4).

The basic principle of such operations is to use parenchyma-sparing resections, similar to surgery for pulmonary metastases. Pneumonectomy should be avoided, because of the high risk for lethal complictions.

## *Aspergillus bronchitis*

This entity has been described in a short series of heart–lung graft recipients reported by the Stanford group [19]. The usual presentation is an ulcerative tracheobronchitis with abundant fibrin deposits, located in the immediate vicinity of the airway anastomosis and in the proximal segment of the donor airway. Microbiological analysis of the fibrin deposits identifies high concentration of fungal hyphae. One-third of the patients progressed to a fatal invasive aspergillosis. Therefore, early and aggressive treatment is

**Table 4. – Operative mortality and relapse of aspergillosis following surgery**

| First author [Ref.] | Patients n | Operative mortality n | Relapse aspergillosis n |
|---|---|---|---|
| Baron [12] | 12 | 0 | 1 |
| Bernard [13] | 7 | 0 | 0 |
| Lupinetti [15] | 6 | 1 | 3 |
| Robinson [16] | 16 | 5 | 1 |
| Wong [17] | 16 | 1 | 0 |
| Young [18] | 8 | 0 | N.S. |

N.S.: not stated.

mandatory. In the author's experience, a patient with aspergillus bronchitis following right single-lung transplantation succumbed to a broncho-arterial fistula [20].

### *Other forms of aspergillus infections*

Patients may present with a cutaneous abcess at the site of a central venous line or with osteomyelitis of the sternum. All patients recovered with antifungal treatment after surgical debridement [21, 22].

### *Conclusion*

Aspergillus may cause a wide spectrum of diseases within the chest. Adequate management requires knowledge of the feasibilities of surgical management. The management of these, often complicated, patients should be routinely discussed on a multidisciplinary basis.

## Bronchiectasis

Bronchiectasis may result from very different causal factors. An exhaustive classification is presented in table 5, defining two fundamentally different categories, *i.e.* congenital and acquired bronchiectasis. A functional classification has been proposed by Ashour [23], who has observed that the usual acinar bronchiectasis have virtually no systemic vascularisation, whereas the tubular bronchiectases have a relatively important systemic vascularisation. In extreme situations, there may be a significant left to right shunt, which the authors have described as the "acquired patent ductus syndrome". In the latter case, the operation does not only cure the infectious disease, but also corrects the haemodynamic abnormalities.

In the perspective of surgical management, the precise anatomical extent of the bronchiectatis malformations is the most important consideration. Patients may be simply classified as having localised or diffuse bronchiectasis.

The concept of localised bronchiectasis may include bilateral disease, but focussed on precise anatomic territories (usually basal segments on either side, right middle lobe and lingula) alternating with normal surrounding lung tissue [24]. This disease has become rare as a result of the early use of antibiotics in cases of pneumonia, bacterial bronchitis or sinusitis in children. In such patients, precise surgical resection favouring anatomical segmental resections, may significantly improve the patients quality of life (as described

**Table 5. – Classification of bronchiectasis according to the cause of disease**

| Congenital bronchiectasis | Acquired bronchiectasis |
|---|---|
| Polycystic lung disease | Recurrent infection (+/- sinusitis) |
| | Bronchial obstruction |
| | Tumour |
| | Corpus alienum |
| IgA deficiency | Extrinsic compression |
| Hypo $\gamma$-globulinaemia | Tuberculosis |
| Agenesia of cartilage | Post-traumatic stenosis |
| Ciliary syndromes | Diseases of the upper digestive tract |
| | Zencker's diverticulum |
| | Reflux disease |
| Cystic fibrosis | |

IgA: immunoglobulin A.

later in this chapter). Incomplete resection, leaving diseased bronchi, will eventually lead to recurrence of symptoms, and progression to chronic respiratory failure.

Diffuse bronchiectasis may occur as a sporadic disease, but is most often associated with cystic fibrosis in the Western world. Such patients are potential candidates for bilateral lung transplantation and should be carefully followed. Regular courses of antibiotics significantly improves prognosis by delaying the onset of chronic respiratory failure. Deterioration of the respiratory function is ultimately associated with bronchial colonisation with *Staphylococcus aureus* or *Pseudomonas* sp.. Indication for transplantation is to be discussed when life expectancy is estimated to be <2 yrs. Usual indicators of such ominous prognosis are decrease of forced expiratory volume in one second (FEV1) <30%, dependance on antibiotics, weight loss, and hypercarbia [25, 26].

This chapter will focus on indications and results of resection for localised bronchiectasis.

Morphological definition of the precise extent of the disease is the cornerstone of decision making. In this respect, bronchography represents the historic standard. There is no doubt that high resolution CT scans are the new gold standard for diagnosis with sensitivity and specificity rates >95% [27]. Another study demonstrated a false negative and a false positive rate of only 2% and 1% respectively [28].

Surgical treatment should be considered in the presence of gross (recurrent) haemoptysis, and recurrent infection with or without abcess formation. In addition, failure of nonsurgical management and poor compliance to treatment are reasonable indications. The surgical option should also be discussed in children with relapsing infection [24, 29–32].

The basic type of resection is anatomical segmentectomy. Lower lobe disease is amenable to resection of the basal segments; lingular disease is dealt with segmental resection of the lingula. Middle lobe disease requires middle lobectomy. In multisegmental disease, basal segmental resection may be combined with middle lobectomy or lingular resection. Bilateral operations on a sequential basis have proved to be safe [24]. It should be underlined that anatomical segmentectomies are technically more demanding than standard lobectomies, and that such resections should be performed in large and experienced centres, as has also been demonstrated for lung cancer resection [33]. An important adjunct to the operation is perioperative care. Preoperatively, the patient should be prepared with aggressive physiotherapy and antibiotics chosen according to sputum sample cultures; ideally, the operation should be undertaken in a patient with a "dry bronchial tree" [30].

Reported mortality rates are low, and close to 0 in the most recent publications. Complications are observed in 20–25% of patients and include perioperative bleeding due to adhesions and hyperplasia of bronchial vessels. Also sputum retention, and prolonged air-leak or residual air spaces are frequently encountered. Quite obviously, prevalence of pleural space disease is related to the number of resected segments (table 6).

Table 7 summarises the assessment of the operative risk in some major series. Bilateral

**Table 6. – Complications related to the extent of the resection**

| | Segments | | |
|---|---|---|---|
| | 2 | 4–5 | 6–7 |
| Subjects n | 23 | 32 | 31 |
| Bleeding >600 mL | 13 | 25 | 29 |
| Air-leak >10 days | 8.6 | 18.7 | 25.8 |
| Residual space | 13 | 28.1 | 35.5 |

Data are presented as % unless otherwise stated.

sequential resection does not significantly increase the operative risk: in a series of 16 patients reported by MAZIÈRES *et al.* [24], there was no mortality, whereas complications were observed in 18% of the patients.

Following resection, ~60% of patients may be considered as cured; 30% have a considerable improvement of their symptoms, and 10% remain unchanged. If resection is incomplete, the cure rate decreases to 20%; still 50% of patients will have decreased symptoms, but 30% remain unchanged (table 8). Multivariate logistic resection analysis revealed three positive prognostic factors: cylindrical type of bronchiectasis, absence of sinusitis, and complete resection [31].

This certainly questions the role of incomplete resections. On the one hand, it appears feasable and may transiently improve symptoms; on the other hand, it is unlikely to change the natural history of the disease. Moreover, the increased operative risk of completion pneumonectomy if a further operation is required should be considered and take into account that it may interfere with the later possibility of lung transplantation.

## Multidrug-resistant tuberculosis

Lung surgery has been initially performed for patients suffering from tuberculosis. This disease remains a major challenge in countries with low socio-economic status. In the Western world, public health policies have controlled tuberculosis during recent decades, with an observed progressive decrease of its prevalence until the end of the 1980s. Increase of migration during recent years has again led to a slight increase of the prevalence.

Indications for surgery may be either complications of the natural history of the disease such as a destroyed lung, haemoptysis, bronchial stenosis and chronic bronchopleural fistula, or the presence of multidrug-resistant infection [35]. Resection for multidrug-resistent tuberculosis has two aims: firstly, the operation has a curative intent for the individual patient; and secondly, resection may prevent further spreading of infection in the community.

Patients with multidrug-resistant tuberculosis usually present with thick-walled cavitary disease or a destroyed lobe. The parenchymal cavities contain huge amounts of mycobacteria ($10^7$–109 per g of tissue) [35]. Removal of this bacterial burden is essential for treatment. Preoperatively, an attempt should be made to convert the

**Table 7. – Operative risk of resection for bronchiectasis**

| First author [Ref.] | Subjects n | Mortality % | Morbidity % |
|---|---|---|---|
| DOGAN [34] | 487 | 3.1 | 11 |
| KUTLAY [29] | 166 | 1.7 | 10.5 |
| AGASTHIAN [32] | 134 | 2.2 | 25 |
| PRIETO [30] | 119 | 0 | 15 |
| ASHOUR [23] | 85 | 0 | 17 |
| FUJIMOTO [31] | 90 | 0 | 20 |

**Table 8. – Long-term results in relation to completeness of resection**

| | Total | R0 | R1 |
|---|---|---|---|
| Cured | 59.2 | 65.2 | 21.4 |
| Improved | 29.1 | 25.8 | 50.0 |
| Unchanged | 11.7 | 9.0 | 28.6 |

Data are presented as %; R0: complete resection; R1: incomplete resection.

patient's sputum smear and culture, although this will not be achieved in ~50% of patients, even with appropriate antibiotics. The anti-tuberculous regimen chosen should ideally be given for a 3-month period prior to the operation. At the same time, the patient's nutritional status should be corrected, as they are often nutritionally deprived.

The basic principle of surgery is to remove all cavitary disease. Scattered nodular disease may be left because mycobacterial burden is low ($10^2$–$10^4$ per g of tissue). However, such resections remain technically challenging due to well-vascularised pleural adhesions and hilar fibrosis. Careful operative technique is mandatory. Taping hilar vessels prior to any dissection of lobar branches, is recommended in order to be ready for expeditious clamping, should a vascular injury occur. Scarred lung tissue sets a risk for failing re-expansion, but single stage thoracoplasty should be avoided.

Despite the technical complexity of such resections, the reported mortality rates are low and may vary 0–3% (table 9). The most serious postoperative complication is bronchopleural fistula. Factors favouring this complication are persistent positive sputum, polymicrobial super-infection, malnutrition and diabetes [35]. In case of pneumonectomy, such factors may trigger a fistula rate in excess of 30%. However, after segmentectomy or lobectomy, its incidence is usually <5%. Among other complications, bleeding during or after the operation is the most frequent (table 9).

Surgery remains an effective treatment of multidrug resistant disease, because the sputum conversion rate ranges from 75–96% (table 10). As such, surgery is not only useful to the individual patient, but also helps to control the spread of the disease.

# Destroyed lung

Pneumonectomy for destroyed lung remains a distressing problem which may be regarded as one of the most serious surgical challenges in general thoracic surgery.

Conditions that may lead to destructive lung disease may be classified into the following categories: sequellae of tuberculosis; sequellae of treatment for lung cancer (and more specifically irradiation pneumonitis or bronchial stenosis following bronchoplasty); or congenital malformations or severe unilateral forms of bronchiectasis [40].

Tuberculosis is by far the leading cause in Western series, whereas in Eastern countries, there is a relatively equal balance between tuberculosis and bronchiectasis (table 11).

**Table 9. – Immediate postoperative results after resection for tuberculosis**

| First author [Ref.] | Patients n | Mortality % | Morbidity % |
|---|---|---|---|
| Pomerantz [35] | 172 | 3.3 | 12 |
| Furak [36] | 144 | 1.4 | 46 |
| Sung [37] | 27 | 0 | 26 |
| Van Leuven [38] | 62 | 1.6 | 23 |
| Treasure [39] | 59 | 0 | 10 |

**Table 10. – Sputum conversion following resection for multi-drug resistant tuberculosis**

| First author [Ref.] | Operated n | Converted n | % |
|---|---|---|---|
| Treasure [39] | 19 | 17 | 89 |
| Van Leuven [38] | 24 | 18 | 75 |
| Sung [37] | 27 | 22 | 81 |
| Pomerantz [35] | 91 | 87 | 96 |

**Table 11. – Prevalence of history of tuberculosis in patients with destroyed lung**

| First author [Ref.] | Patients n | Tuberculosis % |
|---|---|---|
| BLYTH [41] | 155 | 72 |
| CONLAN [42] | 124 | 86 |
| HALEZEROGLU [43] | 118 | 40 |
| MASSARD [40] | 25 | 60 |

Destructive lung disease predominates on the left side: 21 out of 27 pneumonectomies in the series of RIZZI *et al.* [44] were left-sided, and 13 out of 18 in the experience of TREASURE and SEAWORTH [39]. ASHOUR *et al.* [45] described the so-called left bronchus syndrome, consisting of a, preferentially, left lung destruction (12 out of 13 in their experience) associated with an important left-to-right shunt through bronchial-to-pulmonary arterial flow. According to the latter authors, anatomical features are likely to explain the predominance of disease on the left side: the narrower calibre of the bronchus is further surrounded by the aortic arch; thus, enlarged lymph nodes favour bronchial compression, resulting in retention of secretions and infection. Besides, hyperplasia of mediastinal lymph nodes might be more important in African and Asian patients. POMERANTZ *et al.* [46] confirmed a left predominance in patients with *Mycobacterium tuberculosis* infection (21 out of 23), whereas this did not apply to patients with atypical mycobacterial infection (only eight out of 17 were left-sided). From the authors previously published work, 60% of destroyed lungs were left-sided; this predominance was confirmed for both tuberculosis and bronchiectasis [40].

Pneumonectomy is usually indicated for recurrent infections. In some patients, however, surgery may be required because of a massive shunting through hyperplastic bronchial vessels; the latter has been referred to as the acquired patent ductus syndrome [23, 46]. In very sick patients, unfit for a prolonged operation with risk of strong bleeding, there could be an indication for the so-called "physiological pneumonectomy". Through a transsternal approach, the surgeon divides the pulmonary artery and the bronchus, leaving the lung in place; complementary resection may be performed a couple of months later, if the patient's condition has improved.

All authors agree that pneumonectomy for chronic infection is a real technical challenge. REED [47] reported a mean operative time of 5.7 h, a mean blood loss of 2.083 mL, and a mean transfusion of 6.23 units; bleeding was in excess of 1,000 mL in nine out of 13 patients, and three patients encountered a tear of the *vena cava* during hilar dissection. Intraoperatively, difficulties may arise from pleural adhesions, perihilar scarring, and hyperplasia of both hilar nodes and bronchial vessels. Considerable blood loss should always be anticipated. Aprotinine may control diffuse oozing, intrapericardial dissection of the hilar structures or bronchus-first approach are helpful when hilar fibrosis precludes a standard dissection. Hilar dissection is particularly demanding during completion pneumonectomy. In the Mayo Clinic (MN, USA) experience, four patients with irradiation pneumonitis died intraoperatively from hilar bleeding [48].

Given the high risk for bronchopleural fistula, especially in the presence of granulomatous infection, the bronchial stump should always be butressed with a flap of viable and well vascularised tissue [49]. Transsternal approach has been recommended to allow for easier dissection of the hilar vessels, and for expeditive installation of cardiopulmonary bypass in case of central vascular injury [47]. However, the transsternal approach offers a poor exposure of the posterior area of the pleural sac, where adhesions are usually the tightest.

Reported operative mortality rates range form 2–5% (table 1), however, when completion pneumonectomy in patients with previous irradiation therapy, is necessary,

**Table 12. – Operative risk of pneumonectomy for chronic infection**

| First author [Ref.] | Patients n | Deaths % | Complications % | Empyema/fistula |
|---|---|---|---|---|
| Blyth [41] | 155 | 1.2 | 23 | 16.7 |
| Conlan [42] | 124 | 2.4 | | 20.9 |
| Halezeroglu [43] | 118 | 5.9 | 12 | 13.2 |
| Massard [40] | 25 | 4.0 | | 44.0 |

mortality may exceed 25% [48]. Radiation fibrosis leads to sclerosis of bronchial vessels, and explains poor bronchial healing. Furthermore, the particularly dense adhesions may lead to traumatic surgery.

Major perioperative threats are secundary bleeding, empyema and bronchopleural fistula. The prevalence is high and at least 25% (table 12). Intraoperative and postoperative bleeding is easily explained by the usually dense and well vascularised adhesions, and in addition by the hypertrophy of bronchial vessels associated with chronic infection. Empyema is an expected complication in septic lung surgery. In the authors own series, a significant increase of empyema has been observed in patients with a history of tuberculosis, in the presence of aspergilloma, and when gross intraoperative spillage has occurred [40]. The excessively high rate of empyema and/or fistula in that series may be related to the association of sequellae of tuberculosis with aspergilloma: five out of seven patients within this context developed empyema postoperatively [40]. Bronchial fistula is a consequence of bronchial devascularisation during dissection and merely reflects the complexity of the operation. However, some fistulae also occur as spontaneous drainage of an otherwise unrecognised empyema. Again, tuberculosis, aspergilloma and intraoperative spillage are factors of increased risk; furthermore, right-sided operations are associated with a higher fistula rate, which is also reported after cancer surgery. Pomerantz *et al.* [46] pointed to an increased risk for fistula in case of surgery for atypical mycobacterial infection: they observed only one fistula among 23 patients with *M. tuberculosis* infection, and eight among 17 patients with atypical mycobacterial infection [45]. Positive sputum at the time of operation is a well recognised risk factor [42, 45]. Halezeroglu *et al.* [43] confirmed that preoperative empyema, tuberculosis and right-sided operations are associated with an increased risk for complications. It is interesting to underline that the series reported by Halezeroglu *et al.* [43] has the lowest complication rate while containing 40% of patients with tuberculosis (table 11).

## Conclusion

Suppurative lung disease does not represent a single disease entity, but a whole spectrum of disorders. The common denominator is that such procedures are technically demanding and that patient's general health status has already suffered from chronic infection. Such patients require expert management and should be cared for exclusively in highly specialised thoracic surgical units.

## Summary

Surgery for suppurative lung disease is often technically demanding and the patient may have an increased operative risk because their general health status has mostly suffered from the infectious disease status. Thoracic aspergillosis is by far the most common fungal disease of the lung and the pleura, requiring surgical care in Western Europe. For a long time, only the saprophytic aspergilloma has received surgical interest, but in the last decade it has become clear that surgical management may also improve the outcome of selected patients with invasive aspergillosis. Patients with bronchiectasis should be considered for surgery when the disease is localised and when they present with haemoptysis and/or recurrent infections with failure of medical treatment and poor compliance to this treatment. The basic principle of surgery in multidrug-resistant tuberculosis is to remove all cavitary disease after the antibiotic regimen has already been given for a 3-month period; the operation has a curative intent and prevents spreading of these multidrug-resistant mycobacteria in the community. Pneumonectomy for destroyed lung is mostly indicated because of recurrent infections; it remains a distressing problem which may be regarded as one of the most serious challenges in general thoracic surgery.

**Keywords:** Aspergillosis, bronchiectasis, destroyed lung, lung surgery, multidrug-resistant tuberculosis.

# References

1. Belcher JR, Plummer NS. Surgery in bronchopumonary aspergillosis. *Br J Dis Chest* 1960; 54: 335–341.
2. Massard G, Roeslin N, Wihlm JM, Dumont P, Witz JP, Morand G. Pleuropulmonary aspergilloma. Clinical spectrum and results of surgical treatment. *Ann Thorac Surg* 1992; 54: 1159–1164.
3. Daly RC, Pairolero PC, Piehler JM, Trastek VF, Payne WS, Bernatz PE. Pulmonary aspergilloma. Results of surgical treatment. *J Thorac Cardiovasc Surg* 1986; 92: 981–988.
4. Battaglini JW, Murray GF, Keagy BA, Starek PJ, Wilcox BR. Surgical management of symptomatic pulmonary aspergilloma. *Ann Thorac Surg* 1985; 39: 512–516.
5. Stamatis G, Greschuchna D. Surgery for pulmonary aspergilloma and pleural aspergillosis. *Thorac Cardiovasc Surgeon* 1988; 36: 356–360.
6. Shirakusa T, Ueda H, Suito T, *et al.* Surgical treatment of pulmonary aspergilloma and aspergillus empyema. *Ann Thorac Surg* 1989; 48: 779–782.
7. Regnard JF, Icard P, Nicolisi M, *et al.* Aspergilloma: a series of 89 surgical cases. *Ann Thorac Surg* 2000; 69: 898–903.
8. Chatzimichalis A, Massard G, Barsotti P, Kessler R, Wihlm JM. Surgery for aspergilloma: a reappraisal. *Ann Thorac Surg* 1998; 65: 927–929.
9. Massard G, Dabbagh A, Wihlm JM, *et al.* Pneumonectomy for chronic infection is a high risk procedure. *Ann Thorac Surg* 1996; 62: 1033–1038.
10. Kibbler CC, Milkins SR, Bhamra A, Spiteri MA, Noone P, Prentice HG. Apparent pulmonary mycetoma following invasive aspergillosis in neutropenic patients. *Thorax* 1988; 43: 108–112.
11. McGovern EM, Trastek VF, Pairolero PC, Payne WS. Completion pneumonectomy: indications, complications and results. *Ann Thorac Surg* 1988; 46: 141–146.
12. Baron O, Guilaumé B, Moreau P, *et al.* Aggressive surgical management in localised pulmonary mycotic and nonmycotic infections for neutropenic patients with acute leukaemia. *J Thorac Cardiovasc Surg* 1998; 115: 63–69.
13. Bernard A, Caillot D, Couailler JF, Casasnovas O, Guy H, Favre JP. Surgical management of pulmonary aspergillosis in neutropenic patients. *Ann Thorac Surg* 1997; 64: 1441–1447.
14. Saito H, Anaissie EJ, Morice RC, Dekmezian R, Bodey GP. Bronchoalveolar lavage in the diagnosis of pulmonary infiltrates in patient with acute leukaemia. *Chest* 1988; 94: 745–749.

15. Lupinetti FM, Behrendt DM, Giller RH, *et al.* Pulmonary resection for fungal infection in children undergoing bone marrow transplantation. *J Thorac Cardiovasc Surg* 1992; 104: 684–687.
16. Robinson LA, Reed EC, Galbraith TA, Alonso A, Moulton A, Fleming WH. Pulmonary resection for invasive Aspergillus infections in immunocompromised patients. *J Thorac Cardiovasc Surg* 1995; 109: 1182–1197.
17. Wong K, Waters CM, Walesby RK. Surgical management of invasive pulmonary aspergillosis in immunocompromised patients. *Eur J Cardiothorac Surg* 1992; 6: 138–143.
18. Young VK, Maghur HA, Luke DA, McGovern EM. Operation for cavitating invasive pulmonary aspergillosis in immunocompromized patients. *Ann Thorac Surg* 1992; 53: 621–624.
19. Kramer MR, Denning DW, Marshall SE, *et al.* Ulcerative tracheobronchitis after lung transplantation. A new form of invasive aspergillosis. *Am Rev Respir Dis* 1991; 144: 552–556.
20. Kessler R, Massard G, Warter A, Wihlm JM, Weitzenblum E. Bronchial_pulmonary artery fistula after unilateral lung transplantation: a case report. *J Heart Lung Transplant* 1997; 16: 674–677.
21. Walker WA, Pate JW. Primary aspergillus osteomyelitis of the sternum. *Ann Thorac Surg* 1991; 52: 868–870.
22. Buescher TM, Moritz DM, Killyon GW. Resection of chest wall and central veins for invasive cutaneous aspergillus infection in an immunocompromized patient. *Chest* 1994; 105: 1283–1285.
23. Ashour M. Hemodynamic alterations in bronchiectasis: a base for a new subclassification of the disease. *J Thorac Cardiovasc Surg* 1996; 112: 328–334.
24. Mazières J, Murris M, Didier A, *et al.* Limited operation for severe multisegmental bilateral bronchiectasis. *Ann Thorac Surg* 2003; 75: 382–387.
25. Egan TM, Detterbeck TM, Mill MR, *et al.* Long term results of lung transplantation for cystic fibrosis. *Eur J Cardiothorac Surg* 2002; 22: 602–609.
26. Vricella L, Karamichalis JM, Ahmad S, Robbins RC, Whyte RI, Reitz BA. Lung and heart-lung transplantation in patients with end-stage cystic fibrosis: the Stanford experience. *Ann Thorac Surg* 2002; 74: 13–18.
27. Munro NC, Cooke JC, Currie DC, Strickland B, Cole PJ. Comparison of thin section computed tomography with bronchography for identifying bronchiectatic segments in patients with chronic sputum production. *Thorax* 1990; 45: 135–139.
28. Young K, Aspestrand F, Kolbenstedt A. High resolution CT and bronchography in the assessment of bronchiectasis. *Acta Radiol* 1991; 32: 439–441.
29. Kutlay H, Cangir AK, Enön S, *et al.* Surgical treatment in bronchiectasis: analysis of 166 patients. *Eur J Cardiothorac Surg* 2002; 21: 634–637.
30. Prieto D, Bernardo J, Matos MJ, Eugenio L, Antunes M. Surgery for bronchiectasis. *Eur J Cardiothorac Surg* 2001; 20: 19–24.
31. Fujimoto T, Hillejan L, Stamatis G. Current strategy for surgical management of bronchiectasis. *Ann Thorac Surg* 2001; 72: 1711–1715.
32. Aghastian T, Deschamps C, Trastek VF, Allen MS, Pairolero PC. Surgical management of bronchiectasis. *Ann Thorac Surg* 1996; 62: 976–978.
33. Birkmeyer JD, Siewers AE, Finlayson EVA, *et al.* Hospital volume and surgical mortality in the United States. *N Engl J Med* 2002; 346: 1128–1137.
34. Dogan R, Alp M, Kaya S, *et al.* Surgical treatment of bronchiectasis: a collective review of 487 cases. *Thorac Cardiovasc Surg* 1989; 37: 183–186.
35. Pomerantz BI, Cleveland JC, Olson HK, Pomerantz M. Pulmonary resection for multi-drug resistant tuberculosis. *J Thorac Cardiovasc Surg* 2001; 121: 448–453.
36. Furak J, Trojan I, Szöke T, *et al.* Surgical intervention for pulmonary tuberculosis: analysis of indications and perioperative data relating to diagnostic and therapeutic resections. *Eur J Cardiothorac Surg* 2001; 20: 722–727.
37. Sung SW, Kang CH, Kim YT, Han SK, Shim YS, Kim JH. Surgery increased the chance of cure in multidrug resistant pulmonary tuberculosis. *Eur J Cardiothorac Surg* 1999; 16: 187–193.
38. Van Leuven M, De Groot M, Shean KP, Von Oppell UO, Willcox PA. Pulmonary resection as an

adjunct in the treatment of multiple drug resistant tuberculosis. *Ann Thorac Surg* 1997; 63: 1368–1372.

39. Treasure RL, Seaworth BJ. Current role of surgery in mycobacterium tuberculosis. *Ann thorac Surg* 1995; 59: 1405–1407.
40. Massard G, Dabbagh A, Wihlm JM, *et al.* Pneumonectomy for chjonic infection is a high-risk procedure. *Ann Thorac Surg* 1996; 62: 1033–1038.
41. Blyth DF. Pneumonectomy for inflammatory lung disease. *Eur J Cardiothorac Surg* 2000; 18: 429–434.
42. Conlan AA, Lukanich JM, Shutz J, Hurwitz SS. Elective pneumonectomy for benign lung disease: modern day mortality and morbidity. *J Thorac Cardiovasc Surg* 1995; 110: 1118–1124.
43. Halezeroglu S, Keles M, Uysal A, *et al.* Factors affecting postoperative morbidity and mortality in destroyed lung. *Ann Thorac Surg* 1997; 64: 1635–1638.
44. Rizzi A, Rocco G, Robustellini M, Rossi G, Della Pona C, Massera F. Results of surgical management of tuberculosis: experience in 206 patients undergoing operation. *Ann Thorac Surg* 1995; 59: 896–900.
45. Ashour M, Pandya L, Mezraqji A, *et al.* Unilateral posttuberculosis lung destruction: the left bronchus syndrome. *Thorax* 1990; 45: 210–212.
46. Pomerantz M, Madsen I, Gobble M, Iseman M. Surgical management of resistant mycobacterial pulmonary infection. *Ann Thorac Surg* 1991; 52: 1108–1112.
47. Reed CE. Pneumonectomy for chronic infection: fraught with danger? *Ann Thorac Surg* 1995; 59: 408–411.
48. McGovern EM, Trastek VF, Pairolero PC, Payne WS. Completion pneumonectomy: indications, complications and results. *Ann Thorac Surg* 1988; 46: 141–146.
49. Anderson TM, Miller JI. Use of pleura, azygos vein, pericardium, and muscle flaps in tracheobronchial surgery. *Ann Thorac Surg* 1995; 60: 729–733.

*CHAPTER 12*

# Surgical treatment of pleural infections: the surgeon's point of view

*H.B. Ris, E. Pezzetta, T. Krueger, D. Lardinois*

*Dept of Thoracic Surgery, Centre Hospitalier Universitaire Vaudois, Lausanne, Switzerland.*

*Correspondence: H.B. Ris, Service de Chirurgie Thoracique, Centre Hospitalier Universitaire Vaudois, CH-1011, Lausanne, Switzerland.*

Pleural empyema is a serious disease involving a large number of patients per year. It may lead to severe and disabling consequences if unrecognised or incorrectly treated. The main symptoms are related to uncontrolled infection (pain, weight loss, asthenia and temperature), and to restriction and ventilation-perfusion mismatch (dyspnoea). The mainstay of treatment of pleural empyema is therefore two-fold: prevention of ongoing and recurrent infection and prevention of late restriction [1–3]. Many surgical and nonsurgical treatment options are available for the treatment of pleural empyema (table 1). The choice of the appropriate intervention depends on the nature of the underlying disease, the chronicity of the empyema, and the patient's overall condition [4].

## Nature of underlying disease

Various underlying diseases may cause a pleural empyema. The recognition of the underlying disease is important since this may considerably influence the treatment strategy. Computed tomography (CT) scans are of utmost importance in estimating the chronicity of empyema and detecting its underlying cause and should be performed in every situation with suspected empyema. The current authors have analysed 282 consecutive patients with surgically treated American Thoracic Society (ATS) stage II and III [2] pleural empyema over a 10-yr period with respect to the surgical treatment applied and the underlying cause of empyema (table 2) [1]. Parapneumonic empyema (62%) was by far the most frequent indication in this series followed by postoperative (13%) and post-traumatic empyema (9%); empyema related to pulmonary embolism (6%) and tuberculosis (mixed empyema 6%); tumours or lung abscess (2%), pleural aspergillosis (2%), and pleural actinomycosis (0.4%).

**Table 1. – Options for the treatment of pleural empyema**

| |
|---|
| Antibiotics |
| Thoracocentesis, chest tube |
| Fibrinolysis |
| VATS debridement |
| Decortication |
| Myoplasty (intrathoracic muscle transfer) |
| Thoracoplasty |
| Open window thoracostomy (pleurostomy) |

VATS: video-assisted thoracoscopic surgery.

Eur Respir Mon, 2004, 29, 181–198. Printed in UK - all rights reserved. Copyright ERS Journals Ltd 2004; European Respiratory Monograph; ISSN 1025-448x. ISBN 1-904097-33-2.

**Table 2. – Underlying cause of pleural empyema in a consecutive series of 282 patients with surgically treated stage II and III empyema 1992–2002**

| Underlying cause | Patients | |
|---|---|---|
| | n | % |
| Parapneumonic | 175 | 62 |
| Postoperative | 38 | 13 |
| Post-traumatic | 24 | 9 |
| Pulmonary embolism (infarction) | 18 | 6 |
| Pleural tuberculosis | 16 | 6 |
| Abscess, tumour | 5 | 2 |
| Pleural aspergillosis | 5 | 2 |
| Pleural actinomycosis | 1 | 0.4 |

## *Parapneumonic empyema*

Parapneumonic empyema and its different stages have been well described, as have stage-related treatments. Parapneumonic effusions in the exudative stage may be treated by antibiotics, thoracocentesis, or tube thoracostomy. Complicated loculated effusions usually require other treatments such as fibrinolytic irrigation through chest tubes [5–9] or video-assisted thoracoscopic surgery (VATS) debridement [10–18]. Chronic parapneumonic empyema will usually require open decortication [1, 19, 20]. However, the extent of the parenchymal disease may require deviation from the planned treatment strategy. For instance, a patient with complicated fibrinopurulent empyema may not tolerate VATS debridement or open decortication in the presence of severe pneumonia with extensive bilateral infiltrations. In these situations, an early surgical intervention should be postponed unless the pneumonia has been resolved [21]. Repeated CT scans are of great importance to delineate the extent of the pleural and parenchymal pathology and to determine the evolution of the parenchymal alterations during conservative treatment [22].

## *Postoperative empyema*

Postoperative empyema poses a major challenge with respect to diagnosis and treatment [23]. It may arise after extrathoracic (abdominal, urological) or intrathoracic (cardiac, pulmonary) interventions. Abdominal surgery associated with peritonitis may lead to empyema by infection of accompanying pleural effusions, and urological interventions by contamination of the pleural cavity by a percutaneous nephrostomy, which might pass inadvertently through the pleural space. Severe descending mediastinitis, associated with bilateral empyema and pericarditis, may be observed after infections or interventions of the oropharynx, requiring early and extensive mediastinal debridement and bilateral decortication as a life-saving procedure [24]. Cardiac surgery may lead to empyema, which is often associated with sternum osteomyelitis and mediastinitis. Debridement of the mediastinum and the sternum associated with complex soft tissue reconstructions might be required in addition to debridement or decortication of the pleural cavities in these situations [25–27]. Empyema is not frequently observed after lung resection, however, its treatment may be difficult if it does occur. It is usually related to the inability of the remaining lung to fully re-expand and to the presence of a bronchopleural fistula. A postresectional empyema must be suspected if a pleural effusion occurs in the presence of fever and other signs of infection (leucocytosis, rise of C reactive protein:CRP). Bronchoscopy should be performed in order to rule out a bronchopleural fistula in conjuction with CT guided pigtail drainage of the pleural effusion, with pH measurements and microbiological examinations of the collected fluid. Intravenous administration of broad-spectrum antibiotics is initiated as soon as samples from the effusion have been harvested for microbiological analysis. The antibiotics are then adapted accordingly. In the absence of a bronchopleural fistula, daily instillation of a fibrinolytic agent (*e.g.* urokinase 100,000 IU per day ) may be performed through the pigtail until resolution of the empyema. Instillation of fibrinolytic agents has proven to be efficient in fibrinopurulent empyema [5–9]. Most postresectional emypema can be treated in this way in the absence of a bronchopleural fistula provided the lung is fully re-expanded after drainage without detectable postresectional residual space. However, if an infected post-resectional residual space persists despite drainage (which may be associated with a bronchopleural fistula), re-operation should be considered and decortication should be performed in association with space obliteration procedures such as thoracoplasty [28], or intrathoracic transposition of omentum [29–31] or extrathoracic muscle flaps [32–35].

Postpneumonectomy empyema occurs in ~3% of patients and deserves special consideration. The mortality of this dreadful complication has been considerably reduced due to modern management [23, 30, 36–38]. Postpneumonectomy empyema is often associated with a bronchopleural fistula and may be observed from several days up to several years after pneumonectomy. Several factors have been associated with the development of a postpneumonectomy empyema such as preoperative mediastinal irradiation, diabetes, active bronchial infection during operation, cardiac insufficiency, prolonged postoperative mechanical ventilation and the abscence of bronchial stump reinforcement by healthy tissues [39–43]. Postpneumonectomy empyema typically occurs 2 weeks after the operation with fever and signs of infection. Productive cough with abundant expectorations are observed in the presence of an associated bronchopleural fistula together with a drop of the air-fluid level on the operated side at standard chest radiographs (fig. 1). Postpneumonectomy empyema requires immediate chest drainage in order to prevent spillage of the contralateral lung by the fluid emerging from the postpneumonectomy cavity. Bronchoscopy is then performed to confirm or rule out a fistula and the appropriate treatment is chosen according to the presence or absence of a

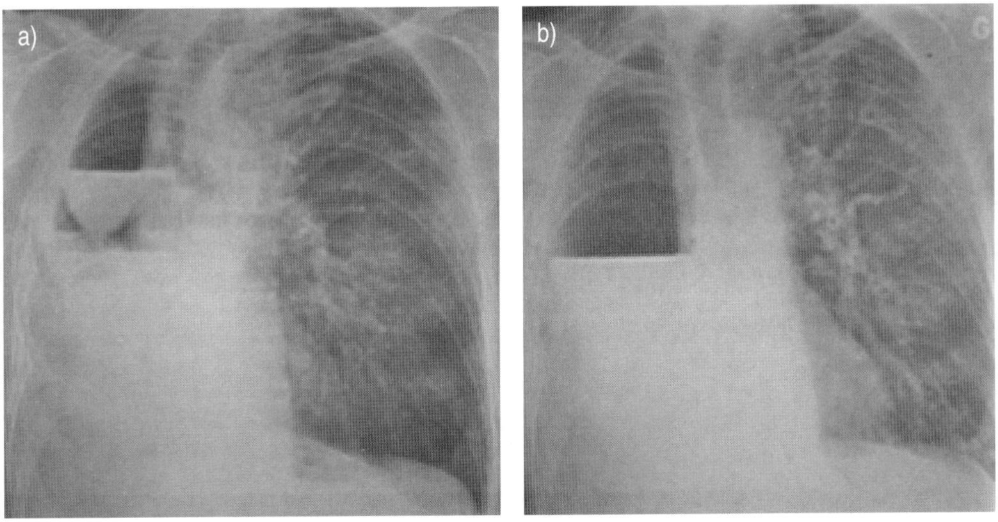


Fig. 1. – Drop of air-fluid level on standard chest RX after pneumonectomy suggesting postpneumonectomy empyema and bronchopleural fistula.

bronchopleural fistula (fig. 2). A thoracoscopic debridement followed by obliteration of the cavity by use of an antibiotic solution, according to CLAGETT and GERACI [44], may be performed in the absence of a fistula. In the presence of a small bronchopleural fistula (<1 mm), an endobronchial closure may be attempted using fibrin glue or a block of spongiosa [45, 46]. Larger fistulas usually require a re-thoracotomy, debridement of the cavity, closure of the fistula and reinforcement of the mediastinum by omentum, or an extra thoracic muscle flap transposed within the chest cavity [36, 38]. Intrathoracic muscle transposition of the latissimus dorsi or serratus anterior muscle has shown to be efficient in these situations [32–35]. These muscles may also be used for closure of the bronchial stump and reconstruction of the airway, where the use of a primary suture may be too risky [35] (fig. 3). After closure and reinforcement of the bronchial stump, the cavity is packed with betadine-soaked towels. The towels are changed every 48 h until the cavity and the mediastinum are covered by granulation tissue, which normally takes 2–3 weeks. This can be done by either a temporary open window thoracostomy or by re-adapting the skin between these interventions [47]. The cavity is then filled (obliterated) by Dab's solution (0.5 g neomycin, 0.1 g polymyxin B, 80 mg garamycin per litre of sodium chloride) [44]. This technique allowed permanent control of intrathoracic infection in ~88% of the patients, provided that the fistula remained closed [37].

## *Post-traumatic empyema*

Post-traumatic empyema in the current authors' series was seen in 9% of the patients. It may occur after blunt or penetrating chest trauma as a result of an infected haemothorax. Prompt drainage with large-bore chest tubes is important in cases of post-traumatic haemothorax in order to prevent empyema. Incorrect drainage and persistent

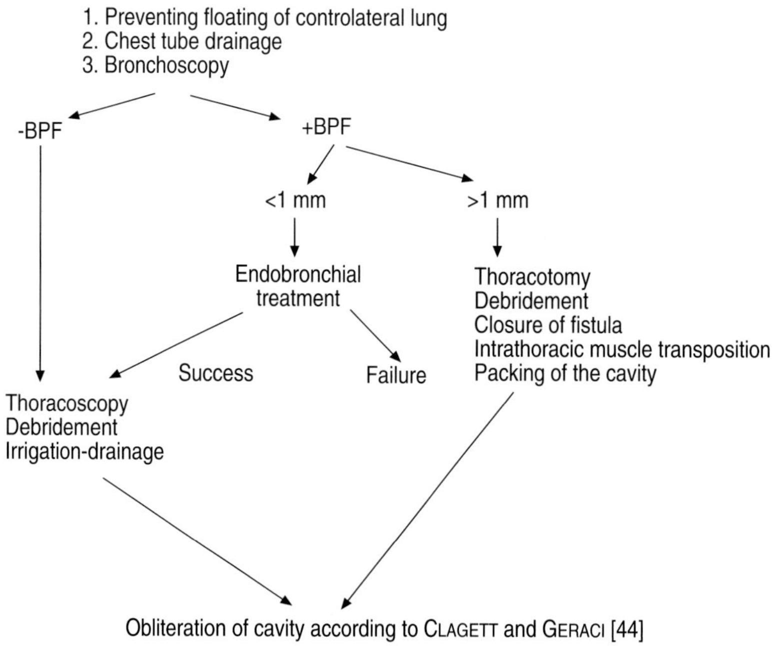


Fig. 2. – Algorithm for the diagnosis and treatment of postpneumonectomy empyema. BPF: bronchopleural fistula.

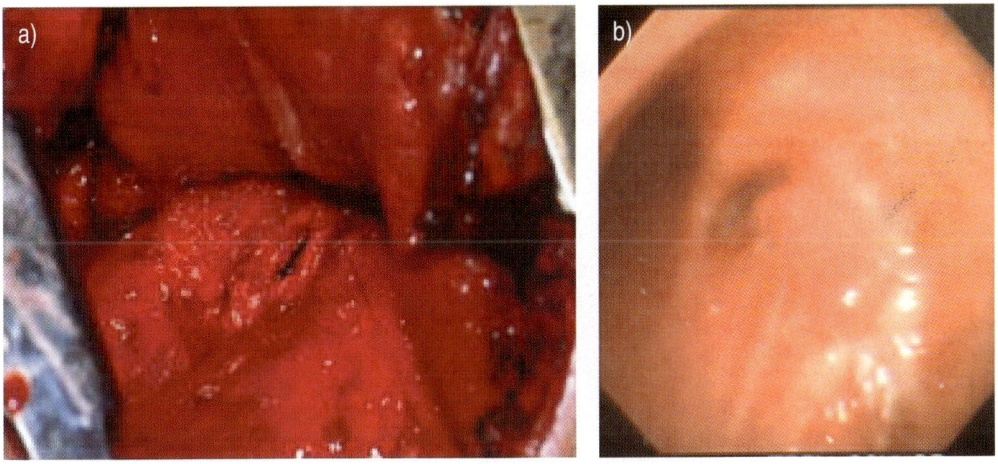

Fig. 3. – a) Repair of right-sided postpneumonectomy empyema with bronchial stump insufficiency. A pedicled intrathoracic serratus anterior muscle flap was transposed into the chest cavity and sutured into the defect airway without attempting primary closure. b) Endoscopic control after 2 months.

haemothorax may lead to empyema in ~20% of patients in certain series [48]. Persistent or recurrent effusion after drainage for post-traumatic haemothorax should be evacuated using thoracoscopy rather than by insertion of a new chest tube in order to prevent empyema. The reinsertion of a chest tube *versus* thoracoscopic clot removal was compared in a prospective, randomised study for recurrent or persistent haemothorax; empyema developed in 40 and 0% of the patients, respectively [49]. Post-traumatic empyema may also be associated with a flail chest; early treatment of respiratory insufficiency by peridural anaesthesia, intubation or surgical chest wall stabilisation by osteosynthesis is mandatory in order to prevent life-threatening septic complications [50].

## *Empyema related to pulmonary embolism*

Empyema related to pulmonary embolism is a rare event when compared with the incidence of pulmonary emboli; however, it was observed in 6% of the current authors' series of patients with surgically treated stage II and III empyema. Peripherally located pulmonary emboli may lead to absceding pulmonary infarction, with perforation and formation of empyema (fig. 4). Denominators for infarction after pulmonary embolism were investigated in 69 patients with pulmonary emboli [51], 36 patients without infarction were compared with 33 patients who developed infarction. The diameter of the occluded arteries, a peripheral location of pulmonary emboli and congestive heart failure were significant predictors for infarction. Treatment consists of thoracotomy, decortication, and resection of the absceding lung infarction by a parenchyma-sparing technique (wedge resection, segmentectomy, rarely lobectomy). These operations have to be performed under anticoagulation (20,000 IU Liquemin$\cdot$24 $h^{-1}$) in order to prevent recurrent pulmonary embolism. In a series of 78 patients requiring resection for cavitary pulmonary lesions 1990–1998, seven (9%) were performed for absceding pulmonary infarction [52]. In patients with empyema and massive, centrally located or bilateral emboli, preoperative deployment of a temporary *vena cava* filter should be considered. In case of inoperability due to haemodynamic instability, the insertion of CT guided pigtail drainage into the pleural cavity should be performed followed by the instillation of urokinase (100,000 IU$\cdot$24 $h^{-1}$) until the patient's condition has been stabilised.

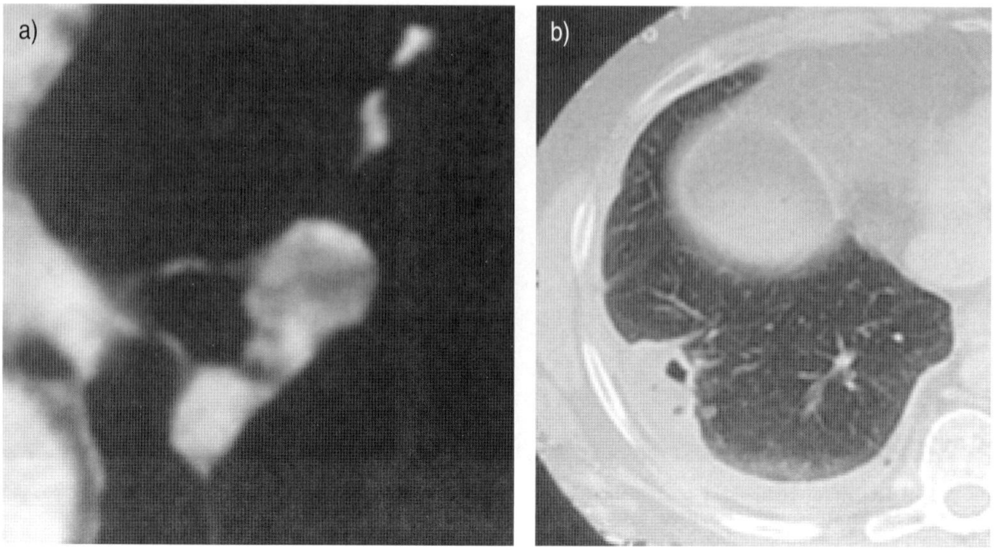


Fig. 4. – Pulmonary emboli (a) causing absceding peripheral lung infarction (b) with penetration into the pleural space and formation of empyema.

## *Empyema related to tumour and lung abscess*

Empyema related to tumour and lung abscess were found in 2% of the patients in the current authors' series, requiring surgery for stage II and III empyema. Absceding tumours and abscess perforating into the pleura may look similar on preoperative CT scans (fig. 5). Both need specific considerations with respect to further diagnosis and treatment. Tissue diagnosis and microbiological examinations may be obtained by bronchoscopy or transthoracic fine-needle aspiration of the pulmonary lesion. Lung abscesses causing empyema usually require thoracotomy, decortication and resection of the abscess by means of wedge resection, segmentectomy or lobectomy [52]. Reinforcement of the bronchial stump and the mediastinum using soft tissue coverage is necessary if a pneumonectomy is required in order to prevent bronchopleural fistula and recurrent infection. Lung tumours require diagnostic investigations and therapeutic

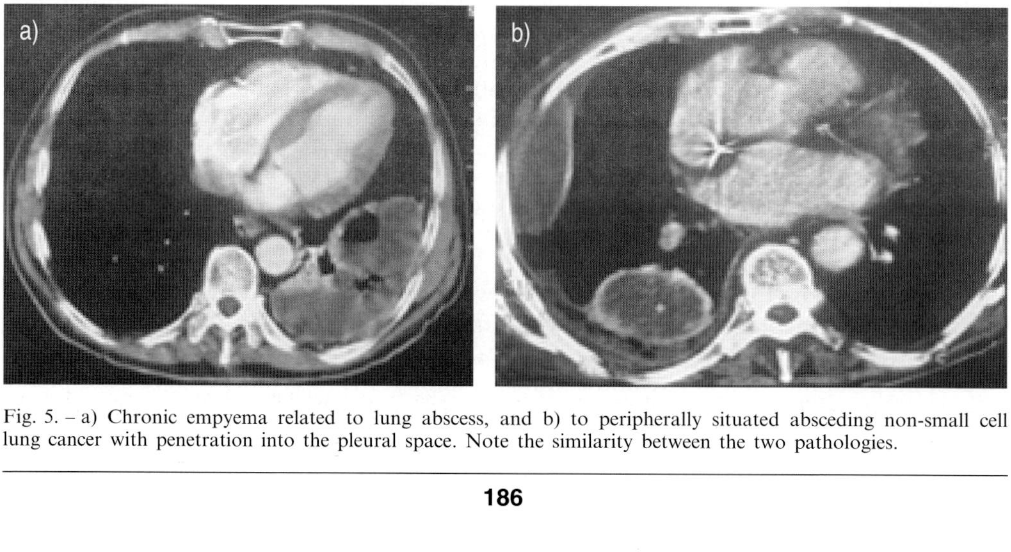


Fig. 5. – a) Chronic empyema related to lung abscess, and b) to peripherally situated absceding non-small cell lung cancer with penetration into the pleural space. Note the similarity between the two pathologies.

considerations according to their histology and stage. However, patients with absceding tumours and empyema are usually not candidates for chemotherapy. They may require resection and decortication, even in advanced disease, in order to prepare the field for chemotherapy, provided a complete resection can be performed. Nonresectable tumours associated with empyema are a difficult clinical problem as no chemotherapy can be offered to those patients; CT guided pleural pigtail insertion and fibrinolysis may be attempted in combination with endobronchial treatment and stenting of the airway. Unfortunately, the tumour often prevents re-expansion of the lung despite these manoeuvres. In patients with a reasonable life expectancy (*i.e.* without wide-spread systemic tumour dissemination), thoracotomy, debridement and intrathoracic muscle transfer may be considered. Quality of life is usually increased by this intervention in addition to the benefit of local control of infection and the possibility to consider chemotherapy [35].

## *Tuberculous empyema*

Tuberculous empyema occurred in 6% of the authors' current series. Tuberculous empyema with entrapped lung (which does not re-expand after chest-tube drainage or thoracocentesis) requires, in addition to appropriate tuberculostatic therapy, thoracoscopic debridement or decortication just as a normal stage II and III empyema does [53]. This approach has been investigated in 26 patients in a recently published report [54]. Exudative empyema (n=4) was treated either by thoracocentesis or chest-tube drainage, fibrinopurulent empyema by VATS debridement (n=4) and the organising stage by decortication (n=16), in combination with lung resection if required. All patients fully recovered with a mean duration of drainage of 18 days. All 16 patients in the series were treated by thoracoscopic debridement or decortication according to the stage of empyema in addition to an appropriate tuberculostatic treatment. All patients recovered without further infection or complications. Re-expansion of the lung is also the key to success for the treatment of tuberculous empyema.

Tuberculosis may lead to a destroyed lung associated with pleural empyema, especially in the presence of multidrug-resistant tuberculosis. In these situations, thoracotomy, decortication and resection of the lung should be performed, followed by mediastinal reinforcement and obliteration of any residual pleural space by intrathoracic muscle transposition (fig. 6) [35, 53].

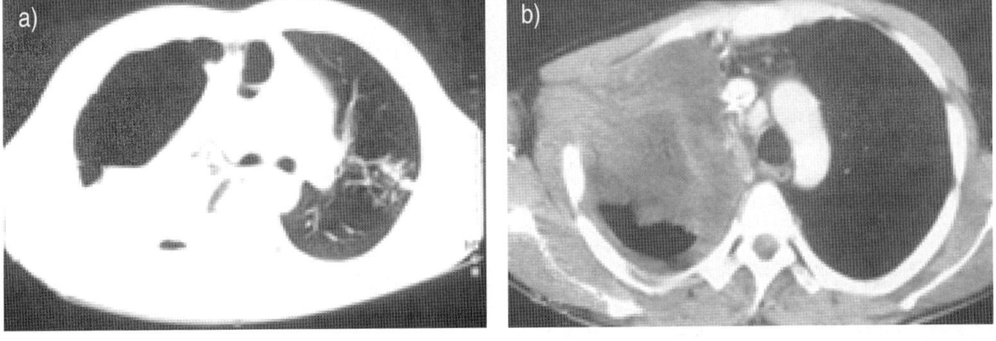


Fig. 6. – Tension pyopneumothorax related to absceding multidrug-resistant tuberculosis with perforation into the pleural space (a), requiring decortication, lobectomy, bronchial stump reinforcement and obliteration of the residual pleural space (b) using intrathoracic latissimus dorsi muscle transfer.

## *Pleural aspergillosis and actinomycosis*

Pleural aspergillosis and actinomycosis was observed in six patients in the current authors' series. Fungal empyema thoracis is recognised as an emerging clinical entity, which has been stressed in a recent report [55]. The reason for this is an increasing number of patients with immunocompromising conditions and fungal cultures from pleural effusions, most of whom have acquired nosocomial infections. Pleural aspergillosis is usually seen in immunocompromised patients with an infected pleural cavity and a persistent bronchopleural fistula after thoracic interventions. This may occur after pneumonectomy, lobectomy or decortication (fig. 7). Half of the patients presented with symptoms such as haemoptysis, pain or massive bleeding from subclavian artery erosion. Treatment consists of debridement of the cavity and obliteration of the infected pleural space by means of intrathoracic muscle transposition in combination with thoracoplasty (table 3). Limited and tailored extrapleural thoracoplasty with extrafascial apicolysis remains the intervention of choice [37]. Post-resectional pleural aspergillosis is indeed one of the rare indications for thoracoplasty at date; however, postoperative morbidity and mortality remain high for this indication [56].

Invasive aspergillosis in immunocompromised patients may not only cause local infiltration of the pleura but also of the chest wall (fig. 8). In these situations, *en bloc* resection of the involved parenchyma (usually by lobectomy) together with the infiltrated chest wall may be performed in good-risk patients followed by reconstruction of the chest wall by a pedicled muscle flap in order to avoid synthetic material [57].

Pleural actinomycosis is rare and requires prompt decortication by thoracotomy since this disease has the propensity to invade the chest wall as well as the site of chest-tube drainage.

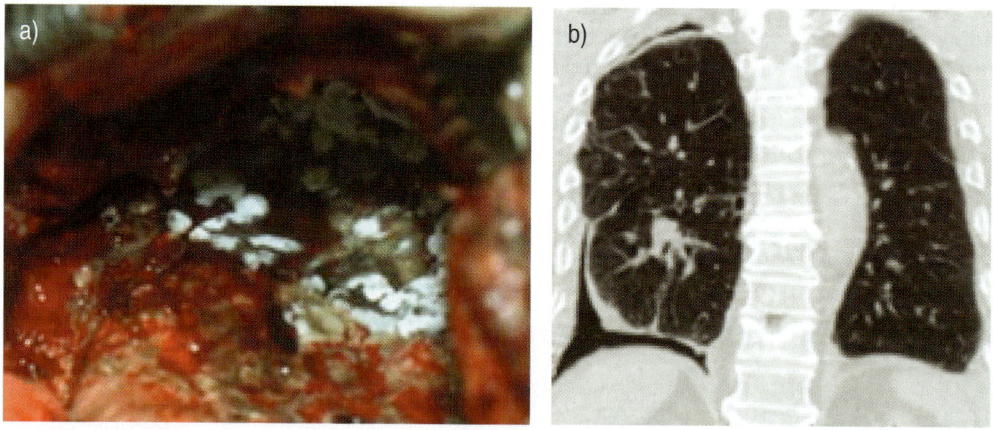


Fig. 7. – a) Pleural aspergillosis within a chronically infected postpneumonectomy cavity and b) within a chronically infected residual space after decortication in an immunocompromised patient.

**Table 3. – Indications for intrathoracic muscle transfer±thoracoplasty in patients with empyema**

| |
|---|
| Postpneumonectomy empyema with bronchopleural fistula |
| MDR tuberculosis with destroyed lung |
| Pleural aspergillosis |
| Invasive aspergillosis invading the chest wall |
| Pleuropulmonal actinomycosis requiring pneumonectomy |
| Absceding tumours with empyema requiring pneumonectomy after induction treatment |

MDR: multidrug resistance.

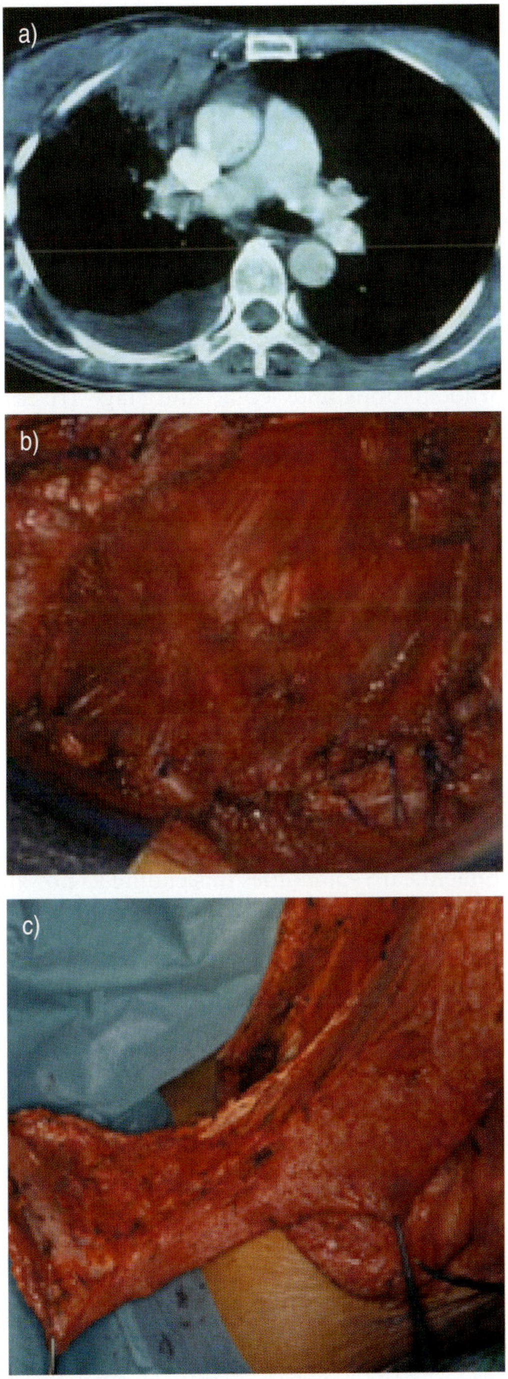


Fig. 8. – a) Invasive aspergillosis in a immunocompromised patient invading the anterior chest wall which requires an *en bloc* resection with lobectomy and chest wall, b) reconstruction of the chest wall and obliteration of the remaining residual pleural space, c) by the use of a pedicled latissimus dorsi flap including its thoracolumbal fascia.

# Chronicity of empyema

As defined by the ATS in 1962, parapneumonic empyema may pass from its exudative form (stage I) through a fibrinopurulent phase (stage II) before becoming organised (stage III) [2]. As a consequence, the treatment modality must be adapted accordingly [1]. Although these principles of treatment have been outlined in the past [3], conservative treatment is often overemphasised in daily practice.

CT scans not only give useful information about the underlying cause of empyema and the state of the parenchyma, they also enable physicians to estimate, to a certain degree, the stage of empyema. Stage I parapneumonic effusions do not present with loculations, septae, enhancement of the parietal pleura and signs of chest wall restriction (narrowing of the intercostal spaces and loss of volume of the chest cavity) (fig. 9a). These signs are typical of a more chronic stage of empyema. Stage II empyema is characterised on a CT scan by the presence of loculations and septae and stage III empyema is identified, in addition to this, by the enhancement of the parietal pleura and signs of restriction (fig. 9b).

## *Stage I empyema*

Stage I parapneumonic effusions are usually treated by antibiotics and thoracocentesis or chest-tube drainage. However, a recent study has challenged the usefulness of chest-tube drainage in complicated parapneumonic effusions in 100 consecutive patients [58]. Successful outcomes were achieved in 53% patients and failure requiring surgery in a further 47% of the patients. Predicting factors for failure of chest-tube drainage were loculated effusions on CT scans and a leucocyte count >6,400 $mL^{-1}$. Failure of complete re-expansion of the lung after chest-tube drainage should raise the suspicion of a more advanced stage of empyema than anticipated.

The fibrinopurulent empyema (ATS stage II) is characterised by the appearance of loculated effusions on a CT scan and intrapleural pH measurements <7.1. However, intrapleural pH measurements are sometimes misleading as not all loculations may show the same stage of empyema. CT scans in combination with clinical symptoms (fever, leucocytosis, rise of CRP) are more reliable in this respect. Thoracoscopic exploration reveals purulent collections and fibrin septae (fig. 10). This stage of empyema is not likely to be successfully treated by chest-tube drainage alone since the clearance of the involved

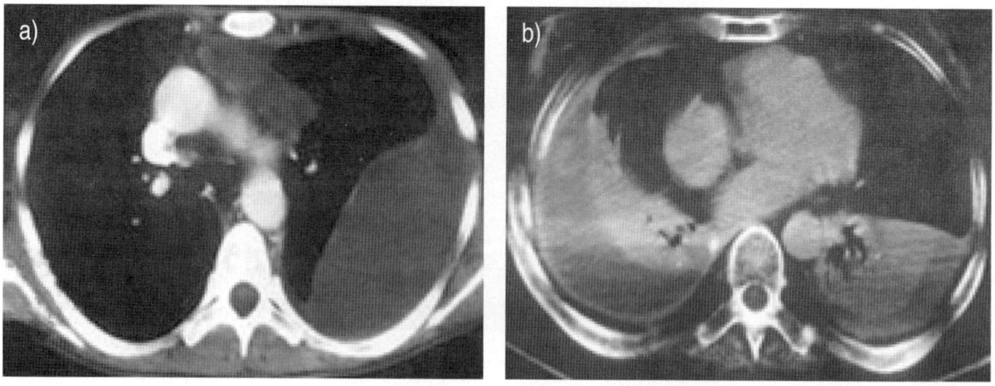


Fig. 9. – a) Stage I parapneumonic empyema, without loculations, septae, pleural enhancement and restrictions. b) Stage III parapneumonic empyema, with pleural enhancement and signs of restriction (narrowing of the intercostal spaces).

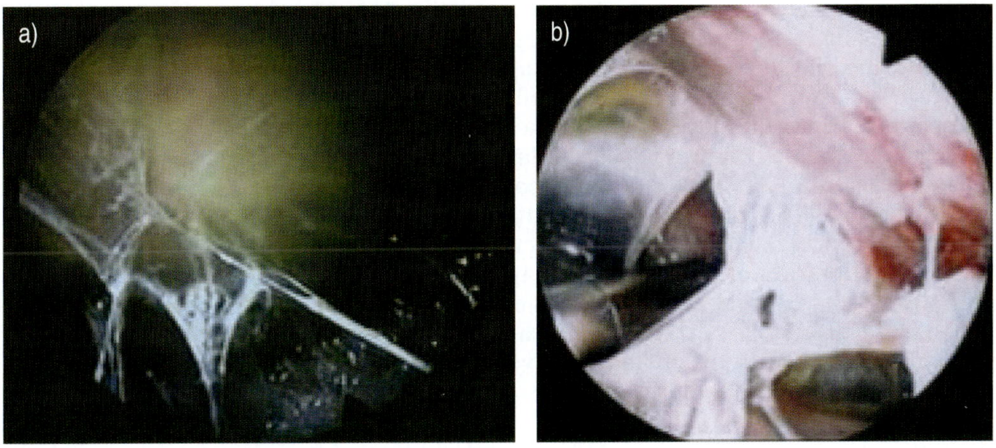

Fig. 10. – a) Typical thoracoscopic aspect of stage II fibrinopurulent empyema with purulent effusion, fibrin deposits and septae. b) Mixed tuberculous stage II empyema with the reddish and granular aspect of the parietal pleura.

chest cavity from infection by chest tubes is hindered by the presence of fibrin deposits and septae. A recently published randomised trial compared intrapleural urokinase instillation with saline instillation *via* a chest tube for complicated parapneumonic empyema in 49 patients. The authors found a significant difference in duration of fever, amount of drained fluid at 5 days, hospitalisation time and decortication rate in favour of urokinase instillation. [59]. In another study, multiloculated pleural empyema was treated in 14 patients using CT guided pigtail catheter drainage. Deterioration of septic symptoms was observed in all patients and all of them required decortication which led to the disappearance of the septic symptoms within 24–48 h after the operation [60].

Treatment options for stage II empyema consist of the instillation of fibrinolytic agents, thoracoscopic (VATS) debridement or early decortication by thoracotomy. Nowadays, early open decortication has been abandoned in many centres in favour of VATS debridement or fibrinolysis. A recently published study compared, in a prospective randomised trial, VATS debridement with the instillation of urokinase in stage II empyema [61]. The authors found a significant difference in the control of the infection, the duration of drainage and hospitalisation, the costs and decortication rate, all in favour of VATS debridement. However, caution in the interpretation of these results is required due to the small sample size of the study.

Debridement using VATS has been assessed in various studies for the treatment of stage II empyema [10–18]. The results after VATS debridement suggest that appropriate control of infection may be obtained, but the long-term results regarding restoration of pulmonary function after VATS debridement still await further confirmation. The present authors' validated, in an earlier report, VATS debridement for stage II empyema and have demonstrated its usefulness [13, 18]. However, pulmonary function testing 6 months after the operation revealed some degree of restriction in ~30% of the patients. This indicates that VATS debridement is probably not indicated in stage III empyema. In the current authors' opinions, VATS does not allow formal decortication to be performed. Entrapment of the lung may persist after VATS debridement of a stage III empyema which may lead to late restriction. Conversion thoracotomy and decortication should be liberally used if a more chronic form of empyema is found during thoracoscopic exploration than anticipated [18]. The present authors' have actualised data emerging from a consecutive series of 276 patients with stage II and III empyema requiring VATS debridement or decortication (fig. 11). There were 276 patients, 192 males and 84 females with a mean age at operation of 55 yrs. Primary open decortication was performed in 96 patients due to an apparently chronic stage III empyema. In 180 patients a VATS approach was attempted but 82 of these patients required conversion thoracotomy (since the stage of empyema was more advanced than anticipated) and 98 patients were treated by VATS. A 30-day mortality rate was observed in 2% of the patients after VATS and 4% after decortication. Postoperative complications were observed after VATS and open decortication in 8 and 8.3% of the patients, respectively, with a reoperation rate for bleeding or recurrent infections in 2.7 and 3.4%, respectively. The median duration of chest tube drainage and hospitalisation were 4.1 and 11.6 days after VATS, and 6.4 and 14.4 days after open decortication, respectively. These results demonstrate that VATS debridement is a valid option for treating stage II empyema; however, a liberal attitude towards conversion thoracotomy is justified if a stage III empyema is found at exploration. The conversion thoracotomy rate during VATS exploration for empyema has been analysed in several reports. WALLER *et al.* [62] have found that 41% of 39 patients could be succesfully treated by VATS which is similar to the present authors' results (54%). In contrast, CASSINA *et al.* [63] demonstrated that VATS was successful in 82% of 45 patients. This discrepancy in the results emerging from these reports may be explained by differences in patient selection and stage of their empyema.

## *Stage II empyema*

Stage II empyema is a transitory stage between the exudative and chronic form of empyema. It may represent, in fact, only a short period of time in the evolution of an empyema. For instance, the current authors' have found that VATS debridement is unlikely to be successful if an empyema is >2–3 weeks old, after the onset of the disease [18]. Fibrinolysis and VATS are valid options for the treatment of stage II empyema but they are not effective in the organising stage. They represent two concurring techniques avaliable for a narrow therapeutic window in the treatment of empyema. This means that usually VATS cannot be considered in a sequential manner once fibrinolysis has failed. The data acually availabe in the literature indicate that VATS is preferred in good-risk paients and fibrinolysis may be an excellent option in patients who would not tolerate a surgical intervention. For instance, fibrinolytic irrigation is an excellent option for a complicated parapneumonic effusion in the presence of major pneumonic consolidation of the parenchyma; every surgical intervention (if still necessary after fibrinolysis) should be postponed until the radiological signs of pneumonia have been resolved.

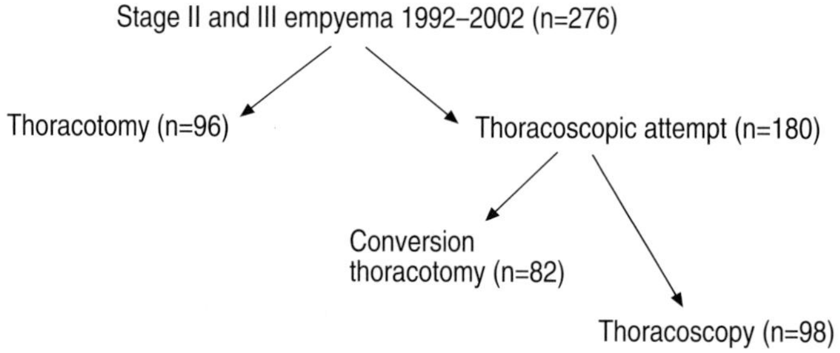


Fig. 11. – The role of video-assisted thoracic surgery in 276 consecutive patients with stage II and III empyema requiring surgery between 1992–2002.

## *Stage III empyema*

Stage III empyema is characterised by loculated effusion with pleural enhancement and signs of restriction on a CT scan in combination with temperature, weight loss and elevated CRP (fig. 9b). Organisation of the peel from the underlying (visceral) pleura usually starts 2–3 weeks after the onset of infection and requires formal decortication by thoracotomy in order to free the trapped lung and to prevent recurrence and restriction (fig. 12). The effect of decortication on lung function was assessed on 26 patients before and 35 weeks after decortication for chronic empyema in a recently published study [64]. The authors found a significant increase in lung perfusion after decortication, on the right side from 25 to 45% and on the left side from 18 to 34%. Predicted vital capacity increased from 62 to 80% and forced expiratory volume in one second (FEV1) from 50 to 70% after the operation. Similar results were obtained by SWOBODA *et al.* [65]. However, the prolonged presence of chronic empyema may result in irreversible restriction and loss of pulmonary function (fig. 13) indicating that decortication should be performed as soon as possible after empyema has been diagnosed.

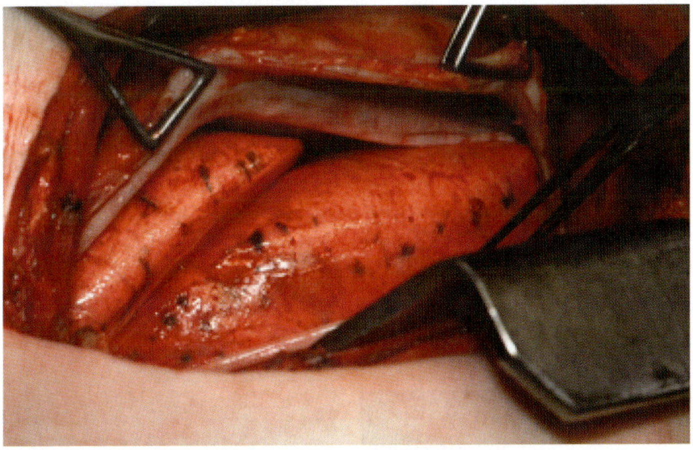

Fig. 12. – Open decortication for chronic stage III empyema. Note the liberation of the entrapped lung by visceral decortication, which prevents ongoing or recurrent infection and late restriction.

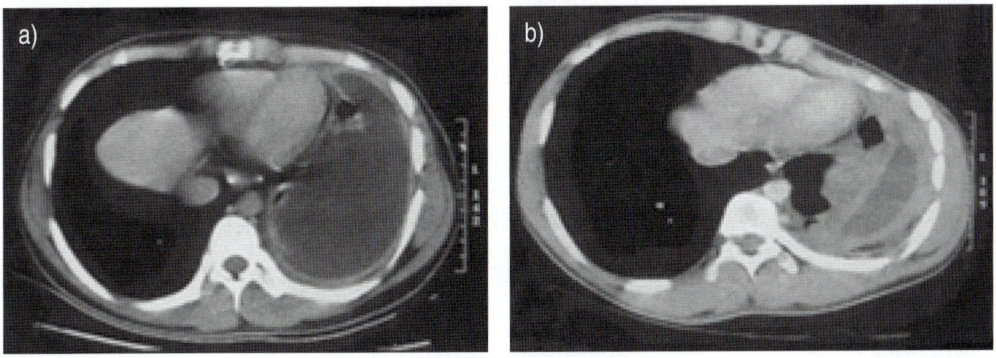


Fig. 13. – a) Stage III pleural empyema treated several months by antibiotics alone. b) The same patient 1 yr after conservative treatment with severe restriction and irreversible loss of pulmonary function.

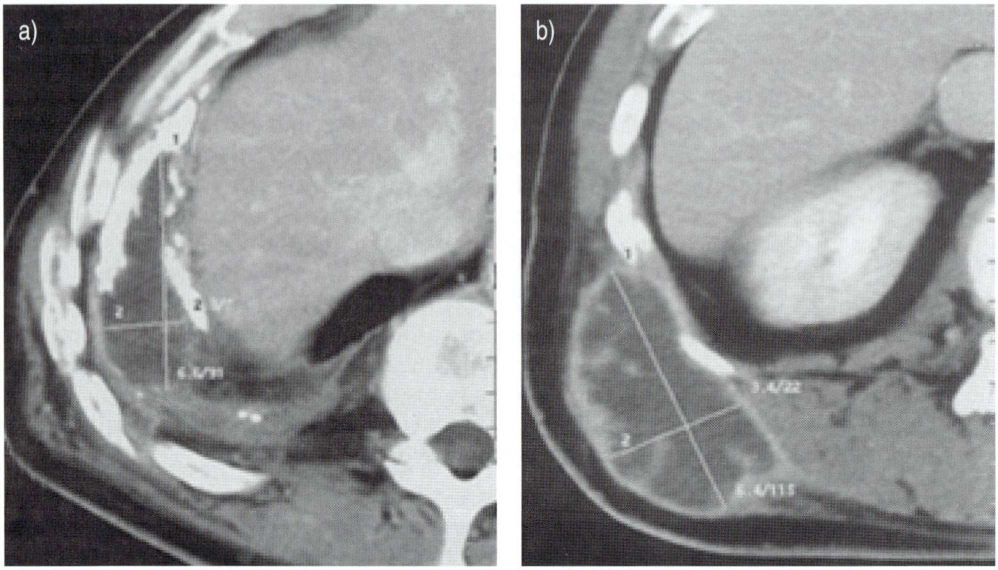


Fig. 14. – a) Chronic calcified tuberculous empyema, b) penetrating the chest wall (empyema necessitatis).

# Patient's overall condition

Special considerations are required in the presence of old, post-tuberculous empyema with calcifications (fig. 14). The calcifications maintain chronic infection and infections cannot heal in the presence of calcifications. Patients are usually elderly, malnourished and present with complex comorbidities which preclude formal decortication. Surgical

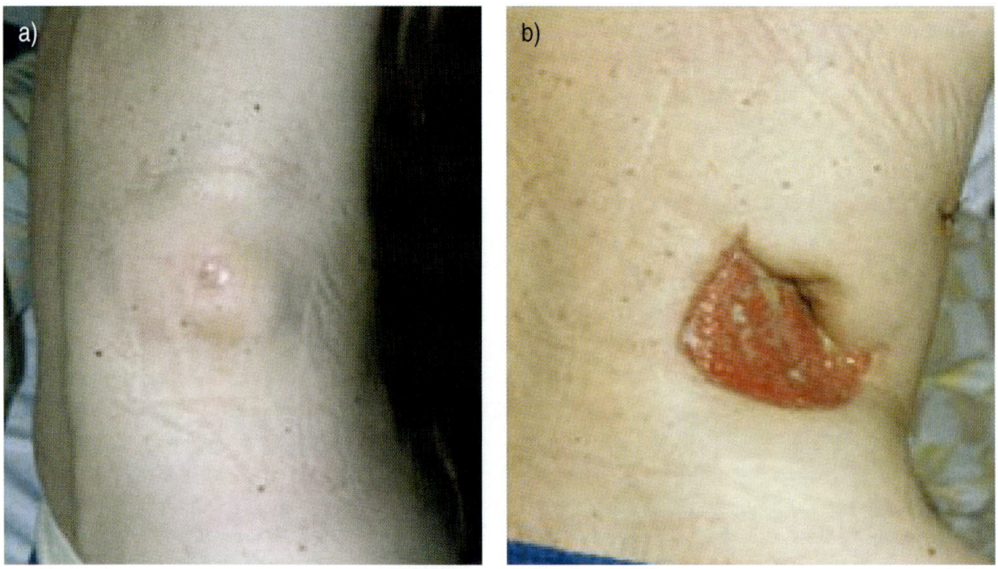


Fig. 15. – a) Empyema necessitatis, b) treated by permanent pleurostomy.

**Table 4. – Indications of open window thoracostomy (pleurostomy) in patients with empyema**

| Transitory | Permanent |
|---|---|
| Postpneumonectomy empyema prior to the obliteration of the cavity | Chronic empyema necessitatis in malnourished, sick patients |

removal of those calcifications may be a formidable operation and possibly be accompanied, even in the presence of good-risk patients, by a high risk of bleeding and persistent residual spaces. This situation may be one of the rare indications for the creation of a permanent thoracic window as described by ELOESSER [66] and SHAMJI *et al.* [67] (fig. 15, table 4).

Open window thoracostomy (pleurostomy), thoracoplasty and intrathoracic muscle transfer were initially designed to control chronic tuberculous infections and are still valid surgical options in the treatment of special kinds of chronic empyema. These procedures have in fact relived a renaissance in recent years due to an increase in the number of complex intrathoracic diseases observed in a growing number of immunocompromised patients.


## Summary

The mainstay of treatment of pleural empyema is the treatment of ongoing infection and the prevention of recurrent infection and late restriction. The choice of the appropriate intervention depends on the nature of the underlying disease, the chronicity of the empyema, and the patient's overall condition. Computed tomography (CT) scans are important in estimating the chronicity of empyema and detecting its underlying cause. The different treatment strategies, with respect to chronicity and underlying cause of empyema, will be discussed on behalf of 282 consecutive patients with surgically treated American Thoracic Society (ATS) stage II and III pleural empyema over a 10-yr period at the present authors' institution; CHUV, Lausanne, Switzerland.

ATS stage I parapneumonic effusions are usually treated with antibiotics and thoracocentesis or a chest-tube drainage. However, recent studies have challenged the usefulness of chest-tube drainage alone in complicated parapneumonic effusions and a high failure rate has been reported, especially in multilocolulated effusions. Treatment of stage II empyema consists of fibrinolysis *via* a chest tube or thoracoscopic (video-assisted thoracoscopic surgery; VATS) debridement. VATS is preferred in good-risk paients whilst fibrinolysis is an excellent option in patients who do not tolerate surgery. Fibrinolysis and VATS are valid options in the treatment of fibrinopurulent empyema but they are not effective in its organising stage. Stage III empyema requires formal decortication by thoracotomy in order to prevent recurrence and restriction. Alterations of lung perfusion and respiration mechanics induced by chronic empyema may be restored if decortication is promptly performed once empyema has been diagnosed.

Open window thoracostomy, thoracoplasty and intrathoracic muscle transfer are still valid surgical options in the treatment of special kinds of empyema. These procedures have in fact relived a renaissance in recent years due to an increase of complex intrathoracic diseases observed in a growing number of immunocompromised patients.

**Keywords:** Decortication empyema, fibrinolysis, parapneumonic effusion.

## References


1. Thurer RJ. Decortication in thoracic Empyema: Indications and surgical technique. *Chest Surg Clin N Am* 1996; 6: 461–490.
2. Andrews NC, Parker EF, Shaw RP, *et al.* Management of non-tuberculous empyema. *Am Rev Respir Dis* 1962; 85: 935–936.
3. Graham EA. Some fundamental considerations in the treatment of empyema thoracis. St Louis, CV Mosby, 1925: pp. 7–110.
4. Ferguson MK. Surgical management of intrapleural infections. *Semin Resp Infect* 1999; 14: 73–81.
5. Lahorra JM, Haaga JR, Stellato T, Flanigan T, Graham R. Safety of intracavitary uriokinase with percutaneous abcess drainage. *Am J Roentgenol* 1993; 160: 171–174.
6. Moulton JS, Moore PT, Mencini RA. Treatment of loculated pleural effusions with transcatheter intracavitary urokinase. *AM J Roentgenol* 1989; 153: 941–945.
7. Robinson LA, Moulton AL, Fleming WH, Alonso A, Galbraith TA. Intrapleural fibrinolytic treatment of multiloculated thoracic empyema. *Ann Thorac Surg* 1994; 57: 803–814.
8. Taylor RFH, Rubens MB, Pearson MC, Barnes MC. Intrapleural streptokinase in the management of empyema. *Thorax* 1994; 49: 856–859.
9. Bryant ER, Salmon CJ. Pleural empyema. *Clin Infect Dis* 1996; 22: 747–764.
10. Hutter JA, Harari D, Braimbridge MV. The management of empyema thoracic by thoracoscopy and irrigation. *Ann Thorac Surg* 1985; 39: 517–520.
11. Kerr JA, Rodgers BM. Thoracoscopy in the management of empyema in children. *J Pediatr Surg* 1993; 28: 1128–1132.
12. Ferguson MK. Thoracoscopy for empyema, bronchopleural fistula and chylothorax. *Ann Thorac Surg* 1993; 56: 644–645.
13. Striffeler H, Ris HB, Würsten HU, Im Hof V, Stirnemann P, Althaus U. Video-assisted thoracoscopic treatment of pleural empyema. A new therapeutic approach. *Eur J Cardiothorac Surg* 1994; 8: 585–588.
14. Hurley JP, McCarthy J, Wood AE. Retrospective analysis of the utility of video-assissted thoracic surgery in 100 consecutive procedures. *Eur J Cardiothorac Surg* 1994; 8: 589–592.
15. Liu HP, Chang CH, Lin PJ, Hsieh HC, Chang JP, Hsieh MJ. Video-assissted thoracic surgery. The Chang Gung experience. *J Thorac Cardiovasc Surg* 1994; 108: 834–840.
16. Mackinlay TA, Lyons GA, Chimondeguy DJ, Piedras MA, Angamaro G, Emery J. VATS debridement versus thoracotomy in the treatment of loculated postpneumonia empyema. *Ann Thorac Surg* 1996; 61: 1626–1630.
17. Weissberg D, Refaely Y. Pleural empyema: 24-year experience. *Ann Thorac Surg* 1996; 62: 1026–1029.
18. Striffeler H, Furrer M, Im Hof V, Gugger M, Ris HB. Video-assisted thoracoscopic treatment of pleural empyema: a cosecutive series of 67 cases. *Ann Thorac Surg* 1998; 65: 319–323.
19. Delorme E. Nouveau traitement des empyèmes chroniques. *Gas d'hop* 1894; 67: 94.
20. Fowler GR. A case of thoracoplasty for the removal of a large cicatricial fibrous growth from the interior of the chest, the result of an old empyema. *Med Rec* 1893; 44: 838.
21. Debesse B, Bellamy J, Dumouchel A, *et al.* Drainage pleural et éradication du foyer pulmonaire. Traitment standard des pleurésies purulentes aigues à germes banales. *Rév fr Mal Resp* 1983: 1245–1246.
22. Lee-Chiong TL, Matthay RA. Current diagnostic methods and medical management of thoracic empyemas. *Chest Surg Clin N Am* 1996; 6: 419–438.

23. Pairolero PC, Deschamps C, Allen MS, Trastek VF. Postoperative empyema. *Chest Surg Clin N Am* 1992; 2: 813–822.
24. Ris HB, Banic A, Furrer M, Caversaccio M, Cerny A, Zbären P. Descending necrotizing mediastinitis: Debridement via clamshell approach. *Ann Thorac Surg* 1996; 62: 1650–1654.
25. Banic A, Ris HB, Striffeler H, Erni D. Free latissimus dorsi flaps for chest wall repair after complete resection of infected sternum. *Ann Thorac Surg* 1995; 60: 1028–1032.
26. Choi JB, Han JO. Comparison of omental and pectoralis flaps for poststernotomy mediastinisis. *Ann Thorac Surg* 1999; 96: 1126–1127.
27. Moor EV, Neuman RA, Weinberg A, Wexler MR. Transposition of the great omentum for infected sternotomy wounds in cardiac surgery. Report of 16 cases. *Scand J Plast Reconstr Surg Hand Surg* 1999; 3: 25–29.
28. Heuer GH. Observations on the treatment of chronic empyema. *Ann Surg* 1920; 70: 80.
29. Shirakusa T, Ueda H, Takata S. Use of pedicled omental flap in the treatment of empyema. *Ann Thorac Surg* 1990; 50: 420–424.
30. Saito H, Tatsuzawa T, Kikkawa H. Transpericardial bronchial closure with omentopexy for postpneumonectomy bronchopleural fistula. *Ann Thorac Surg* 1989; 47: 312–313.
31. Mathisen DJ, Grillo HC, Vlahakes GJ, Dagett WM. The omentum in the management of complicated cardiothoracic problems. *J Thorac Cardiovasc Surg* 1988; 95: 677–684.
32. Arnold PG, Pairolero PC. Intrathoracic muscle flaps. A 10-year experience in the treatment of life-threatening infections. *Plast Reconstr Surg* 1989; 84: 92–99.
33. Arnold PG, Pairolero PC. Intrathoracic muscle flaps. An account of their use in the management of 100 consecutive patients. *Ann Surg* 1990; 211: 656–662.
34. Robinson S. The treatment of chronic non-tuberculous empyema. *Coll Papers Mayo Clin* 1915; 7: 618–644.
35. Widmer MK, Krueger T, Lardinois D, Banic A, Ris HB. A comparative evaluation of intrathoracic latissimus dorsi and serratus anterior muscle transposition. *Eur J Cardiothorac Surg* 2000; 8: 435–439.
36. Deschamps C, Pairolero PC, Allen MS, Trastek VF. Management of psotpneumonectomy empyema and brochopleural fistula. *Chest Surg Clin N Am* 1996; 3: 519–527.
37. Ris HB, Meyer A, Krueger T, Aubert JD. Infections après chirurgie thoracique. *In*: Charbonneau P, Praz G, Glauser M, ed. Pathologies infectieuses en réanimation. Paris, Elsevier, 2002; pp. 222–240.
38. Allen MS, Deschamp C, Trastek VF, Pairolero PC. Bronchopleural fistula. *Chest Surg Clin N Am* 1992; 2: 823–837.
39. Lardinois D, Horsch A, Krüger T, Dusmet M, Ris HB. Mediastinal reinforcement after induction therapy and pneumonectomy: comparison of intercostal muscle versus diaphragm flap. *Eur J Cardiothorac Surg* 2002; 21: 74–78.
40. Grant DR, Finley RJ. Empyema: analysis of treatment techniques. *Can J Surg* 1985; 28: 449–451.
41. Klepetko W, Taghavi S, Pereszlenyi A, Birsan T, Groetzner J, Kupilik N. Impact of different coverage techniques on incidence of postpneumonectomy stump fistula. *Eur J Cardiothorac Surg* 1999; 15: 758–763.
42. Hollaus PH, Huber M, Lax F, Wurnig PN, Bohm G, Pridun NS. Closure of brtonchopleural fistula after pneumonectomy with pedicled intercostal muscle flap. *Eur J Cardiothorac Surg* 1999; 16: 181–186.
43. Rendina EA, Venuta F, Ricci P, Fadda GF, Bognolo DA, Ricci C. Protection and revascularisation of bronchial anastomoses by the intercostal pedicle flap. *J Thorac Cardiovasc Surg* 1994; 107: 1251–1254.
44. Clagett OT, Geraci JE. A procedure for the management of postpneumonectomy empyema. *J Thorac Cardiovasc Surg* 1963; 45: 141–145.
45. Eng J, Sabanathan S. Tissue adhesive in bronchial closure. *Ann Thorac Surg* 1989; 48: 683–685.
46. Baumann WR, Ulmer JL, Ambrose PG, Garvey MJ, Jones DT. Closure of a bronchopleural fistula using decalcified human spongiosa and a fibrin sealant. *Ann Thorac Surg* 1997; 6: 230–233.

47. Schneiter D, Kestenholz P, Dutly A, *et al.* Prevention of recurrent empyema after pneumonectomy for chronic infection. *Eur J Cardiothorac Surg* 2002; 21: 644–648.
48. Deneuville M. Morbidity of percutaneous tube thoracostomy in trauma patients. *Eur J Cardiothorac Surg* 2002; 22: 673–678.
49. Meyer DM, Jessen ME, Wait MA, Estrera AS. Early evacuation of traumatic retained hemothoraces using thoracoscopy: a prospective, randomized trial. *Ann Thorac Surg* 1997; 64: 1396–1400.
50. Lardinois D, Krueger T, Dusmet M, Ghisletta N, Gugger M, Ris HB. Pulmonary function testing after operative stabilisation of the chest wall for flail chest. *Eur J Cardiothorac Surg* 2001; 20: 496–501.
51. Katsumura Y, Ohtsubo KT. Correlation between clinical and pathological features of pulmonary thromboemboli and the development of infarcts. *Respirology* 1998; 3: 203–206.
52. Ris HB, Stocker JM, Im Hof V. Pulmonary abcesses and bronchiectasis. *Schweiz Med Wochenschr* 1999; 129: 547–555.
53. Lardinois D, Furrer M, Mouton W, Ris HB. Aspects chirurgicals de la tuberculose: évolution dans les ving dernières années. *Schweiz Med Wochenschr* 1997; 127: 1961–1968.
54. AL-Kattan KM. Management of tuberculous empyema. *Eur J Cardiothroac Surg* 2000; 17: 251–254.
55. Ko SC, Chen KY, Hsueh PR, Luh KT, Yang PC. Fungal empyema thoracis: an emerging clinical entity. *Chest* 2000; 117: 1672–1678.
56. Massard G, Roeslin N, Wihlm JM, Dumont P, Witz JP, Morand G. Pleuropulmonary aspergilloma: clinical spectrum and results of surgical treatment. *Ann Thorac Surg* 1992; 54: 1159–1164.
57. Raffoul W, Dusmet M, Landry M, Ris HB. A novel technique for the reconstruction of infected full-thickness chest wall defects. *Ann Thorac Surg* 2001; 72: 1720–1724.
58. Huang HC, Chang HY, Chen CW, Lee CH, Hsiue TR. Predicting factors for outcome of tube thoracostomy in complicated parapneumonic effusion for empyema. *Chest* 1999; 115: 751–756.
59. Tuncozgur B, Ustunsoy H, Sivrikoz MC, *et al.* Intrapleural urokinase in the management of parapneumonic empyema: a randomised controlled trial. *Int J Clin Pract* 2001; 55: 658–660.
60. Maier A, Domej W, Anegg U, *et al.* Computed tomography or ultrasonically guided pigtail catheter drainage in multiloculated pleural empyema: a recommended procedure? *Respirology* 2000; 5: 119–124.
61. Wait MA, Shama S, Hohn J, Dal Nogare A. A randomized trial of empyema therapy. *Chest* 1997; 111: 1548–1551.
62. Waller DA, Rengarajan A. Thoracoscopic decortication: a role for video-assisted surgery in chronic postpneumonic pleural empyema. *Ann Thorac Surg* 2001; 71: 1813–1816.
63. Cassina PC, Hauser M, Hillejan L, Greschuna D, Stamatis G. Video-assisted thoracoscopy in the treatment of pleural empyema surgery-based management and outcome. *J Thorac Cardiovasc Surg* 1999; 117: 234–238.
64. Rzyman W, Skokowski J, Romanowicz G, Lass P, Dziadziuszko R. Decortication in chronic pleural empyema-effect on lung function. *Eur J Cardiothorac Surg* 2002; 21: 502–507.
65. Swoboda L, Laule K, Blattmann H, Hasse J. Decortication in chronic empyema: Investigation of lung function based on perfusion scintigraphy. *Thorac Cardiovasc Surg* 1990; 38: 359–361.
66. Eloesser L. An operation for tuberculous empyema. *Surg Gynecol Obstet* 1935; 60: 1096–1097.
67. Shamji FM, Ginsberg RJ, Cooper JD, Spratt EH, Goldberg M, Waters PF. Open window thoracostomy in the management of postpneumonectomy empyema with or without bronchopleural fistula. *J Thorac Cardiovasc Surg* 1983; 86: 818–822.

*CHAPTER 13*

# Treatment of parapneumonic pleural effusion and empyema: conservative view

*R. Loddenkemper*, D. Kaiser#, W. Frank¶*

**Dept of Pneumology II, #Dept of Thoracic Surgery, Lungenklinik Heckeshorn, Berlin, and ¶Dept of Pneumology, Johanniter Hospital in the Flaeming, Treuenbrietzen, Germany.*

*Correspondence: R. Loddenkemper, Lungenklinik Heckeshorn, Zum Heckeshorn 33, D-14109, Berlin, Germany.*

Pleural infections are almost always associated with pleural effusions, and the combined incidence of empyema and parapneumonic effusions (PPE) accounts for ~20% of all effusions [1]. It is estimated that PPE develop in up to 57% of patients hospitalised with bacterial pneumonia [2, 3]. Patients with AIDS will probably develop more often pleural complications due to pneumonia [4].

Besides pneumonia, empyema occurs secondary to surgery in 2.5–21% and trauma in 1–6%. Other causes include: oesophageal perforation (1.5%); pneumothorax (2.5%); iatrogenic interventions (thoracentesis, drainage, pleuroscopy: 1–9%); and miscellaneous (*e.g.* septicaemia: 12.5%) (table 1).

Pleural infections can be caused by a variety of microbial pathogens (table 2). The diagnosis is usually established by symptoms, imaging techniques, examination of the pleural fluid (or other material like blood or bronchial secretions) [8]. In some pleural infections (*e.g.* tuberculosis), additional biopsy methods *e.g.* closed needle biopsy or medical thoracoscopy, may become necessary for diagnosis [9, 10], or seldomly, a surgical approach. But tuberculous empyema has become a rare event in industrialised countries, due to the low incidence of tuberculosis and the early treatment with antituberculous drugs.

**Table 1. – Causes of empyema in different series**

| Cause | Source of data | | | Total |
|---|---|---|---|---|
| | R.W. Light# | D. Kaiser¶ | W. Frank+ | |
| Parapneumonic | 55 | 63 | 82.5 | 62.0 |
| Thoracic surgery | 21 | 14 | 2.5 | 15.5 |
| Trauma | 6 | 1 | 1 | 2.5 |
| Oesophageal perforation | 5 | 0 | 1 | 1.5 |
| Spontaneous pneumothorax | 2 | 2 | 4 | 2.5 |
| Thoracentesis and others | 1 | 6 | 9 | 4.5 |
| Subdiaphragmatic infection | 1 | 0 | 0 | 0.5 |
| Sepsis | 1 | 1 | 0 | 1.0 |
| Miscellaneous or unknown | 7 | 13 | 0 | 10.0 |

Data presented as % unless otherwise stated, total patients n=997. #: n=319, data taken from YEH [5] 1963, SNIDER and SALEH [6] 1968, and SMITH [7] 1991; ¶: n=598, personal communication (Dept of Thoracic Surgery, Lungenklinik Heckeshorn, Berlin, Germany) 1985–2000; +: n=80, personal communication (Dept of Pneumology, Treuenbrietzen, Germany) 1995–2002.

Eur Respir Mon, 2004, 29, 199–207. Printed in UK - all rights reserved. Copyright ERS Journals Ltd 2004; European Respiratory Monograph; ISSN 1025-448x. ISBN 1-904097-33-2.

**Table 2. – Pathogens causing infectious pleural effusions**

| Pathogenic organism | Type |
|---|---|
| Bacteria | Gram-positive aerobes |
| | Gram-negative aerobes |
| | Anaerobes |
| | Special: |
| | *Mycobacterium tuberculosis* |
| | *Actinomyces* |
| | *Nocardia* |
| | *Mycoplasma pneumonii* |
| | *Coxiella burneti* |
| Fungi | Aspergillus |
| | Cryptococcus |
| Parasites | Echinococcus |
| | Paragonimus |
| Virus | Adenovirus |
| | Hepatitis |
| | Infective mononucleosis |
| | Hantavirus |

# Treatment

In this overview, only the treatment of PPE due to bacteria will be discussed. Therapeutic goals and options including: relief of symptoms *e.g.* fever, pain, dyspnoea; the removal of the causative pathogen; the prevention of the recurrence by systemic and local treatment; and the prevention of loss of function, mainly due to pleural fibrosis and lung trappings; are summarised in table 3.

The treatment of PPE and empyema must always include antibiotics. The selection of antibiotics depends primarily on whether the pneumonia is community-acquired or nosocomial. The treatment should follow the established guidelines for treatment of community-acquired and nosocomial pneumonia, by using particular antibiotics that show good penetration of the pleural fluid (penicillins, cephalosporins, clindamycin, aztreonam, and chinolones). An empirical scheme is given in table 4. The therapy should be adjusted to the bacteriological findings (pathogen) and susceptibility test results, in particular if there is not satisfactory clinical and radiological response.

Antibiotic treatment, including supportive measures, is sufficient in the early pleuritis sicca stage and in the exudative stage. In the majority of patients in the fibrinopurulent

**Table 3. – Treatment goals and options in pleural infections**

| Therapeutic goals | Treatment |
|---|---|
| Relief of symptoms (fever, pain, dyspnoea) | Anti-inflammatory drugs |
| | Analgesic drugs |
| | Therapeutic thoracentesis |
| Removal of cause(s) | Antibiotics |
| | Drainage |
| | Surgery |
| Prevention of loss of function | Early drainage |
| | Corticosteroids in tuberculosis (?) |
| | Decortication |
| Prevention of recurrence | Definitive cure by antibiotics and/or by surgery |

?: not proven.

**Table 4. – Antibiotic treatments**

| Empyema complicating | Common isolates | Empirical therapy |
|---|---|---|
| Community-acquired pneumonia | Pneumococci<br>*Streptococcus* spp.<br>*Staphylococcus aureus*<br>*Haemophilus influenzae*<br>Anaerobes | β-lactam/β-lactamase inhibitor combination<br>2nd/3rd-generation cephalosporin plus clindamycin<br>Moxifloxacin |
| Nosocomial pneumonia | Enterobacteriaceae<br>*Pseudomonas* spp.<br>*S. aureus*<br>*Acinetobacter* spp.<br>*Bacteroides* spp.<br>*Fusobacterium* spp. | 3rd and 4th-generation cephalosporins plus clindamycin<br>Piperacillin/Tazobactam (+aminoglycoside for *Pseudomonas aeruginosa*)<br>Carbapenems<br>Linezolid (Methicillin resistant *S. aureus*) |

Table modified from [11].

stage (stage II), additional local treatment must be applied, since this stage may create several intrapleural problems, *e.g.* large effusions with bacterial invasion, loculations by creation of fibrinous membranes ("sails"), and/or pleural thickening ("peels") by fibrin deposition.

The local treatment options can be separated into medical (conservative) and surgical ones (table 5). Arguments in favour of conservative treatment are: 1) it is less invasive; and 2) it can be applied even in severely sick patients (sepsis, on ventilator, in the intensive care unit, immunosuppressive disease/treatment, other severe concomitant diseases).

The optimal management of PPE and empyema in the stage II is still controversial, with a lack of controlled studies, whereas the organisational stage (stage III) is reserved almost exclusively for surgical interventions, since this stage shows continued fibroblast migration and the production of pleural fibrosis with lung trapping. These events prevent the lung from expanding, or cause contraction of the hemithorax resulting in deformation and reduction in mobility, or induce the creation of loculations surrounded by dense fibrous walls and refractory localised empyema (table 6).

Treatment goals in stage II PPE, besides eradication of the causative pathogen, include: evacuation of all (infected) pleural fluid; prevention or breakdown of (multi-) loculations; and prevention of lung trapping by fibrin deposition on the visceral and parietal pleura. This is rarely achieved by antibiotic treatment alone, but needs pleural space drainage in almost all cases.

Features suggesting additional local treatment in PPE because they signal a higher risk for poor outcomes include: clinical features, imaging characteristics, and pleural fluid findings (table 7).

**Table 5. – Local pleural treatment options**

| Treatment Options | |
|---|---|
| Medical | Surgical |
| (Serial) therapeutic thoracenteses<br>(Image guided) small bore tubes#<br>Standard chest tubes#<br>Medical thoracoscopy (pleuroscopy)# | VATS (surgical thoracoscopy)<br>Standard thoracotomy<br>Open drainage (fenestration) |

#: ±fibrinolytic agents/±irrigation; VATS: video-assisted thoracoscopic surgery.

**Table 6. – Medical or surgical treatment in parapneumonic effusions and empyema?**

| Stage | Definition | Treatment |
|---|---|---|
| 0 | Pleuritis sicca stage | Medical domain |
| I | Exudative stage | Medical domain |
| II | Fibrinopurulent stage | Grey zone |
| III | Organisational stage | Surgical domain |

# Evidence-based guidelines

The American College of Chest Physicians (ACCP) in 2000 published an evidence-based guideline on medical and surgical treatment of parapneumonic effusions and came to the following recommendations as a consensus statement.

"The studies identified through a careful literature review as relevant to the medical and surgical management of PPE have significant methodological limitations. Despite these limitations in the data, there did appear to be consistent and possibly clinically meaningful trends for the pooled data and the results of the randomized, controlled trials and the historically controlled series on the primary management approach to PPE. Based on these trends and consensus opinion, the panel recommends the following approach to managing PPE.

- In all patients with acute bacterial pneumonia, the presence of a PPE should be considered. Recommendations based on level C evidence (historically controlled series and case series).
- In patients with PPE, the estimated risk for poor outcome, using the panel recommended approach based on pleural space anatomy, pleural fluid bacteriology, and pleural fluid chemistry, should be the basis for determining whether the PPE should be drained. Recommendation based on level D evidence (expert opinion without explicit critical appraisal or based on physiology, bench research, or "first principles").
- Patients with category 1 or category 2 risk for poor outcome with PPE may not require drainage. Recommendation based on level D evidence.
- Drainage is recommended for management of category 3 or 4 PPE based on pooled data for mortality and the need for second interventions with the no drainage approach. Recommendation based on level C evidence.
- Based on the pooled data for mortality and the need for second interventions, therapeutic thoracentesis or tube thoracostomy alone appear to be insufficient treatment for managing most patients with category 3 or 4 PPE. Recommendation based on level C evidence. However, the panel recognizes that in the individual patient, therapeutic thoracentesis or tube thoracostomy, as planned interim steps before a subsequent drainage procedure, may result in complete resolution of the PPE. Careful evaluation of the patient for several hours is essential in these cases. If resolution occurs, no further intervention is necessary. Recommendation based on level D evidence.
- Fibrinolytics, VATS, and surgery are acceptable approaches for managing patients with category 3 and category 4 PPE based on cumulative data across all studies that indicate that these interventions are associated with the lowest mortality and need for second interventions. Recommendation based on level C evidence."

COLICE *et al.* [12]

**Table 7. – Features suggesting additional local treatment in parapneumonic effusions (higher risk of poor outcome)**

| Features | |
|---|---|
| Clinical | Prolonged symptoms prior to presentation<br>Leucocytosis, anaemia and hypalbuminaemia<br>Failure of response to antibiotic therapy<br>Anaerobic infection<br>Virulence of pathogen |
| Imaging | Chest radiographs/CT:<br>Effusion of >40% of the hemithorax<br>Presence of an air-fluid level<br>Loculation, multiple loculations<br>Pleural thickening<br>Ultrasound:<br>Septation, fibrin strands, necrotic debris |
| Pleural fluid | Putride fluid<br>Positive Gram stain or culture<br>pH<7.30 or 7.20<br>Glucose<40 $mg \cdot dL^{-1}$<br>LDH>1,000 $IU \cdot L^{-1}$ |

CT: computed tomography; LDH: lactic acid dehydrogenase. Table modified from [2].

## Prospective controlled studies on intrapleural fibrinolytics

Up to now, only four controlled and randomised trials on the use of intrapleural fibrinolytics have been reported (table 8). DAVIES *et al.* [13] in a randomised, prospective, controlled trial compared the efficacy of intrapleural streptokinase with normal intrapleural saline flushes in 24 patients. The streptokinase group showed 100% success, whereas the saline group was successful in only three patients (25%). The same results were obtained by BOUROS *et al.* [14], who compared urokinase and saline in 31 patients (success rate: 86.5 *versus* 25%). In 1997, BOUROS *et al.* [15] had already demonstrated a similar success rate of streptokinase and urokinase, which they each used in 25 patients with a success rate of 92%. The patients received either streptokinase (250,000 IU in 100 mL normal saline solution), or urokinase (100,000 IU in 100 mL normal saline) through tube thoracostomy in a double-blinded fashion on a daily basis until the PPE resolved. All patients had undergone inadequate drainage through a chest tube before fibrinolytic treatment.

The only study comparing the conservative treatment of drainage and fibrinolytic therapy with the surgical approach of video-assisted thoracoscopic surgery (VATS) showed a clear advantage of VATS, with a success rate of 91% in eleven patients *versus* 44% with drainage and streptokinase in nine patients [16]. The streptokinase failures were referred to thoracic surgery for additional treatment. The VATS groups had significantly fewer days on chest tube drainage, and shorter hospital stays. There was even a trend

**Table 8. – Percentage success rates of controlled, prospective studies in parapneumonic effusions and empyema**

| Reference | Year | Patients n | Treatment | Success % |
|---|---|---|---|---|
| Davies [13] | 1997 | 24 | SK *versus* NS | 100 *versus* 25 |
| Bouros [14] | 1999 | 31 | UK *verus* NS | 86.5 *versus* 25 |
| Bouros [15] | 1997 | 50 | SK *versus* UK | 92 *versus* 92 |
| Wait [16] | 1997 | 20 | SK *versus* VATS | 44 *versus* 91 |

SK: streptokinase; UK: urokinase; NS: normal saline; VATS: video-assisted thoracic surgery; Table modified from [8].

to lower hospital costs in the VATS group, but it must be taken into account that the sample size was small, the duration of streptokinase treatment was short (three instillations at 24-h intervals), and that chest tube placement was performed by house officers at the bedside and the chest tube position was only judged by standard chest radiography. It seems possible that more frequent or prolonged use of streptokinase would have produced better results. The cost trend was probably only greater for the streptokinase group because the VATS procedure had been added in five cases [2].

## The Lungenklinik Heckeshorn and Johanniter Hospital in the Flaeming approach

The own treatment approach (table 9) consists of drainage (sometimes the insertion of the tube is combined with medical thoracoscopy) *via* double-lumen trocar catheter (20–28 F, length 40 cm), allowing simultaneous irrigation. Irrigation is performed using 1,000 mL of normal saline solution +20 mL of 2% povidone-iodine as antiseptic, one or two times per day until a clear irrigation fluid is recovered [11, 17]. For fibrinolysis, a combination of 200,000 IU streptokinase +50,000 IU of streptodornase (varidase N) is installed, after which the tube is clamped for 4–8 h, depending on the patient's tolerance. The fibrinolytic therapy extends over 5–6 days on average (range: 1–21 days). In the two series comprising of 442 patients with PPE/empyema (table 10), the success rates reached 92 and 89%, respectively. The failure rate was 8 and 11% and the 30 days mortality was 3.3 and 10%, respectively. This was not related to the treatment, but to the severity of the underlying disease with acute respiratory distress syndrome (ARDS), pancreatitis, multi-organ failure, renal failure, and hepatorenal syndrome.

## Role of medical thoracoscopy (pleuroscopy)

There are only a few publications on the use of medical thoracoscopy in the diagnosis and treatment of PPE and empyema. As early as 1925, JACOBAEUS [18] reported on 100 cases of empyema, in which he performed thoracoscopy. BOUTIN *et al.* [19] recommend the use of medical thoracoscopy, and WEISSBERG and REFAELY [20], thoracic surgeons, used the technique in many cases. Recently, SOLER *et al.* [21] have described the successful use of medical thoracoscopy in the treatment of early parapneumonic empyema.

Medical thoracoscopy (pleuroscopy) is a technique which is similar to chest tube insertion and is performed under local anaesthesia. The only difference is that after

**Table 9. – Procedural approach to large-volume irrigation and instillation (fibrinolysis) in the local treatment of empyema (Lungenklinik Heckeshorn)**

| Procedure | |
|---|---|
| Drainage | Thoracoscopic/image-guided double-lumen trocar catheter insertion, 20–28F, length 40 cm. |
| Irrigation | 1,000 mL normal saline solution +20 mL 2% povidone iodine, *q.d./b.i.d.* until clear irrigation fluid recovered. |
| Instillation (fibrinolysis) | 200,000 IU streptokinase+50,000 IU streptodornase, tube clamped 4–8 h (tolerance dependent). |
| Duration | <14 days |
| Side effects | Fever >38°C (42%), pain (10%) |
| Precautions | Postural manoeuvers (diseased side in dependent position), no bronchopleural fistula, no allergy. |

**Table 10. – Outcome in parapneumonic effusions and empyema with conservative treatment**

| Outcome | Source of data | | Total |
|---|---|---|---|
| | D. Kaiser# | W. Frank¶ | |
| Number of patients n | 376 | 66 | 442 |
| Complete remission | 82 | 64 | 79 |
| Partial remission | 10 | 25 | 12 |
| Failure | 8 | 11 | 9 |
| Surgery necessary | 6 | 6.5 | 6 |
| 30-day mortality | 3 | 10.0 | 4 |

Data presented as % unless otherwise stated. #: Personal communication (Dept of Thoracic Surgery, Lungenklinik Heckeshorn, Berlin, Germany) 1985–2000; ¶: personal communication (Dept of Pneumology, Treuenbrietzen, Germany) 1995–2002.

introduction of the trocar, the optique with or without forceps is introduced into the pleural cavity [10]. This allows direct visualisation of loculations and breakdown of fibrinous septa, thus creating one single pleural space. In addition, the pleural surfaces can be inspected concerning their thickness and their consistence, thus allowing a decision on further interventions like instillation of fibrinolytic agents or the indication for surgical decortication. It furthermore allows the correct positioning of the chest tube under visual control.

# Conclusion

In the authors experience, by far the majority of fibrinopurulent effusions/empyemas can be managed successfully by nonsurgical treatment including: antibiotics, pleural drainage (±medical thoracoscopy), intrapleural fibrinolytics, and irrigation. A surgical approach becomes necessary only when medical treatment fails or in the later organisational stage of empyema (fig. 1).

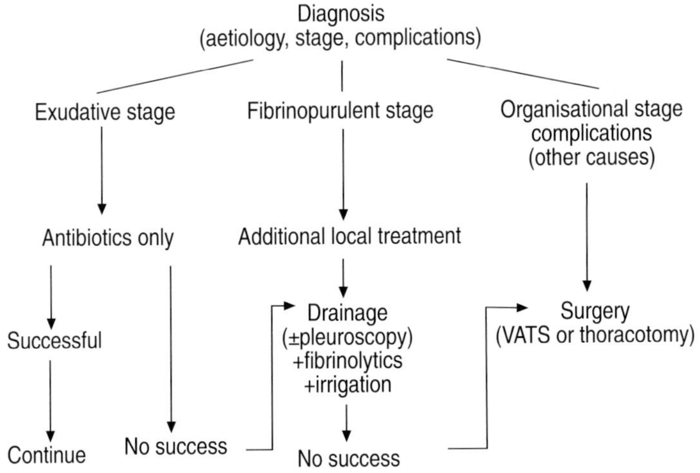


Fig. 1. – Treatment of parapneumonic pleural effusion and empyema.

## Summary

The treatment of parapneumonic effusions (PPE) and empyema must always include antibiotics, which is sufficient in the early pleuritis sicca stage and in the exsudative stage. The fibrinopurulent stage also needs pleural space drainage in almost all cases also. The authors'current treatment approach, which has achieved a success rate of ~90% on >440 patients, consists in drainage *via* double-lumen trocar catheter allowing simultaneous irrigation. Sometimes insertion of the tube is combined with medical thoracoscopy. Intrapleural fibrinolytic therapy is used over 5–6 days on average. In the authors' experience, the majority of fibrinopurulent effusions/ empyemas can be managed successfully by nonsurgical treatment; the latter becomes necessary only when medical treatment fails or in the later organisational stage of empyema.


**Keywords:** Fibrinolysis, fibrinopurulent effusion, medical thoracoscopy, pleural drainage, pleural infection.

## References


1. Light RW. Pleural Diseases. 4th Edn. Philadelphia, Lippincott Williams and Wilkins, 2001; pp. 129–153.
2. Sahn SA. Use of fibrinolytic agents in the management of complicated parapneumonic effusions and empyemas. *Thorax* 1998; 53: Suppl. 2, S65–S72.
3. Heffner JE, McDonald J, Barbieri C, *et al.* Management of parapneumonic effusion. *Arch Surg* 1995; 130: 433–438.
4. Rodriguez Barradas MC, Musher DM, Hamill RJ, *et al.* Unusual manifestations of pneumococcal infection in human immunodeficiency virus-infected individuals: the past revisited. *Clin Infect Dis* 1992; 14: 192–199.
5. Yeh TJ, Hall DP, Ellison RG. Empyema thoracis: a review of 110 cases. *Am Rev Respir Dis* 1963; 88: 785–790.
6. Snider GL, Saleh SS. Empyema of the thorax in adults: review of 105 cases. *Chest* 1968; 54: 12–17.
7. Smith JA, Mullerworth MH, Westlake GW, Tatoulis J. Empyema thoracis: 14-year experience in a teaching center. *Ann Thorac Surg* 1991; 51: 39–42.
8. Bouros D, Hamm H. Infectious pleural effusions. *Eur Respir Mon* 2002; 22: 204–218.
9. Frank W. Tuberculous pleural effusions. *Eur Respir Mon* 2002; 22: 219–233.
10. Loddenkemper R. Thoracoscopy – state of the art. *Eur Respir J* 1998; 11: 213–221.
11. Loddenkemper R, Frank W. Infectious pleurisy (empyema and parapneumonic effusion). *In*: Gibson GJ, Geddes DM, Costabel U, Sterk PJ, Corrin B, eds. Respiratory Medicine Vol. 2. UK, Saunders, 2003; pp. 1920–1924.
12. Colice GL, Curtis A, Deslauriers J, *et al.* Medical and surgical treatment of parapneumonic effusions. *Chest* 2000; 18: 1158–1171.
13. Davies RJO, Traill ZC, Gleeson FV. Randomised controlled trial of intrapleural streptokinase in community acquired pleural infection. *Thorax* 1997; 52: 416–421.
14. Bouros D, Schiza S, Tzanakis N, Chalkiadakis G, Drositis J, Siafakas N. Intrapleural urokinase *versus* normal saline in the treatment of complicated parapneumonic effusions and empyema. *Am J Respir Crit Care Med* 1999; 159: 37–42.
15. Bouros D, Schiza S, Patsourakis G, Chalkiadakis G, Panagou P, Siafakas NM. Intrapleural streptokinase *versus* urokinase in the treatment of complicated parapneumonic effusions. A prospective, double-blind study. *Am J Respir Crit Care Med* 1997; 155: 291–295.

16. Wait MA, Sharma S, Hohn J, Dal Nogare A. A randomized trial of empyema therapy. *Chest* 1997; 111: 1548–1551.
17. Frey DJM, Klapa J, Kaiser D. Spül-Drainage und Fibrinolyse zur Behandlung des metapneumonischen Pleuraempyems [Irrigation drainage and fibrinolysis for treatment of parapneumonic pleural empyema]. *Pneumologie* 1999; 53: 596–604.
18. Jacobaeus HC. Die Thorakoskopie und ihre praktische Bedeutung [Thoracoscopy and its practical importance]. *Ergebn ges Med* 1925; 7: 112–166.
19. Boutin C, Viallat JR, Aelony Y. Practical thoracoscopy. Berlin Heidelberg, Springer, 199; pp. 129–153.
20. Weissberg D, Refaely Y. Pleural empyema. *Ann Thorac Surg* 1996; 62: 1026–1029.
21. Soler M, Wyser C, Bolliger CT, Perruchoud AP. Treatment of early parapneumonic empyema by 'medical' thoracoscopy. *Schweiz Med Wochenschr* 1997; 127: 1748–1753.

*CHAPTER 14*

# Congenital bronchopulmonary malformations in adults

*J. Hasse*

*Correspondence: J. Hasse, Abt. Thoraxchirurgie, Chirurgische Universitätsklinik Freiburg, Joachimsacker str. 33, CH4103, , Boltmingen, Switzerland.*

The clinical impact of congenital diseases of the respiratory system is often extensive and requires early attempts of correction. A high proportion is immediately incurable and ultimately lethal. As a direct result of this relatively few patients present, in adulthood, with known or unexpected bronchopulmonary malformations. Even in larger thoracic centres without paediatric services such malformations are seen only episodically by radiologists, physicians and surgeons. Therefore, in adulthood the differential diagnosis of congenital lesions may sometimes remain unconsidered.

## Embryology

Malformations result from errors and disturbances of the primitive foregut when it starts to divide into two, an anterior respiratory and a posterior oesophageal tube. At the beginning of the 7th week of gestation, these structures are normally separate and the bronchial tree is rudimentarily designated. However, malformations of the major airways and tracheo-oesophageal communication can be dated back to this stage of the embryological development [1–5]. Further branching of the smaller airways takes place until birth. According to GRAY and SKANDALAKIS [4], four generations of alveoli are developing from week 20 to week 40 of gestation, whereas cartilage and glands are definitely developed at week 30. Therefore, the earlier the developmental disturbance occurs, the more severe are the sequelae. Atresia of the trachea and agenesis of the lungs are incompatible with life. Unilateral hypoplasia or agenesis of the lung is associated with a high mortality within the first 5 yrs of life. Among the congenital cysts of the respiratory system the so-called bronchogenic cyst date back to the 6th or 7th week of gestation, whereas pulmonary cysts develop at the 24th week.

Anomalies of lobulation start at the 10th week of gestation and are usually asymptomatic. They present as: azygos lobe, apical upper lobe, segmental bronchus with tracheal origin, or deficient development of fissures without primarily clinical but sometimes surgical relevance. Congenital malformations of the pulmonary circulation occur at the 5th week. Clinically, the absence of a unilateral pulmonary artery, the different types of pulmonary sequestration, and the dystopic origin of the left pulmonary artery from the right one, the so-called pulmonary artery sling, are all of importance.

A brief overview, addressing such pulmonary malformations in adults, that may cross the path of a thoracic surgeon are given below:

- Pulmonary sequestration
- Congenital lobar emphysema
- Congenital cystic adenomatoid malformations
- Bronchogenic cysts

Eur Respir Mon, 2004, 29, 208–222. Printed in UK - all rights reserved. Copyright ERS Journals Ltd 2004; European Respiratory Monograph; ISSN 1025-448x. ISBN 1-904097-33-2.

- Pulmonary hypoplasia, pulmonary artery agenesis
- Primary and secondary tracheal stenosis
- Congenital airway fistulas to the oesophagus
- Pulmonary arteriovenous malformations

# Clinical entities

## *Pulmonary sequestration*

The term sequestration was used by the pathologist Pryce in the late 1940s [6]. He reported on several cases where an intralobar area of the lung was supplied by a lower accessory artery. The acknowledged contemporary definitions of pulmonary sequestration have, in common, the criteria of systemic arterial supply and the absence of airway connection. Pulmonary sequestration is seen as one of the variants of congenital cystic diseases. There are only few clinical reports that exceed a series of >10 adult patients. Van Raemdonck *et al.* [7] compared the differences of manifestation between the adult and the paediatric group. They found a preponderance of the intralobar type in adults and a more balanced ratio between intra- and extralobar ones in children. Similar figures are reported in a review by Hudak [1]. Extralobar sequestration is often associated with other congenital defects *e.g.* diaphragmatic hernia, heart defect, *etc...* and therefore is symptomatic earlier and can be readily diagnosed. Intralobar sequestration, in contrast, is complicated by secondary infection during the course of life and, therefore, is the most known bronchopulmonary malformation in adults. The complications of intralobar sequestration are acute infection with abscess formation and extension to the surrounding parenchyma, thus causing threatening situations including haemoptysis.

The preferential location for intralobar and extralobar sequestrations are the left lower lobe and the left sublobar regions, respectively. In incidentally found lesions of the posterior lower lobe, especially on the left side, the consideration of sequestration should be realised as a possible differential diagnosis. The most reliable diagnostic proof is by aortic catheterisation and selective angiography. Less invasive methods currently preferred are contrast computed tomography (CT) scans, angio-magnetic resonance imaging, or duplex sonography. If the diagnosis has clinically been taken into account, straight forward surgical exploration and confirmation is deemed an appropriate procedure. In the emergency situation this will be the ultimate method.

Few cases have been described in the literature with large systemic arteries, however preserved the bronchial system is. Yamanaka *et al.* [8] reported four such cases. They found aneurysmatic dilation of the anomalous arteries distal to the aortic stem. In all cases radiographically pronounced density was seen due to the enlarged intrapulmonary vasculature of the affected segments or lobes. All patients were adults, their ages ranged from 29–68 yrs. In one case the anomalous lobar artery was anastomosed to the pulmonary artery, in all other cases resection was performed.

Resection is the most widely acknowledged treatment of both, the intra- and the extralobar sequestration, even in patients who are asymptomatic or became asymptomatic after conservative treatment. The rationale behind this attitude is based on the experience of dramatic or fatal complications of untreated sequestration compared with the low morbidity and virtually absent mortality, particularly in patients who are operated on electively. Obviously, surgery in extralobar sequestration is accomplished with total resection of the privately pleuralised abnormal lung. For intralobar sequestration, with regards to inflammatory involvement of the surrounding parenchyma, in many cases lobectomy is advisable. Presently at least the preservation of segment six in lower lobe sequestration is being considered. Van Raemdonck *et al.* [7]

performed sequestrectomy in one-third of 21 intralobar-type cases. In all cases of a parenchyma-saving procedure, perfect venous drainage is a mandatory prerequisite and has to be assured. From a technical point of view, the safe identification and control of the feeding systemic artery is important. These aberrant vessels may expose athero-sclerotic changes already in older children, adolescents and adults and should be handled with particular care [9]. When dealing with acute inflammatory disease, involvement of the pleural space, and often very large inflammatory lymph nodes, any blind dissection is obsolete. If the artery is originating from the abdominal aorta the aberrent vessel stump can retract sub diaphragmatically with difficult control and large blood losses.

Figures 1 and 2 are chest radiographs and CT scans, respectively, showing diffuse cystic changes of the lower left lung in of a 27-yr-old male. This patient presented with a history of alcohol abuse and was acutely septic, despite antibiotic treatment. The patient underwent an emergency thoracotomy, assuming aspiration pneumonia with multiple abscesses. Intra-operatively, an intralobar sequestration was found and the patient recovered uneventfully after a lobectomy. Figure 3 a) shows a retrocardial opacity in an asymptomatic 46-yr-old male. From the CT scan (fig. 3 b) a solid irregular mass is visible. Further diagnostic tests on this patient were negative for malignancy and the differential diagnosis of pulmonary sequestration was made. A thoracotomy was decided without further investigations. The anomalous artery from the descending aorta was found close to the diaphragm and the lesion was removed with the technique of segmental resection.

Few reports on patients with aberrant arterial supply, deriving from the coronary artery system, have been published. In these patients coronary-steal phenomena were found with the clinical symptoms of dyspnoea and unstable angina. In one case only the aberrant vessel was ligated [10]. In two further cases, one of a 66-yr-old Chinese male and

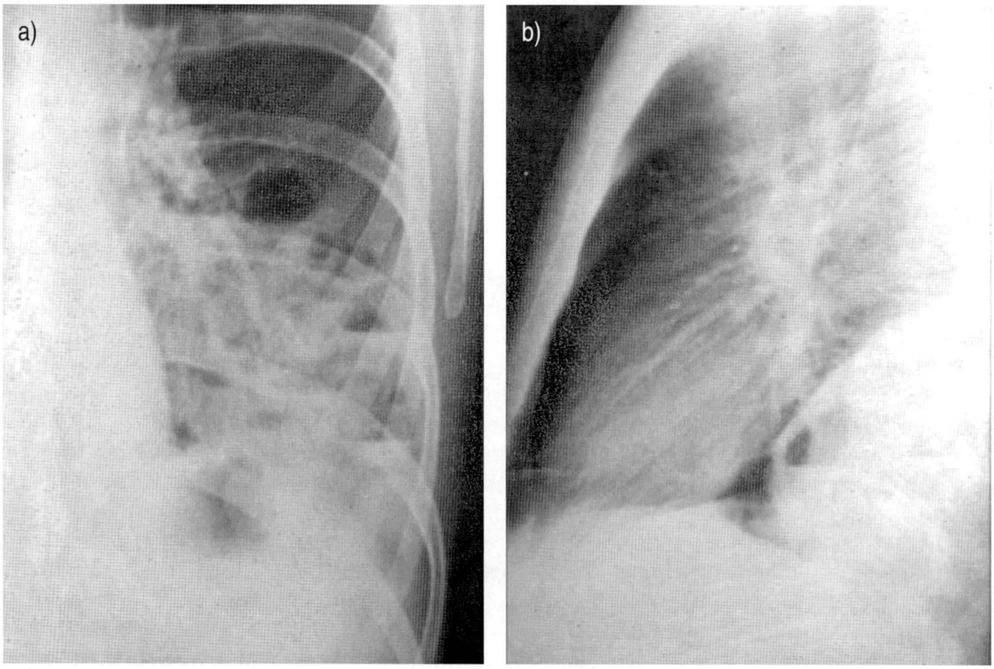


Fig. 1. – Pulmonary sequestration: a) frontal and b) lateral view of the left lower lung field showing multiple cystic lesions with fluid levels in a 27-yr-old male.

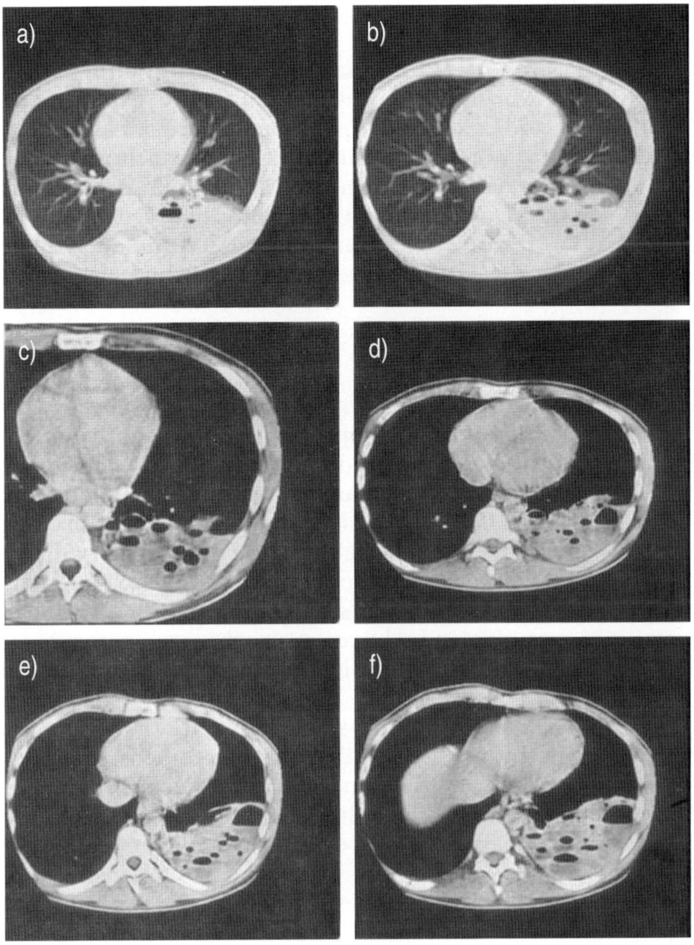


Fig. 2. – Computed tomography scans (a–f) of parenchymal changes occupying the posterior lower lobe in a 27-yr-old male.

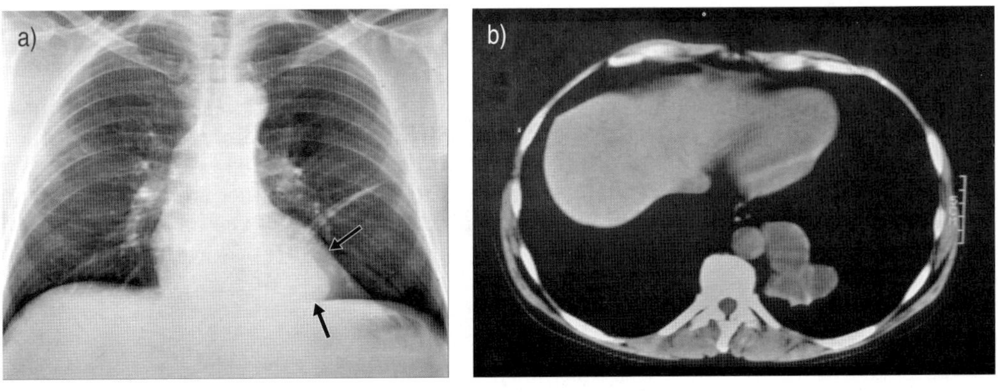


Fig. 3. – Pulmonary sequestration: a) chest radiograph of a 46-yr-old male with an ill-defined lesion enhancing the left heart shadow as shown by the arrows, b) computed tomography scan in the same patient showing solid mass at the posterior base of the left lower lobe.

another of a 51-yr-old Mexican male each with a left lower lobe sequestration, experienced dissolvement of symptoms and were treated conservatively [11, 12]. SIPPEL *et al.* [13] presented a case report of a mediastinal sequestration in which the diagnosis was only established intra-operatively, during diagnostic exploration. The authors described a separate tracheal bronchus that was stapled and an arterial supply from the main pulmonary artery. No findings of eventual tracheobronchoscopy are reported and it is most likely that this case should be categorised as an aberrant accessory tracheal lung or Rokitanski-lobe. CONRAN and STOCKER [14] who analysed 50 cases of extralobar sequestration found a 50% association with congenital cystic adenomatoid malformation. The age range in this histopathological study was from newborn to 65-yrs old.

## *Congenital lobar emphysema*

Congenitally diffuse changes, of at least one entire lobe, often become evident early on after birth or even prenatally. The most probable known entity is congenital lobar emphysema. The over distension of the predominantly affected left upper lobe can lead to atelectasis of the lower lobe and to mediastinal shifting. The underlying anomaly and the classification of this disease is controversially discussed. In certain cases the instability of the upper-lobe bronchus is regarded to be the cause of post-stenotic hyperinflation. In addition, extrinsic compression by a patent duct or an aortic arch anomaly has also been reported as a likely cause [15]. Good results have been reported with early resection in infancy if only one lobe was involved. However, progressive involvement of other parts of the lung has a serious prognosis with a lethal outcome. In the literature, and in the current author's experience, few patients are presenting with lobar emphysema in adulthood [3]. The involvement of only one single lobe but otherwise normal lung tissue, and the absence of chronic bronchitis or other reasons for post-stenotic hyperinflation are leading to the diagnosis lobar emphysema. Less pronounced than in infants, the lobe in adults appears rather pale and a sponge-like structure is seen through the transparent visceral pleura. The resection is a simple operation with immediate improvement of dyspnoea. Figure 4 refers to a 22-yr-old male who complained from dyspnoea on exertion. The chest radiograph showed hypertransparency of the right lower lung field in the frontal view (fig. 4a) and pectus excavatum in the lateral projection (fig 4b). The CT sans (fig. 4c, d) confirmed involvement of the right lower lobe. During the operation it was observed that the lobe was diffusely emphysematous and further histological tests suggested congenital lobar emphysema.

## *Cystic adenomatoid malformations*

In this lesion, adenomatoid proliferation of the bronchioli lead to the development of cysts which contain liquid instead of normal alveoli [1, 16]. Immediately after birth these cysts are trapping air and are presenting with characteristic multiple fluid discs. The type I of this malformation has cysts that are measuring 2–10 cm in diameter, which are restricted to one lobe. Since lower lobes are more commonly involved a chest radiograph may be erroneously taken for diaphragmatic hernia with intrathoracic intestinum. In type II the cysts are numerous and small between 0.5–2 cm in diameter, and in type III they are only identified microscopically. In the author's own experience adults may present, in rare instances, with this unusual malformation.

In newborns and infants with symptoms of acute dyspnoea treatment is by immediate surgery. In one of the author's cases the diagnosis was established prenatally and lobectomy was started 2 h after birth. This otherwise healthy newborn was breast fed the next day and was discharged after 1 week. In adults the diagnosis is confirmed

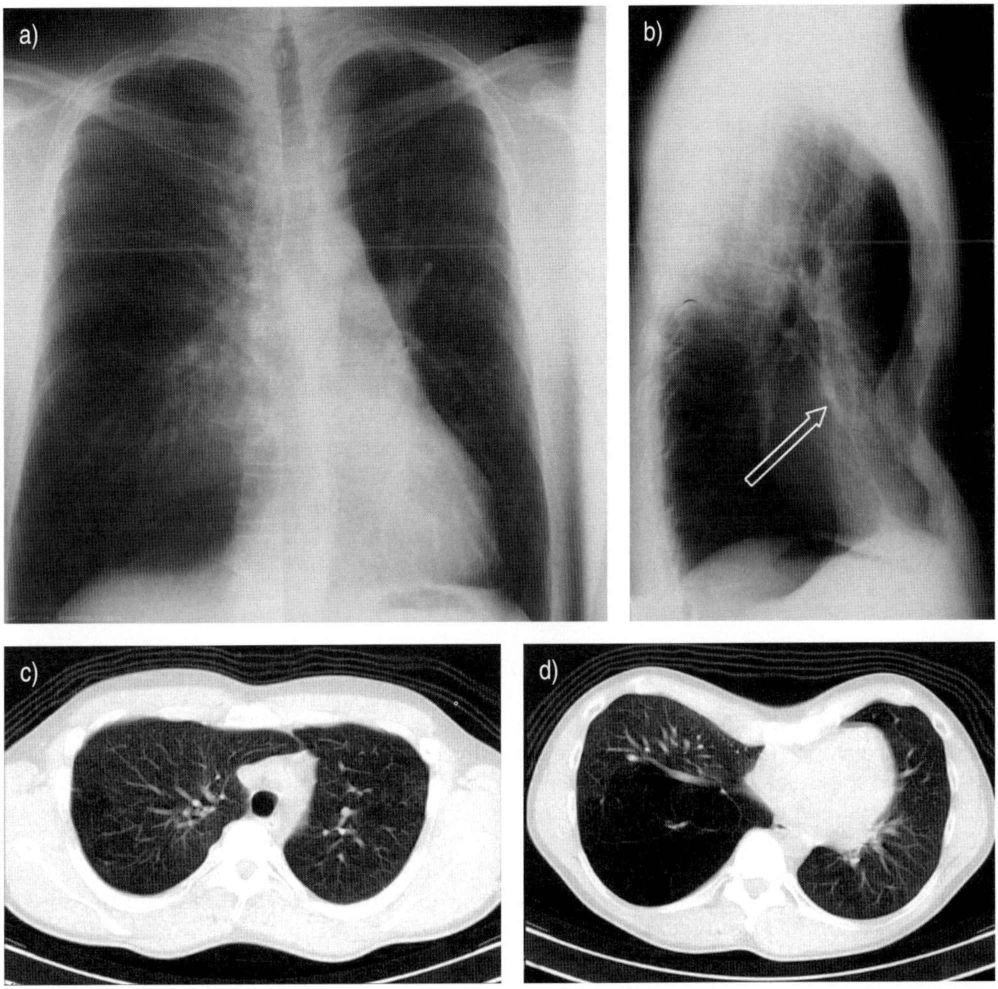


Fig. 4. – Adult congenital lobar emphysema: hyperlucency of the right lower field of the lung in (a) the frontal and (b) sternal pectus recurvation in the lateral projection of chest radiograph, c and d) computed tomography scans of the same patient.

histologically. In the literature the symptoms of recurrent pneumonia complicating the malformation has been reported [3].

## *Bronchogenic cysts*

Bronchogenic duplications occur in the 6th embryological week from the right lateral tracheal wall. By definition, congenital bronchogenic cysts have an inner lining with a respiratory epithelium and can be distinguished from oesophageal cysts by this criterion [2]. The pathology of bronchogenic cysts is variable. The content of bronchogenic cysts may be of clear or of mucoid quality. Bronchogenic cysts are found in a large variety of topographical locations not only in the chest but occasionally in the neck or subdiaphragmatically [17]. Bronchogenic cysts, if asymptomatic, are probably the most frequent congenital malformations diagnosed in adulthood either as incidental findings or for symptoms of pain, dyspnoea, or infection. Extrapulmonary mediastinal cysts are located along the trachea, below the carina but also in other compartments of the mediastinum. Symptoms can arise from compression of the oesophagus and/or major airways.

Intrapulmonary bronchogenic cysts may be connected to the airway system and thereby, may reach large volumes. They may be complicated by infection and haemoptysis [18–21]. In 1996 Ribet *et al.* [19] reported a series of 41 patients with an even distribution between paediatric and adult age. In the adult group there were 25 female and only five male patients. The dominating symptoms in adults, like in children, were: chest pain, infection, and haemoptysis. Nusair *et al.* [20] recently published a case report with massive haemoptysis from a bronchogenic cyst. Duranceau and Deslauriers [21] published a series of 61 mediastinal and 20 intrapulmonary bronchogenic cysts in 1991. A total of 65% of their patients with a mediastinal manifestation, and 85% with intrapulmonary cysts were symptomatic. From these findings and reports of life-threatening complications, surgical treatment is recommended for the confirmation of the diagnosis and for definite treatment. The literature reports a low surgical morbidity with no mortality in most series, even at the time when video-assisted thoracoscopic surgery (VATS) were not yet developed and often a transpleural approach was applied. The surgical treatment of intrapulmonary cysts is by an open approach and involves in segmental resection or lobectomy. The exposure of mediastinal cysts is often possible with a VATS. Complete removal of the cystic wall does prevent any reoccurrence.

## *Pulmonary hypoplasia and pulmonary artery agenesis*

Unilateral hypoplasia of the lung carries a high risk of early death [1, 16], 50% of the children are either stillborn or die in their first years of life. Right lung hypoplasia without cystic changes is associated with the Scimitar syndrome and is occasionally asymptomatic; sometimes it is only diagnosed in adulthood [22]. In general, adults are rarely seen with the anomaly of hypoplasia. The hypoplastic lung is small with a reduced calibre of the bronchial system. In some cases the hypoplasia seems to be related to a hypoplastic or atretic pulmonary artery. A pneumonectomy is required when the clinical picture is dominated by recurrent infection, chronic purulent sputum, and the risk of severe haemoptysis [23, 24]. The current author's experience of pulmonary hypoplasia involves the cases of two female patients: a 23-yr-old with a right-sided pulmonary hypoplasia (fig. 5) and a 15-yr-old with a left-sided pulmonary hypoplasia. In both cases perfusion scintis revealed the absence of physiological perfusions. Of the above mentioned signs and symptoms in only the elder of both patients haemoptysis was observed which occurred in a mild form. The operative procedure requires meticulous haemostasis of the excessive arterial collaterals connected to bronchial, mediastinal, and diaphragmatic arteries. Although both did well immediately after the operation, in the case of the 15-yr-old female the preoperative existing mediastinal shift was attenuated due to missing development of a serothorax (fig. 6a). The patient experienced severe dyspnoea from tracheobronchial compression against the vertebral column (fig. 6b), *i.e.* postpneumonectomy syndrome. Lasting relief was achieved by positioning of 800 cc silicone implant behind the heart counteracting the mediastinal shift (fig. 6c–d).

## *Primary and secondary tracheal stenoses*

It is only in exceptional circumstances that patients reach adult age with congenital tracheal stenosis without correction. The present author is unaware of slide tracheoplasty for this disease in adults. However, Niwa *et al.* [25] presented a series of six patients

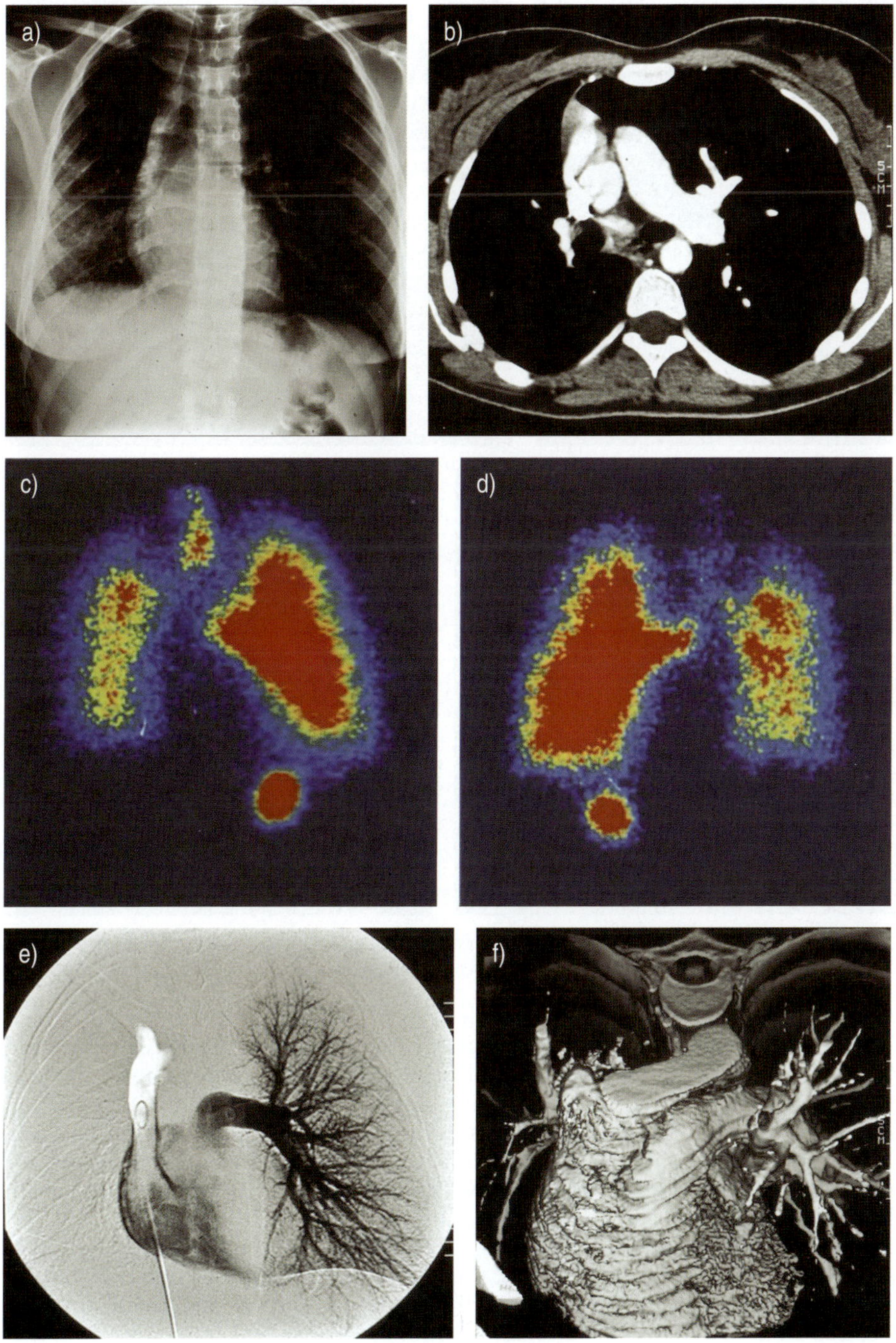


Fig. 5. – Right-sided pulmonary hypoplasia in a 23-yr-old female: a) frontal chest radiograph, b) computed tomography (CT) scan, c–d) scintiscans, e) pulmonary artery angiogram, and f) 3-dimentional CT-reconstruction image showing pulmonary hypoplasia and arterial agenesis.

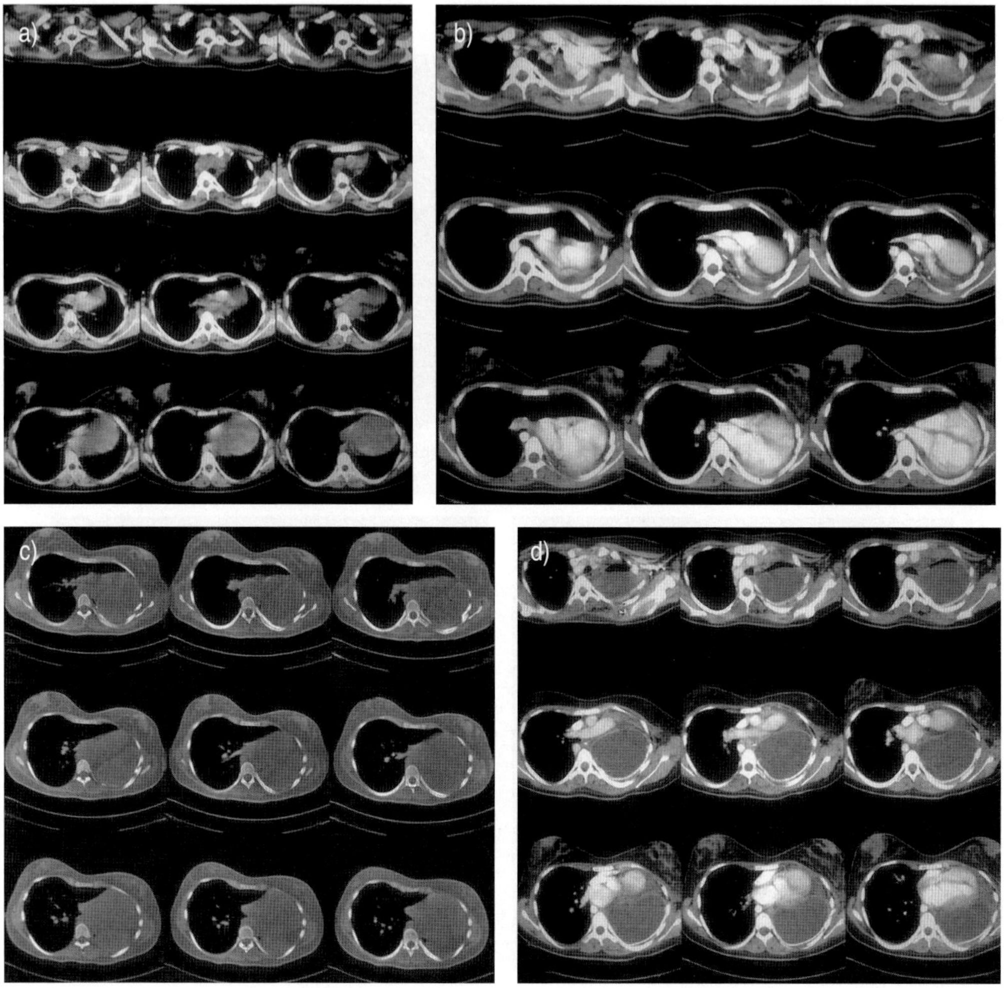


Fig. 6. – Serial computed tomography images of a 15-yr-old female with left-sided pulmonary hyperplasia: a) before pneumonectomy, overriding right lung; b) tracheal compression after further mediastinal shift; c and d) preliminary and definite silicone implants.

successfully undergoing so-called oesophageal tracheoplasty through a right thoracotomy for this condition, three of them adults, one with a long congenital stenosis. Their technique consisted of longitudinal splitting of the tracheal membranous part that was extended into a main bronchus if necessary. Along the advanced tracheal tube the anterior wall of the oesophagus is attached with running sutures first at the left, then on the right side of the split. In one case swallowing discomfort was noticed which was resolved after 6 months.

Secondary tracheal stenosis, besides by bronchogenic cysts, can also be caused by abnormalities of the great vessels, *i.e.* the pulmonary artery sling malformation and aortic arch anomaly [22]. In the presence of a pulmonary artery sling the distal trachea is compressed from behind by the left main pulmonary artery that originates from the right instead from the trunk and passes the distal trachea posteriorly. Usually, this is not tolerated and requires early postnatal correction. Whereas an asymptomatic patient was reported by ZYLAK *et al.* [3], the current author observed a 60-yr-old female who had been treated for asthma since childhood. The latter patient was referred for stent implantation because of severe dyspnoea that only allowed her to rest in a sitting position. On bronchoscopy the subtotal occlusion by the bulging membranous part showed slight pulsation (fig. 7). After angiographical confirmation of the diagnosis occurred, correction was performed by the transposition of the left pulmonary artery to the left circumference of the pulmonary artery trunk with the aid of extracorporeal circulation.

Another female adolescent patient, also treated for asthma since early childhood, presented with a severe stenosis of the distal trachea and right main bronchus. The patient had a history of double aortic arch and ventricular septal defect correction in infancy. The ascending aorta was compressing the tracheobronchial angle. The bronchial ostium of the right upper lobe was displaced ~3 cm from the tracheal angle distally. After a right thoracotomy the ascending aorta was mobilised, including the proximal arch, and the right subclavian artery and circumferential polytetrafluorethylene strips were anchored at the adventitia of the aorta allowing traction towards the superior and anterolateral chest wall (fig. 8). This resulted in a 5–7 mm distance between the tracheal and aortic walls. A recent cardio-respiratory investigation revealed normal lung function tests 13 yrs later.

## *Congenital airway fistulas to the oesophagus*

Most tracheo-oesophageal fistulas are seen in association with atresia of the oesophagus and need repair in the early postnatal period. However, mild developmental disturbance may result in the so-called H-type with a narrow tube-like connection between the lumina of trachea and oesophagus. This condition can remain nearly asymptomatic and might be discovered only in adulthood. The symptoms are often unexplained with recurrent pulmonary infections due to aspiration. Congenital broncho-oesophageal fistulae are most often presented as communications between the lower third of the oesophagus and the lower lobe bronchi, with a preponderance of the right lower lobe.

There are three series [26–28] and a number of case reports [29–31] published in recent literature, which dealt with treatment of broncho-oesophageal fistulas and a single case

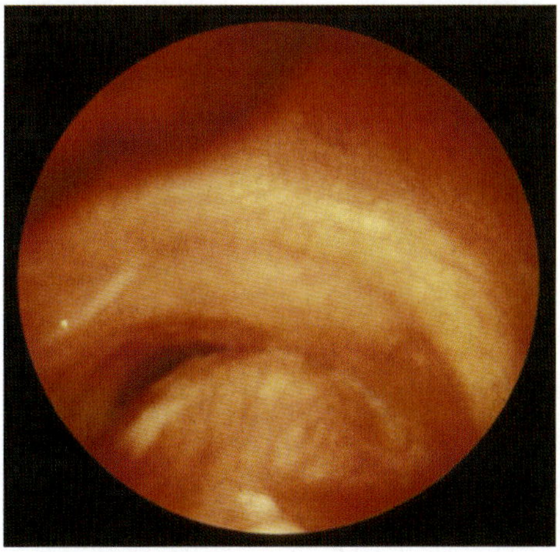

Fig. 7. – Bronchoscopic view of the supracarinal portion of the trachea in a 60-yr-old female with secondary tracheal stenosis, showing subtotal occlusion by malposition of the left pulmonary artery.

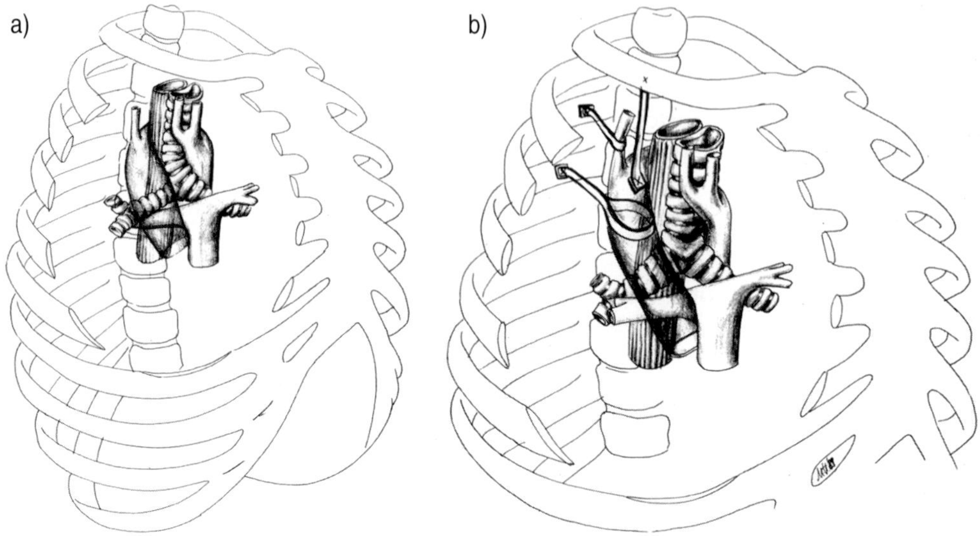


Fig. 8. – Mechanism of right tracheobronchial compression by the ascending aorta (left) and principle of decompression aortopexy.

of tracheo-oesophageal fistula, in adults. This indicates that only small oligosymptomatic fistulas are tolerated without early surgery. The predominant symptoms are: chronic cough, recurrent pulmonary infections, and eventually haemoptysis. The diagnosis and exact localisation is achieved endoscopically with proof of luminal communication by inspection, radiograph contrasts, dyed liquid, or air inflation. The right bronchial system seems to be involved more frequently. During surgery the orifices are closed separately. Interposition of well vascularised tissue flaps is recommended. In the presence of irreversible pulmonary damage, *i.e.* bronchiectasis or carnefication, appropriate resection is performed. In the current author's practice a single case with left-sided congenital fistula was observed and a left lower lobectomy was required (fig. 9).

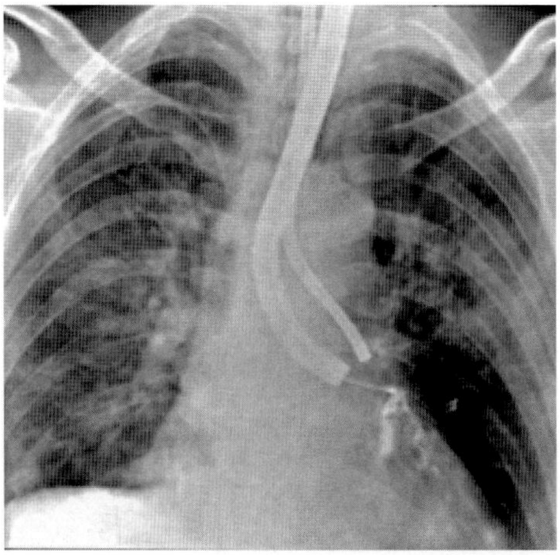

Fig. 9. – Fluoroscopy image during combined oesophageal and bronchial fibre endoscopy proving broncho-oesophageal fistula.

## *Pulmonary arteriovenous malformations*

Arteriovenous communications in the lung parenchyma according to HUDAK [1] represent a congenital malformation of the capillary bed. Increasing diameters of afferent and efferent vessels of the aneurysmatic communication are lead to spheric lesions radiologically and to arterial hypoxaemia *via* pathological right-to-left shunts clinically.

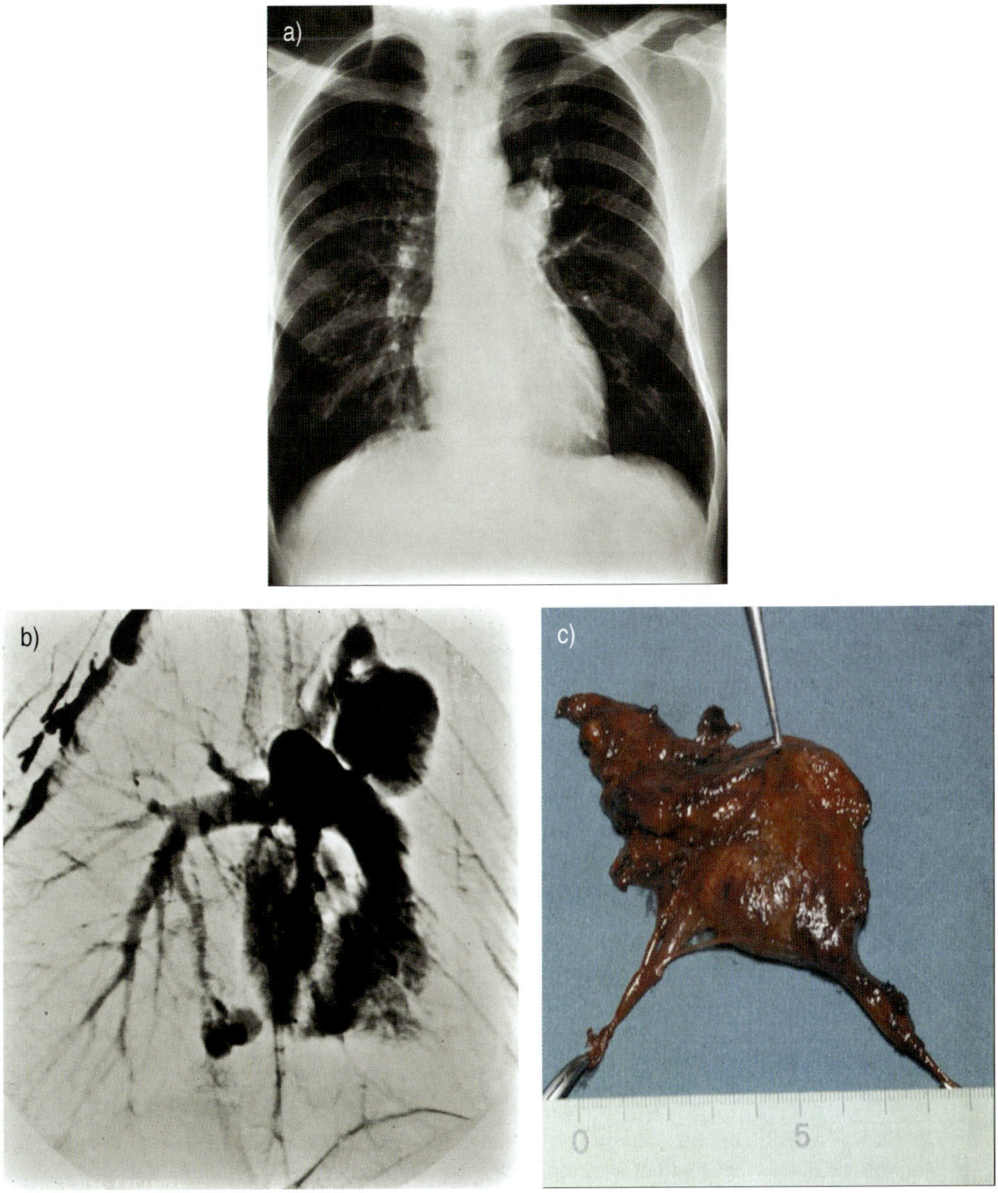


Fig. 10. – Vascular anomaly in a 32-yr-old male whose arterial oxygen tension at rest is 6.65 kPa (50 mmHg): a) chest radiographs with oval lesion to the left of the aortic arch, b) pulmonary artery angiogram showing large aneurysm to the left and a smaller one to the right, and c) anatomical subsegmental resection, specimen showing vascular pedicles.

A total of 70% of cases occur in association with the hereditary Rendu-Osler-Weber disease [32]. Cerebral systemic arterial embolism and massive haemoptysis are the most serious complications. In multiple small aneurysms catheter embolisation is preferred. In large aneurysms surgery is required. The involved segmental or subsegmental vessels are ligated and the lesion is removed anatomically with the surrounding parenchyma following the principles of segmentectomy (fig. 10).

## Conclusions

Some familiarity with congenital malformations of the bronchopulmonary system is indispensable for the thoracic surgeon. Although very few patients will present with congenital lesions in adulthood, the surgeon has the ultimate responsibility for the indication and performance of the appropriate treatment and has to estimate potential risks related to the procedure and related to eventual conservative treatment, respectively. Moreover, congenital malformations that might be reduced to anatomical divergence to the normal, require intra-operative decisions in patients who are operated on for acquired diseases. Where paediatric cases are included in the thoracic surgical service more experiences will be accumulated. Surgical correction is very rewarding, both in the paediatric and in the adult group. Patients who reach adulthood have usually passed a favourable selection. Therefore, in the current author's experience, and in the literature, surgical treatment carries a low risk of morbidity and mortality and should be advocated in the majority of those patients.

## Summary

Congenital malformations of the respiratory system are only occasionally the subject of thoracic surgery in adults. Among the spectrum of clinically relevant diseases pulmonary sequestration and bronchogenic cysts are the most frequent. The purpose of this chapter is to present a brief synopsis of such malformations, their clinical symptoms and, eventually, complications as well as treatments and outcomes based on the recent literature and the current author's experiences. It is shown that in the majority of congenital lesions presenting in adulthood surgery is successful and carries a low risk of morbidity and mortality. Therefore, even in the case of incidental diagnosis of asymptomatic malformations, operative correction is usually indicated.

**Keywords:** Adults, congenital malformations, respiratory system, surgery.

## References

1. Hudak B. Congenital malformations of the lung and airways. *In*: Loughlin GM, Howard E, eds. Respiratory disease in children. Baltimore, William & Wilkins, 1994; pp. 501–532.
2. Luck SR, Reynolds M, Raffensperger JG. Congenital bronchopulmonary malformations. *Curr Probl Surg* 1986; 23: 251–314.
3. Zylak CJ, Eyler WR, Spizarny DL, Stone CH. Developmental lung anomalies in the adult: radiologic-pathologic correlation. *RadioGraphics* 2002; 22: S25–S43.

4. Gray SW, Skandalakis JE. The trachea and lungs. *In*: Gray SW, Skandalakis JE, eds. Embryology for Surgeons. Philadelphia, Saunders, 1972; pp. 293–323.
5. Gray SW, Skandalakis JE. Intrathoracic malformations of foregut derivatives. *In*: Fallis JC, Filler RM, Lemoine G, eds. Pediatric thoracic surgery. New York, Elsevier, 1991; pp. 61–74.
6. Bratu I, Flageole H, Chen MF, *et al.* The multiple facets of pulmonary sequestration. *J Pediatr Surg* 2001; 36: 784–790.
7. Van Raemdonck D, De Boeck K, Devlieger H, *et al.* Pulmonary sequestration: a comparison between pediatric and adult patients. *Eur J Cardio-thorac Surg* 2001; 19: 388–395.
8. Yamanaka A, Hirai T, Fujimoto T, *et al.* Anomalous systemic arterial supply to normal basal segments of the left lower lobe. *Ann Thorac Surg* 1999; 68: 332.
9. Chavrier YPM. Intrapulmonary lesions. *In*: Fallis JC, Filler RM, Lemoine G, eds. Pediatric thoracic surgery. New York, Elsevier, 1991; pp. 75–87.
10. Nakayama Y, Kido M, Minami K, *et al.* Pulmonary sequestration with myocardial ischemia caused by vasospasm and steal. *Ann Thorac Surg* 2000; 70: 304–305.
11. Temes RT, Talbot WA, Carillo YM, *et al.* Sequestration of the lung arising from the circumflex coronary artery. *Ann Thorac Surg* 1998; 65: 257–259.
12. Lewis MM, Tsou EA. 66-year-old man with dyspnea, left lower lobe infiltrate, and abnormal imaging. *Chest* 2000; 117: 1782–1786.
13. Sippel JM, Ravichandran S, Antonovic R, Holden WE. Extralobar pulmonary sequestration presenting as a mediastinal malignancy. *Ann Thorac Surg* 1997; 63: 1169–1171.
14. Conran RM, Stocker JT. Extralobar sequestration with frequently associated congenital cystic adenomatoid malformation, type 2: Report of 50 cases. *Pediatr Dev Pathol* 1999; 2: 454–463.
15. Hasse J, Lincoln JC, Paneth M. Differenzierte chirurgische behandlung bei congenitalem lobärem emphysem [differentiated surgical therapy in congenital lobar emphysema]. *Thoraxchir Vask Chir* 1975; 23: 250–255.
16. Dyon JF, Baudain P, Alibeu JP. Malformations of the lung mass. *In*: Fallis JC, Filler RM, Lemoine G, eds. Pediatric thoracic surgery. New York, Elsevier, 1991; pp. 88–101.
17. Takahashi N, Murakami H, Umeda H, *et al.* Retroperitoneal bronchogenic cyst: a case report. *Nippon Hinyokika Gakkai Zasshi* 2002; 93: 583–587.
18. Takeda SI, Miyoshi S, Minami M, *et al.* Clinical spectrum of mediastinal cysts. *Chest* 2003; 124: 125–132.
19. Ribet ME, Copin MC, Gosselin BH. Bronchogenic cysts of the lung. *Ann Thorac Surg* 1996; 61: 1636–1640.
20. Nusair S, Salameh-Giryes S, Springer C, Izhar U. Congenital bronchial cyst with recurrent submassive hemoptysis. *J Thorac Cardiovasc Surg* 2003; 125: 972–973.
21. Duranceau ACH, Deslauriers J. Foregut cysts of the mediastinum in the adult. *In*: Shields TW. Mediastinal surgery. Philadelphia, Lea & Felbiger, 1991; pp. 305–316.
22. Gray SW, Skandalakis JE. Pulmonary circulation. *In*: Gray SW, Skandalakis JE, eds. Embryology for Surgeons. Philadelphia, Saunders, 1972; pp. 323–358.
23. Bouros D, Parc P, Panagon P, *et al.* The varied manifestation of pulmonary artery agenesis in adulthood. *Chest* 1995; 108: 670–676.
24. Ten Harkel ADJ, Blom HA, Ottenkamp J. Isolated unilateral absence of a pulmonary artery. A case report and review of the literature. *Chest* 2002; 122: 1471–1477.
25. Niwa H, Masaoka A, Yamakawa Y, *et al.* Esophageal tracheobronchoplasty for diseases of the central airway. *J Thorac Cardiovasc Surg* 1996; 112: 124–129.
26. Rämö OJ, Salo JA, Mattila SP. Congenital bronchoesophageal fistula in the adult. *Ann Thorac Surg* 1995; 59: 887–890.
27. Kim JH, Park K-H, Sung S, Rho JR. Congenital bronchoesophageal fistulas in adult patients. *Ann Thorac Surg* 1995; 60: 151–155.
28. Mangi AA, Gaissert HA, Wright CD, *et al.* Benign broncho-esophageal fistula in the adult. *Ann Thorac Surg* 2002; 73: 911–915.

29. Danton MH, McMahon J, McGuigan J, Gibbons JR. Congenital oesophageal respiratory tract fistula presenting in adult life. *Eur Respir J* 1993; 6: 1412–1414.
30. Deb S, Ali MB, Fonnseca P. Congenital bronchoesophageal fistula in an adult. *Chest* 1998; 114: 1784–1786.
31. Dogan R, Farsak B, Yilmaz M, *et al.* Congenital broncho-oesophageal fistula associated with bronchiectasis in adults. Report of two cases and review of the literature. *Respiration* 1999; 66: 361–365.
32. Gossage JR, Kanj G. Pulmonary arteriovenous malformations. A state of the art review. *Am J Respir and Crit Care Med* 1998; 158: 643–661.

<u>*CHAPTER 15*</u>

# Tracheobronchial ruptures in blunt trauma of the thorax: diagnosis and treatment

*P. De Leyn*, J. Jougon#, J-F. Velly#*

**Dept of Thoracic Surgery, University Hospitals Leuven, Belgium. #Dept of Thoracic Surgery, Hôpital du Haut-Lévêque, Bordeaux-Pessac, France.*

*Correspondence: J-F.Velly, Dept of Thoracic Surgery, Hôpital du Haut-Lévêque, 33604 Bordeaux-Pessac, France.*

Injuries of the respiratory tract after blunt trauma of the chest are uncommon. However, these are seen as serious injuries because of their consequences in terms of ventilation coupled with the severity of the thoracic and extrathoracic injuries that are often associated with them. In general they affect young patients, an age group who are at greater risk of accidents, but perhaps a population selected for survival due to the flexibility of their vascular system. Their symptomatology is often obvious; however, it can be difficult to recognise *e.g.* in a multiple trauma context, where early intubation has been required. Diagnosis of these injuries is always carried out by tracheobronchial endoscopy. These injuries generally require emergency surgical treatment. However, the time of the repair should be integrated in the strategy and hierarchy used for the overall management of multiple trauma victims. The results of surgical treatment are good, provided the patient is well controlled in terms of ventilation and haemodynamics.

## Definition

Traumatic injuries to the respiratory tract are defined as wounds or complete ruptures of the wall of the tracheobronchial tree. They are situated between the larynx and the opening of the segmentary bronchi and completely open up the airways to the peritracheobronchial spaces. They may affect one or more of three regions: the mediastinum, the hilar and the fissural regions. This topographical definition corresponds to the immediate or secondary clinical severity: mediastinal or pleural air-leak and loss of, or threat to, respiratory function. This definition also corresponds to a diagnostic and therapeutic reality. This is the part of the tracheobronchial tree that is accessible to endoscopic exploration and surgical repair.

Injuries to sub-segmentary bronchi and more distal bronchi, which can be similar in terms of symptomatology and seriousness, are excluded from this chapter. They belong to the chapter on pulmonary parenchymatous wounds and contusions, since they will heal without surgical intervention provided it is possible to control the physiopathological disorders that arise from them, such as pulmonary contusions, air-leaks and bronchial congestion.

## Incidence and circumstances in which these injuries occur

The incidence of post-traumatic tracheobronchial injuries is difficult to assess since a large number of patients will die from these injuries and associated injuries before they

Eur Respir Mon, 2004, 29, 223–233. Printed in UK -  European Respiratory Monograph; ISSN 1025-448x. ISBN 1-904097-33-2.

arrive in hospital. Overall, 2–4% of people with severe thoracic trauma present with a tracheobronchial injury. This incidence is subject to clear variability between different authors and periods. It is 2.8% according to BERTELSEN and HOWITZ [1] in a study of 1,157 autopsies of patients who died after thoracic trauma. KELLY *et al.* [2], in 1985, reported only six cases of blunt trauma in a review of 106 ruptures of the tracheobronchial tree, after wounds to the thorax or to the neck.

The incidence of these injuries in European series [3–5] varies from 0.3–4.5% (table 1). This incidence rose significantly during the 1980s due to the increase in the number of accidents on public roads and also to the improved management of trauma victims. At the present time the number of these injuries seems to be stable, or even falling. Mortality caused by these injuries is estimated to be 30% [6]. However, 90% of patients who arrive at hospital can be cured [7, 8].

# Pathogenesis

Various different mechanisms can cause these injuries:

## *Traffic accidents*

On the occasion of a blunt trauma, the most frequent situation in Europe is being hit by a car in the thoracic or cervico-thoracic region in the event of a frontal impact. The flexibility of the chest wall in young people who suffer trauma creates the possibility of tracheobronchial compression by the sternum against the spinal column even without clinically detectable parietal injuries. The crushing of the anterior chest wall can result in: a direct fracture of the cartilages of the trachea or a complete rupture of the carina or of the main bronchi; due to a sharp transverse shearing actions as described by DE LA ROCHA [9] (fig. 1).

## *Sharpe deceleration*

Another mechanism is a scissoring action in connection with a sharp deceleration, affecting tracheobronchial structures with different kinetic characteristics, a mechanism similar to that involved in ruptures of the aortic arch.

## *Vertical shearing*

A further cause is a sharp vertical shearing action, usually on the occasion of a hyperextension of the head and neck, which is the mechanism most often involved in laryngo-tracheal disruption.

## *Intrathoracic overpressure*

Intrathoracic overpressure against a closed glottis gives rise to tears in the airway wall at its weak points; the posterior part of the trachea or the attachment of the membranous trachea and the cartilaginous rings.

**Table 1. – Incidence of tracheobronchial injuries in thoracic trauma in Europe**

| First author [Ref.] | Thoracic trauma n | Tracheobronchial injuries % |
|---|---|---|
| COURAUD [3] | 550 | 5.5 |
| RIBET [4] | 2000 | 4 |
| GALAN [5] | 696 | 0.3 |

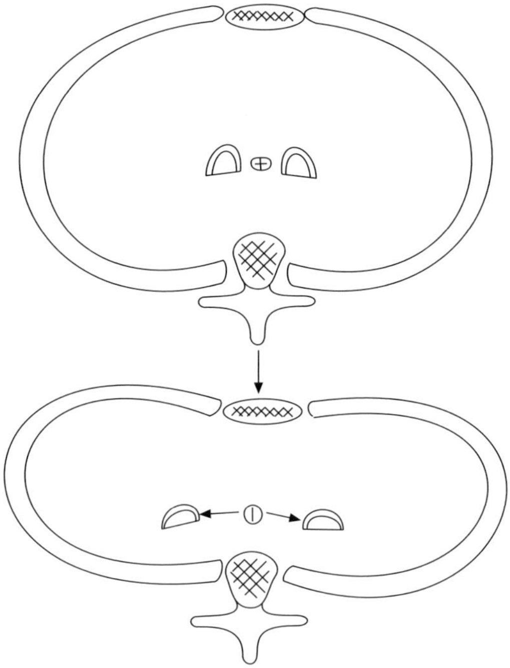

Fig. 1. – Antero-posterior trauma. Tear of the carina or the main bronchi by a sharp transverse shearing action.

### *Open trauma*

An open trauma may be involved; penetrating wounds with extremely variable aetiologies, giving rise to tracheobronchial trauma due to a direct or indirect effect, depending on the nature and the ballistic characteristics of the penetrating agent. These are often associated with other serious thoracic injuries. These type of injuries are frequently encountered in big cities *e.g.* in North America [6, 10].

### *Direct trauma*

Finally, these injuries may occur as the result of direct trauma, which is most frequently iatrogenic: endoluminal injury to the tracheobronchial wall during intubation, exploratory or therapeutic endoscopy, or due to a blast trauma. (which is quite rare).

## Types of injuries

Clearly, three main types of tracheobronchial injuries may be encountered (fig. 2).

### *A tear of the posterior membranous trachea*

This is the first type of tracheobronchial injury. The level and length of tear can be very variable, both in the membranous trachea itself, or at the lateral insertion. These tears may involve the trachea at any level, or the main bronchi, but also the carina, sometimes with multiple complex tears in this region.

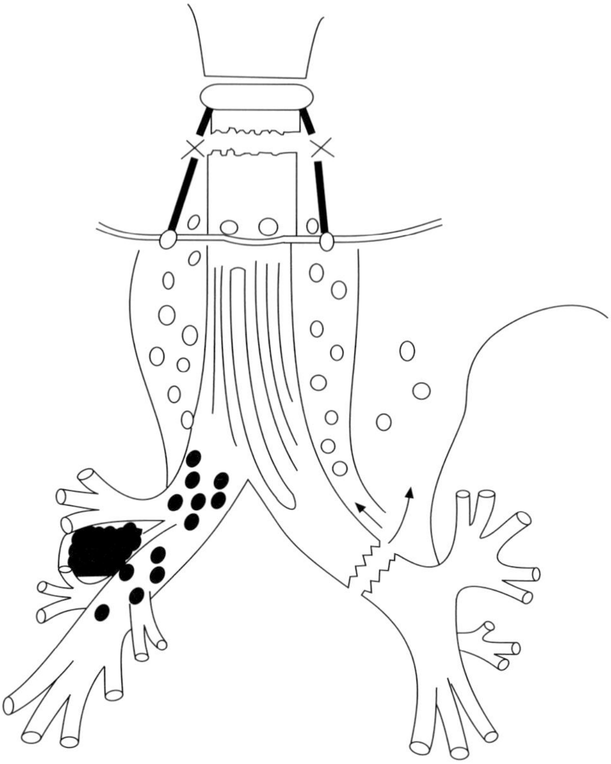

Fig. 2. – Three types of tracheobronchial injuries may be encountered: fissure, fracture and rupture.

### *Fracture of one or more cartilaginous arches*

The second type of tracheobronchial injury is a fracture of one or more cartilaginous arches at the level of the trachea or major bronchi, a fracture which is not circumferential but involving the whole wall.

### *Circumferential rupture*

A complete and circumferential rupture of the entire wall of the tracheobronchial tree, with retraction of the margins of the rupture and more or less rapid interposition of the peritracheobronchial tissues is the last type of injury.

These three basic injuries may be associated with each other, leading to complex damages in the form of tears, lacerations or bursts in the tracheobronchial tree which are difficult to repair. Therefore, they are often associated with damage to the neighbouring tissues, vascular pulmonary tissues or, less frequently, the oesophagus wall.

## Physiopathological consequences

The physiopathological consequences include air-leaks into the peritracheobronchial spaces. Initially, in the mediastinum, this will give mediastinal emphysema (radiological diagnosis), then rapidly subcutaneous emphysema, first in the anterior cervical area superior to the manubrium, then more or less extensively in subcutaneous and submucosal spaces. When the pleura is ruptured, air will leak in one or both pleural cavities giving uni- or bilateral pneumothorax with often tension pneumothorax. Haemorrhage in the tracheobronchial lumen may occur with more or less significant obstruction, leading sometimes to a real haemorrhagic flood.

Injury to the airway may produce a partial or complete reduction of the calibre of the tracheobronchial lumen, and possibly a very high sub-glottal interruption, in cases of laryngo-tracheal disruption. These complete ruptures may allow continuity to be maintained in the airways through the mediastinal tissues for a certain period [9, 11], thus allowing the patients to arrive in hospital alive.

In addition, airway injuries will lead to septic contamination, starting from the respiratory tract. The associated injuries depend on the mechanism and the violence of the trauma:

- Spinal and extrathoracic injuries are very common in multiple trauma patients.
- In the peri-tracheobronchial area, cardiac injuries, aortic and supra-aortic vessels injuries, vascular pulmonary injuries occur in 5–10% of cases. Recurrent nerve injuries are frequent in case of laryngotracheal disruption. Oesophageal wounds are encountered in 12% of cases [12].

## Topography of tracheobronchial injuries

Traditionally, 80% of injuries resulting from blunt trauma are located in the area of the carina. They are situated 2–2.5 cm around the bifurcation [7, 13], a fragile area, which is easily subject to distortion and tearing. Conversely, 80% of injuries resulting from direct instrumental injury, hyperextension or strangulation are situated at the level of the top one-third of the trachea and the laryngotracheal junction. The incidence of complete, circumferential ruptures with retraction of the two tracheal or bronchial extremities is equivalent to that of total tears involving the whole wall, which are longitudinal or circular but not circumferential [8].

The incidence of laryngotracheal injuries in comparison with tracheal or bronchial injuries increased gradually between 1960–1980, and then stabilised [14]. This is the result of strangulation phenomena caused by safety belts on the occasion of "submarining" movements during the trauma. The stabilisation and more over the actual decrease in the number of these very specific injuries can be attributed to improvements in this safety system.

## Symptomatology

Symptoms are frequently early and severe. Classically, severe multiple traumas cause damage to the first two ribs, cervical contusion or strangulation are pictures that should arise suspicion of tracheobronchial injury. This injury can easily be suspected clinically from the initial post-traumatic period in the majority of patients with: acute dyspnoea; cervico-mediastinal emphysema; and uni- or bilateral pneumothorax, which is often pressure pneumothorax, haemopneumothorax, haemoptysis and dysphonia.

However, a tracheobronchial injury should always be suspected in cases of serious chest traumas. However, there is not necessarily an anatomoclinical parallelism between the injuries to the thoracic viscera and those to the chest wall. So, the use of artificial ventilation without pleural drainage may, under these conditions, cause the creation of a hypertensive and pressure pneumothorax leading the patient to death as soon as they are taken in charge.

The rapidity and severity of the onset of respiratory distress often requires emergency treatment for the dyspnoea and air-leak by means of pleural drainage, intubation below the level of a tracheal injury, or selective intubation. The initial symptomatology may sometimes be discrete, retarded or masked by pleuro-pulmonary antecedents, by associated injuries or by resuscitation measures which have been carried out in extreme emergency situations.

Diagnosis can be delayed and is sometimes made very late [11]. Therefore, it is necessary to be attentive to a drain which is bubbling significantly and persistently, and which is not succeeding in re-expanding the pulmonary parenchyma. Atelectasis, either lobar or affecting a whole lung, may be evidence of the complete obstruction of the respiratory tract by peribronchial tissues in the presence of a circumferential rupture. Acute dyspnoea on detubation may be a sign of a high tracheal rupture, associated with recurrent nerve palsy, masked by the intubation which has been inserted at an early stage.

## Diagnosis

Diagnosis is made by endoscopy. The combination of pneumothorax, hypertensive mediastinal emphysema and underlying difficulty in ventilation should give grounds to carry out a fibroscopy or bronchoscopy to look for a tracheobronchial wound or rupture. Although they are rare, wounds to the oesophagus can be associated with tracheobronchial rupture and this justifys the need for systematic oesophagoscopy to be performed. A bronchoscopy should be organised as quickly as possible. It makes it possible to confirm the diagnosis of a tracheobronchial rupture, while also provides the anatomical location of the injuries.

The characteristics and position of the intubation required to maintain balanced ventilation and the need for surgical repair can then be detailed. The treatment strategy can be decided depending on the level of the tracheobronchial injuries and the extent of associated injuries. This examination will be carried out using flexible fibroscopy or rigid bronchoscopy or using both methods.

Fibroscopy allows a dynamic laryngeal examination in search of a recurrent nerve problem in nonintubated patients, and enables a full bronchial exploration to be undertaken. It also allows good distal exploration and does not require either general anaesthetic or any hyperextension of the head on the cervical spine.

Bronchoscopy allows a precise examination of the laryngotracheal axis, the carina and the bronchi, up to the lobar level. It can also be used to catheterise a complete tracheal or bronchial rupture. It is effective in cases of major endoluminal haemorrhage but requires a general anaesthetic and sometimes, depending on the shape of the face and tongue, the mobilisation of the cervical spine.

## Treatment and results

As soon as the symptomatology of thoracic or cervical trauma gives rise to the suspicion of injury to the respiratory tree, it is vital that endoscopic diagnosis and initial palliative care are performed, simultaneously, to avoid errors that might give rise to visceral anoxia and death. This may require pleural drainage, repermeabilisation of the trachea by intubation below the injury and protection of the underlying lungs or the controlateral lung from being flooded with blood from a rupture of the respiratory tree. Carrying out these procedures alleviates the respiratory syndrome and thereby provides enough time to carry out such imaging investigations as appear to be necessary *e.g.*

oesophagoscopy or transoesophageal echography to ascertain if there is an aortic injury, and a computed tomography scan (CT) scan of the thorax and an angiograph. The intervention should be planned depending on the location and type of injuries, the time that has passed since the accident occurred and any associated traumatic injuries.

Data in the literature indicate that when surgical treatment has been carried out under good conditions, where the acute respiratory defect is controlled and stabilised, it has been possible to heal 90% of patients.

## Therapeutic resources

The methods of treatment are most often surgical. Simple suturing is suitable for tears and partial ruptures. This involves minimal trimming of the edges of the injury and suturing without tension. It is used for fresh injuries which are not yet infected. It will be done using slow resorption thread in one plane and at separate points along the cartilaginous arches. A running suture may be used in cases of a posterior linear wound. The suture should be protected by covering with peritracheobronchial tissues or using a flap of pericardial tissue or intercostal muscle. It may be reinforced by the application of biological glue.

End-to-end anastomosis of the respiratory tract is carried out, avoiding extensive dissections to expose edges which give rise to ischaemia and necrosis. It is used for fresh injuries which are not infected and which can be mobilised. It is required at the level of the trachea and the main bronchi.

Resection of the pulmonary territory, underlying the injury, can be a lobar resection at most since pneumonectomies carried out under traumatic conditions are usually lethal.

The methods of treatment are sometimes nonsurgical and may use simple conservative measures: monitoring, or temporary intubation, possibly with the need of laser photocoagulation on granulomas or on a residual hypertrophic scar.

## Indications for surgical repair

Indications for surgical repair are shown in table 2. These depend on the site of the injuries, the amount of time that has passed and the severity of the associated injuries. The site of the injury determines the choice of the repair technique and the route of entry.

### *The repair technique*

For lesions of the trachea suturing is usually mandatory. However, in some selected cases a conservative treatment may be discussed. At the level of the main bronchi,

**Table 2. – Planning the repair**

| Situation | Action |
|---|---|
| The location | |
| Trachea | Repair |
| Main bronchi | Surgical repair without resection as far as possible |
| Lobar bronchi | Resection or repair if non stenosing suture |
| Distal bronchi | Endoscopy and laser |
| Diagnostic delay | Prepare and disinfect |
| Associated injuries | Simultaneous tracheobronchial repair |
| | Delay acceptable under physiopathological control |

surgical repair has to be done as far as possible according to the fact that a pneumonectomy in this situation is not suitable. Lobectomy or segmentectomy is indicated for injuries situated at this level since this intervention has little adverse effect on respiratory function while suturing of small-calibre bronchi may results in stenosis. If the injury is distal to the segmentary orifices or in case of a longitudinal tear of the membraneous part of the trachea it may be possible to refrain from surgery and to treat conservatively provided the air leaks are perfectly controlled by drainage or blocked by mediastinal tissues and the patient is under careful survey in a thoracic unit.

### *Route of entry*

The route of entry varies. Cervicotomy, possibly extended to partial split of the manubrium or full sternotomy is indicated for injuries of the cervical trachea and the superior, supra-aortic part of the thoracic trachea. Right thoracotomy is used for all injuries of the thoracic trachea, the carina and the right main bronchus. It is also recommended for repair of injuries of the initial part of the left main bronchus involving the first 2 or 3 cm. Left thoracotomy is indicated for repair of injuries to the distal part of the left main bronchus and its bifurcation. Certain injuries which extend from the carina to the left bifurcation may give rise to a double right and left incision. Finally, extended complex bilateral injuries with major difficulties of ventilation pre and perioperatively have been repaired under extracorporeal circulatory assistance, provided this is not contraindicated by injuries associated with the multiple trauma.

### *The amount of time passed*

The period between the injury and the ability of surgical repair should be taken into account. Until 3–4 days post injury, dissection is still easy and repair can be carried out on tissues that can be easily mobilised and that are not too inflamed or infected. Longer delays often result in inflammation and sepsis of the tracheobronchial stumps or of the edges of the mucosa laceration associated with a more localised infection of the mediastinal tissues surrounding the tracheobronchial rupture. Since there is no indication for immediate surgery, it is always preferable to delay the repair for a few days using anti-inflammatory and antibiotic treatments. This will reduce the risk of infection at the site of the operation and the very high risk of leakage when the anastomose is carried out on fragile mucosa. This preparation will also reduce the incidence of subsequent stenosing hypertrophic scars.

The technique of reanastomosis or suturing under these delayed conditions has no specific original features; side-to-side anastomosis with clean edges after cutting by separate points using absorbable thread.

### *Associated trauma injuries*

Associated trauma injuries have to be taken into account in the hierarchy of repairs. In cases involving associated multiple injuries, simultaneous surgical repairs are usually recommended. Nevertheless, some serious associated injuries may be adversely affected by the tracheobronchial repair and may give grounds to delay when intubation of the tracheal segment, underlying the rupture, has taken place and when the respiratory problems have been brought completely under control.

## Original problems involving laryngotracheal disruption

Among the various types of ruptures of the respiratory tract, depending on their location, post-traumatic laryngotracheal disruption deserves separate treatment due to its frequency and the diagnostic and therapeutic problems that it raises [14, 15]. This is a common injury and its relative frequency increased until the early 1980s because among the causes (anterior contusion of the neck, strangulation) safety belts were also found to be responsible for this injury

The anatomical injuries have a very characteristic association of laryngotracheal disruption with retraction of the distal tracheal extremity into the superior mediastinum when it is complete. The two recurrent nerves may be torn and stretched. Sometimes only one is affected, if the disruption is partial and the retraction has not taken place. Other findings are a vertical fracture of the cricoid ring into one, two and three parts and retraction of the laryngeal mucosa, exposing the cricoid cartilage to a granulomatous reaction or chondritis. This phenomenon is particularly accentuated in complete detachments. It may be more or less pronounced in other cases. The symptoms are always very acute and often require palliative emergency action: intubation or tracheotomy.

Depending on the case, the diagnosis is made in view of two completely different clinical pictures. The first situation is during the immediate post-traumatic period, in a situation of asphyxiation: acute dyspnoea, aphonia, haemoptysis, erosion of the skin on the anterior surface of the neck, cervico-mediastinal emphysema and pneumothorax, all indicate to an injury of the cervical trachea which is identified and located using endoscopy. The second situation is when the diagnosis is delayed, and is made on symptoms of stenosis such as acute dyspnoea following any attempts at extubation or total stenosis of the respiratory tract above a tracheotomy. A careful analysis of each component of the laryngeal lesions on the CT scan, then at the time of the preoperative bronchoscopy and during the following intervention, will enable the physician to reconstruct the pathogenesis and, above all, to realise which treatment is adapted to each functional consequence of the injury.

Surgical treatment by reanastomosis is the basic treatment for disruptions. It is required in all cases where there is a distance between the fragments. This treatment should take into account the complexity of the injury and should correct each of its components [14, 16]. The tracheal retraction is easily corrected. The superiorly retracted laryngeal mucosa is more difficult to bring down. Therefore, it is useful to make a small circumferential sub-perichondral resection of the lower border of the cricoid ring. This action reveals a short edge of mucosa which makes it possible to make a good quality anastomosis [17]. The recurrent nerve section, when it is bilateral, gives rise to glottic paralysis in adduction and therefore a functional obstacle above the anastomosis. Treatment of this obstacle is vital. This is achieved by performing a vertical posterior cricotomy, separated and supported by a modelling laryngeal intubation (nasotracheal tube or Montgomery T tube) for 3 weeks, gives rise to a posterior glottal enlargement in the same way as a Rethi operation. The posterior cricotomy sometimes exists spontaneously at the level of a fracture, so all that is needed is to enlarge it and to keep it separated.

Therefore, these stenoses need, as ideal surgical repair, a resection followed by a Pearson operation type tracheo-subglottal reanastomosis [17], which may or may not be supplemented by glottal modelling after posterior cricotomy. Failing this, or in the event of inadequate glottal abduction, resulting in persistent effort dyspnoea, laser resection of a vocal cord may improve the respiratory functional situation and make it comfortable, while slightly accentuating the phonatory sequelae. The overall result of this treatment for such injuries is very positive for serious traumatic injury.

## Conclusion

Traumas affecting the tracheobronchial tree are still serious injuries, despite progress in respiratory resuscitation, despite the inceased number of specialised services available for treatment of multiple trauma victims, and despite the improvements in resources for collection and transportation of injured patients. Although gasometric changes generally respond remarkably well to physiopathological treatments, mortality is still high with a death rate of 10–20%. However, most deaths are more closely associated with the severity of coincident visceral injuries in multiple trauma victims or anoxic visceral injuries prior to treatment rather than to the lack of control of injuries affecting the respiratory tract.

The prognosis essentially depends on good initial control of respiratory distress through the use of appropriate and early resuscitation measures. However, legal measures which have been introduced such as compulsory wearing of safety belts, speed limits on road traffic and controls on levels of blood alcohol, will undoubtedly help to reduce the number of these traumas in current treatment units.

## Summary

Management of tracheobronchial ruptures after blunt thoracic trauma requires a good knowledge of original mechanisms and of immediate or secondary physiological consequences of these lesions. An urgent and precise endoscopic diagnosis is mandatory. Immediate surgical treatment is the rule, taking into account, however, the schedule of other surgical repairs in case of polytrauma. The technical problems of surgical repair are nowadays overcome and prognosis mainly depends on the initial control of respiratory failure and complications.

**Keywords:** Bronchial puncture, bronchial rupture, laryngo-tracheal disruption, multiple bronchial traumas, tracheobroncheal injury.

## References

1. Bertelsen S, Howitz P. Injuries of the trachea and bronchi. *Thorax* 1972; 27: 188–194.
2. Kelly JP, Webb WR, Moulder PV, Everson C, Buah BH, Lindsey ES. Managment of airway trauma I: tracheobronchial injuries. *Ann Thorac Surg* 1985; 40: 551–555.
3. Couraud L, Bruneteau A, Durandeau A. Les ruptures traumatiques de la trachée et des bronches. Réflexions sur leur traitement. A propos d'une expérience personnelle de 15 cas. *Bordeaux Medical* 1973; 13: 2828–2864.
4. Ribet M, Woelffle D, Bolleingier D, Hassoun A, Pruvot FR, Giard-Lefevre S. La contusion pulmonaire diffuse. *La Presse Méd* 1987; 16: 578–581.
5. Galan G, Penalver JC, Paris F, *et al.* Blunt chest injuries in 1696 patients. *Eur J Cardio-thorac Surg* 1992; 6: 284–287.
6. Lo Cicero III J, Mattox KL. Epidemiology of chest trauma. *Surg Clin North Am* 1989; 69: 19–24.
7. Dor J, Foster E, Le Brigand H. Rupture traumatiques des bronches et de la trachée thoracique. Doin, Paris, 1964; 228–231.
8. Velly JF, Martigne C, Moreau JM, Dubrez J, Kerdi S, Couraud L. Post traumatic tracheobronchial injuries. *Eur J Cardio-Thorac Surg* 1991; 5: 352–355.

9. De la Rocha AG, Kayler D. Traumatic rupture of the tracheobronchial tree. *Can J Surg* 1985; 28: 68–71.
10. Hood RM, Boyd AD, Culliford AT. Thoracic Trauma. Philadelphia, W.B. Saunders Company, 1989;
11. Kelly JP, Webb WR, Moulder PV, Moustouaas NM, Lirtzman M. Management of airway trauma II: combined injuries of the trachea and esophagus. *Ann Thorac Surg* 1987; 43: 160–163.
12. Besson A, Saegesser F. A Colour Atlas of Chest Trauma and Associated Injuries. (vol 2). London, Wolfe Medical Publications Ltd, 1983.
13. Deslauriers J. Bronchial rupture. *In*: Grillo HC, Eschapasse H, eds. International Trends in General Thoracic Surgery (vol 2). Major challenges. Philadelphia, Saunders, 1987; pp. 246–254.
14. Couraud L, Velly JF. Post traumatic disruption of the laryngo-tracheal junction. *Eur J Cardio-thorac surg* 1989; 3: 441–444.
15. Gussack GS, Jurkovich GJ, Luterman A. Laryngotracheal trauma: a protocol approach to a rare injury. *Laryngoscope* 1986; 96: 660–665.
16. Mathisen DJ, Grillo HC. Laryngo tracheal trauma. Acute and chronic. *In*: Grillo HC, Eschapasse H, eds. International Trends in General Thoracic Surgery (vol 2). Major challenges. Philadelphia, Saunders, 1987; pp. 177–123.
17. Pearson FG, Cooper JD, Nelems JM, Van Nostrahd AW. Primary tracheal anastomosis after resection of the cricoïd cartilage with preservation of recurrent laryngeal nerves. *J Thorac Cardiovasc Surg* 1975; 70: 806–816.

CHAPTER 16

# Airway injury and sequelae: conservative view

M. Noppen

Correspondence: M. Noppen, Head of Clinic, Interventional Endoscopy Clinic, Academic Hospital AZ-VUB, 101, Laarbeeklaan, B-1090, Brussels, Belgium.

Surgical repair is widely considered the golden standard in the treatment of airway injury of benign origin [1]. Corrective tracheobronchial surgery, however, requires considerable surgical expertise and rigorous procedures, *e.g.* avoiding tracheal devascularisation or anastomotic tension, and is not available everywhere. Therefore, transfer of these patients to experienced thoracic surgical centres seems imperative [1, 2].

Furthermore, an extensive preoperative evaluation of the level and extent of the lesion, including preoperative bronchoscopy and extensive radiological evaluation [1], should determine how operable the lesion is.

Finally, the patients' general condition (including respiratory, cardiovascular and neurological status) should allow for corrective tracheal or tracheobronchial surgery, which, even in carefully selected patients and in experienced centres, is associated with an immediate postoperative mortality of 1.5–5%, and with a long-term failure rate of up to 15% [1–3].

Hence, this type of surgery can rarely be performed immediately after the causative injury has occurred (with the exception of a traumatic airway rupture [4]), and preoperative stabilisation of the patients is often necessary. This explains why, in large surgical series, between 26–71% of patients had to be treated conservatively prior to surgery [5]. Moreover, in a considerable number of patients, corrective surgery remains impossible or contra-indicated because of patient or lesion related inoperability.

During recent decades, various bronchoscopic techniques have been developed and increasingly used for the treatment of malignant, and benign central airway lesions [6, 7], including: mechanical and balloon dilation; neodymium-yttrium aluminum garnett (Nd:YAG)-laser and electrocautery resection; and airway stenting. Hence these techniques can be applied for temporary treatment awaiting definitive surgical repair, or for permanent treatment when surgery is impossible or refused.

Conservative bronchoscopic treatment, therefore, should be considered as an adjunct to, and not as a competitor of, surgical repair. The most frequently encountered lesions which are candidates for conservative treatment include: postintubation tracheal stenosis (PITS); burn lesions of the airways; airway fistulae; iatrogenic and traumatic airway rupture; and tracheobronchomalacia.

## Postintubation tracheal stenosis

PITS remains the most common indication for tracheal resection and reconstruction, despite identification of its causes and the development of techniques and strategies for its avoidance [8]. Prospective studies have reported an incidence of postintubation/post-tracheostomy tracheal stenosis of 10–19% [3]. Although symptomatic stenoses

Eur Respir Mon, 2004, 29, 234–245. Printed in UK - all rights reserved. Copyright ERS Journals Ltd 2004; European Respiratory Monograph; ISSN 1025-448x. ISBN 1-904097-33-2.

occurs after <1% of intubations; in a recent prospective study, symptomatic PITS requiring treatment, occurred in 1:1,000 patients admitted to intensive care unit (ICU) [9]. The widespread use of endotracheal tubes with low pressure/high volume cuffs has lead to a 10-fold reduction in the incidence of PITS.

PITS is generally thought to occur most often after prolonged periods of intubation, however, the mean number of days of intubation in a series of PITS patients was only 12±10 days (range 2–40 days) [10].

The occurrence of PITS seems unrelated to the type of endotracheal intubation (oral or transnasal), the urgency of intubation, or to the number of reintubations undertaken by a patient [9, 10].

High endotracheal tube cuff pressures can lead to local ischaemia of the tracheal mucosa, leading to ulceration and cartilage denudation. Local inflammation and supper infection may lead to a progressive loss of cartilaginous support [11]. Tracheostomy is a supplementary factor leading to tracheal wall instability by causing direct damage to the cartilage. Stenotic lesions then occur because of cicatricial fibrosis of the mucosa and tracheal wall with or without tracheal wall instability (focal tracheomalacia).

PITS lesions include: web-like stenoses (fig. 1), which are short (<1 cm) diaphragm-like concentric retractile fibrosis of the mucosa, with a maintained tracheal cartilaginous structure; complex stenoses (fig. 2), these are longer (>1 cm) lesions consisting of various degrees of mucosal fibrous lesions associated with a component of tracheomalacia; and "A-type" or pseudoglottic stenosis (fig. 3), which involve fracture of cartilaginous ring/s following tracheotomy.

PITS has to be considered in every patient following intubation or tracheostomy, presenting with (progressive) dyspnoea or stridor. Most patients become symptomatic within 3 months after extubation [9, 10]. Patients typically may be asymptomatic at rest and stridorous at effort [5]. In more than half of cases, other diagnoses of dyspnoea are erroneously made prior to definitive diagnoses of PITS, including: asthma, cardiac insufficiency and pulmonary embolism. The diagnosis of PITS may be suggested by the presence of a flattened inspiratory and/or expiratory flow-volume curve loop, and is confirmed by flexible bronchoscopy. In symptomatic PITS patients, the residual tracheal lumen is in general <5 mm in diameter, representing a ≥75% of stenosis [9].

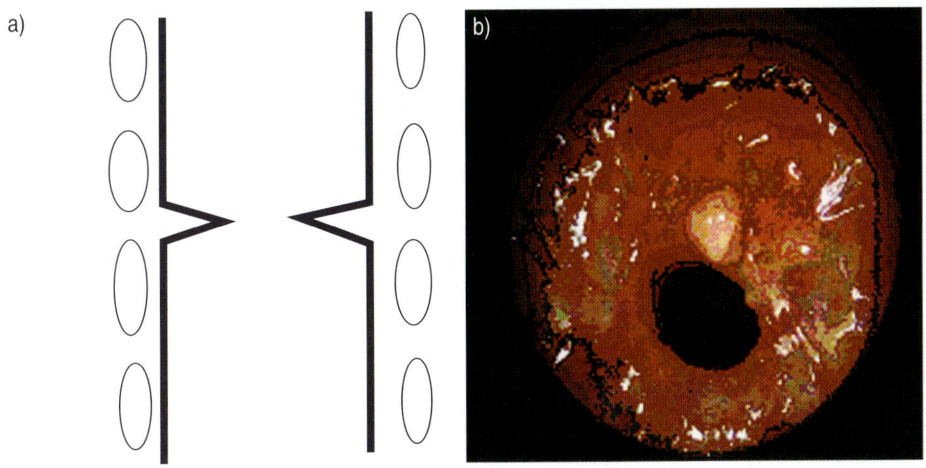


Fig. 1. – a) Figurative and b) photographic examples of postintubation tracheal stenose, showing web-like postintubation tracheal stenosis.

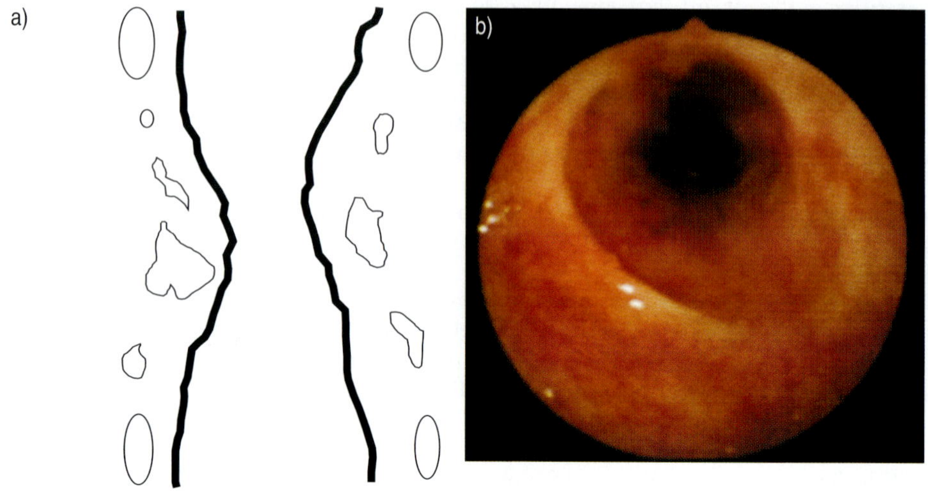


Fig. 2. – a) Figurative and b) photographic examples of complex stenosis.

Definitive treatment of PITS consists of surgical resection of the diseased tracheal segment, followed by primary reconstruction, by means of end-to-end anostomosis.

Laryngotracheal [12] or carinal [1] tracheal release techniques may be necessary, especially in case of resection of long segments. Satisfactory or good results may be obtained in 85–95% of cases in highly specialised centres [1, 3, 5, 13], and in carefully selected patients. Surgical mortality is reported to be 1–5% [3, 5], depending upon the type of lesion and the underlying condition of the patient. Because the majority of patients with PITS have a history of recent ICU-stay and associated comorbidity, immediate surgery after diagnosis of PITS very often is contra-indicated. In prospective studies, up to two-thirds of patients had to be treated by conservative techniques, prior to eventual surgery [5, 9].

Therefore, in contrast with some surgical series, where highly selected patients are included, and with some medical series where surgical treatment often is underscored,

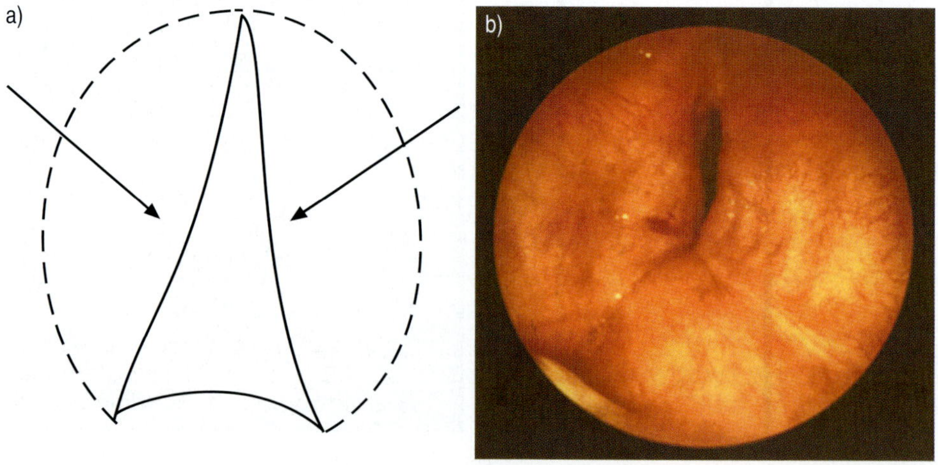


Fig. 3. – a) Figurative and b) photographic examples of pseudoglottic stenosis.

real-world management of these patients most often requires a combined and cooperative approach.

A prospective multidisciplinary treatment algorithm for symptomatic PITS adapting this philosophy has recently been proposed by MARQUETTE *et al.* [9].

In case of "simple" web-like stenoses, mechanical dilation, if necessary by radial Nd:YAG-laser or high frequency electrocautery incision, is proposed, and repeated up to two times [14] in case of recurrence.

In cases of tracheal stabilisation, no further treatment is required and follow-up is proposed. In cases of a third recurrence the patient is operated upon, when possible, or stented with a removable silicone prosthesis in case of inoperability.

In cases involving complex stenoses, a removable silicone stent is inserted during the first interventional bronchoscopy because of the inefficacy of dilation alone with very high recurrence rates in these cases. In MARQUETTE *et al.* [9] series, the silicone stents were removed 6 months after placement. In cases of stabilisation of the trachea, a follow-up is proposed. In cases of recurrent of stenosis, a stent is reinserted if inoperable, or reconstructive surgery is proposed. This multicentre, cooperative multidisciplinary study in 32 consecutive patients has yielded a successful (0% treatment mortality) outcome using conservative treatment only in one-third of patients. Whereas certain minor points in this approach remain subject to discussion (*e.g.* a larger period of stenting up to 18 months may be even more successful [15]) or other types of polymer prostheses may be more appropriate in certain circumstances [16, 17]), this type of multidisciplinary approach probably represents the optimal management strategy.

Pseudoglottic stenoses are less common and poorer candidates for stenting with fixed-diameter silicone stents. In these cases, insertion of self expandable prostheses (*e.g.* nitinol: Ultraflex®) may be preferable.

Finally, a fourth cause of tracheal obstruction (rather than stenosis) can occur in the post-extubation period this is obstructive (fibrinous) tracheal pseudomembranes (OTP) [18], occurring within hours or days after extubation. Typically, patients present with rapidly progressive or acute dyspnoea or stridor shortly after detubation.

Bronchoscopy, typically reveals tracheal obstruction by whitish pseudomembranes dehiscent from the tracheal wall. They consist of fibrinous material and necrotic tracheal mucosa. Treatment consists of "curettage" and mechanical debridement with the tip of the rigid bronchoscope restoring tracheal patency. Thereafter, tracheal mucosa recovers completely.

## Burn inhalation injury

Symptomatic tracheal stenosis occurs in 22–28% of inhalation burn survivors requiring intubation or tracheostomy [19, 20].

The risk for stenosis development parallels the duration of intubation or presence of the tracheostomy [21]. Burn inhalation injury is only in part due to direct thermal damage. The respiratory mucosa, being such an effective heat exchanger, prevents injury in most cases except in instances of exposure to steam, where evaporative cooling is prevented (fig. 4).

Thermal inhalation frequently results in laryngotracheal oedema; the respiratory distress that may follow is best managed in its initial stages by endotracheal intubation. In most cases, the oedema subsides within 72 h permitting safe extubation [22]. Short periods of intubation are generally well tolerated. The most common and most severe respiratory tract lesions therefore arise from the chemical reaction to inhalation of the incomplete products of combustion. In severely burned patients, with massive heat

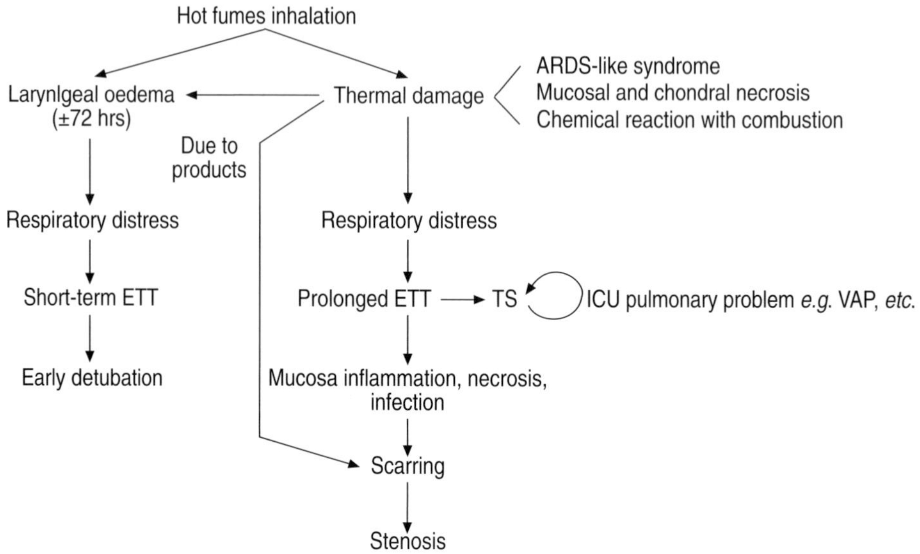


Fig. 4. – Pathophysiology of burn inhalation injury. ETT: endotracheal intubation; TS: tracheal stenosis; ARDS: adult respiratory distress syndrome. ICU: intensive care unit; VAP: ventilator-associated pneumonia.

damage to the upper airway, a conduit through the burned tissue is necessary. Deterioration of respiratory functions may necessitate extended intubation and ventilatory support. Prolonged use of the endotracheal tube can promote necrosis, infection, scarring and eventual stenosis. If prolonged ventilatory support is anticipated, early tracheostomy is indicated. Tracheostomy in burn patients, however, is often performed through burned skin and/or across a damaged tracheal wall, which may lead to complications [21].

Airway complications and early and late sequelae of inhalation burn injury include: extensive scar and granuloma formation; stenosis; tracheocele; and tracheomalacia [23].

In cases where development of severe tracheal stenosis occurs, early primary surgical resection and reconstruction are not the procedures of choice because burn inhalation injury is typically associated with prolonged inflammation (mean, 28 months in one study [24]), and hypertrophic scarring [22, 24, 25]. In these cases, a more expectant and conservative therapeutic approach should be employed, consisting of prolonged endotracheal stenting [22, 24, 25].

## Bronchopleural fistula

The management of bronchopleural fistula is one of the most complex challenges encountered by the chest physician. Bronchopleural fistulae most commonly arise as a complication of lung surgery. It is rare for them to occur after blunt chest trauma, barotrauma, inflammatory lung disorders or chemo- or radiotherapy for lung cancer.

The incidence of bronchopleural fistula following pulmonary resection averages 2–5% ($\leq$1% after lobectomy, up to 12.5% after pneumonectomy) [26, 27]. They almost always occur within 3 months after surgery [28, 29].

Patients with bronchopleural fistula can present in an acute, life-threatening fashion due to pulmonary flooding and/or tension pneumothorax. More often, there is a subacute clinical presentation with cough, expectorations, increasing dyspnoea and fever.

The diagnosis must be suspected when there is a persistent postoperative air-leak (immediate postoperative period) or when there is a new or increasing air-fluid levels or disappearance of pleural fluid on chest radiographs (no chest tube in place; fig. 5). Diagnosis can be confirmed with bronchoscopy (fig. 6), selective bronchography or instillation of methylene blue [27].

When bronchopleural fistula occurs, the healing and repair process is usually associated with substantial morbidity and mortality, prolonged hospitalisation, and great expense. Mortality varies between 18–67%, with aspiration pneumonia being the most frequent cause of death [28, 29].

The first principle of therapy is to address any immediate, life-threatening conditions (pulmonary flooding, tension pneumothorax). This is accomplished by placing the patient with the affected side down and performing adequate pleural drainage.

Since air-leaks through bronchopleural fistulae may range from <1–16 $L \cdot min^{-1}$ [30], a chest tube capable of permitting efficient drainage of this level of airflow is necessary. A chest tube with an adequate diameter to convey these air flows must be chosen (*e.g.* a 32 F chest tube). When mechanical ventilation is necessary, specific ventilator settings and ventilation modes may be required to achieve adequate ventilation and oxygenation [31]. If a major stump dehiscence occurs within the first week after pulmonary resection,

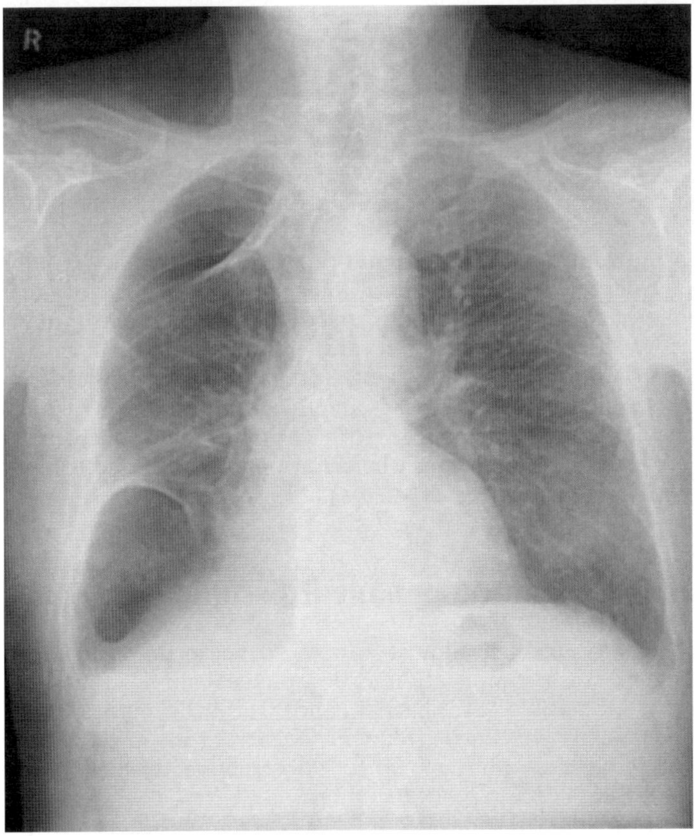


Fig. 5. – Radiographical appearance of postoperative bronchopleural fistula after lobectomy: disappearance of pleural fluid.

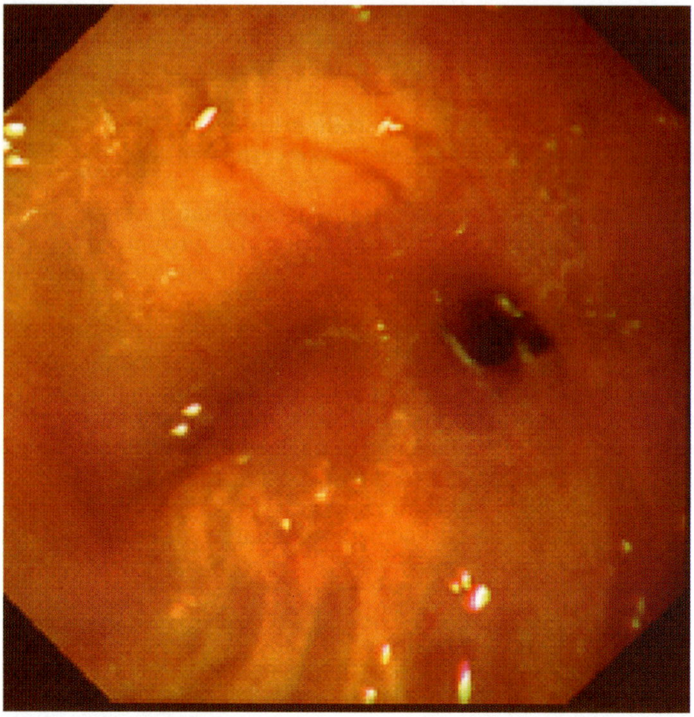

Fig. 6. – Bronchoscopical confirmation of suture dehiscence and bronchopleural fistula.

immediate resuture and reinforcement of the bronchial stump is the procedure of choice [27].

In case of a subacute clinical presentation, patients should initially receive: conservative management with dependent drainage and reduction of the pleural space; antibiotics; nutritional supplementation; and adequate ventilator management when ventilated [27, 31]. After 1–3 weeks, a surgical reintervention can be attempted. If the patient's general condition is poor (as is often the case), or when only a small fistula is present, bronchoscopic treatment appears an efficient alternative. Fistula closure can be achieved in up to 35.6% of patients [28]. Application of silver nitrate, tissue glue, fibrin glue, Gelfoam®, lead plugs, balloon catheterisation and autologous blood patches have all been used with various degrees of success [27].

## Tracheo- and broncho-oesophageal fistula

Oesophageal airway fistulae almost always develop in patients with advanced oesophageal cancer or as a complication of oesophageal surgery. With a 5-yr survival of <1%, recurrent or inoperable oesophageal cancer has a dramatically poor prognosis.

Tracheo-bronchial involvement is frequent, occurring in up to 30% of cases [32]. In patients with inoperable esophageal cancer, obstructive dysphagia often becomes a predominant symptom.

Treatment of dysphagia includes Nd:YAG-laser resection, chemo- or radiotherapy, mechanical dilation, and stenting. The occurrence of respiratory symptoms such as cough, dyspnoea, haemoptysis suggest tracheobronchial involvement. The occurrence of repetitive cough after ingestion of liquids or food, and recurrent aspiration pneumonia suggests the presence of oesophago-airway fistula. The diagnosis can be confirmed by radiological swallow studies and bronchoscopy.

Placement of oesophageal stents can restore oesophageal patency and can also be used with the intention of sealing fistulas between the alimentary and respiratory tract [31, 32]. Because oesophageal sealing may be insufficient, or because of possible direct compromise or invasion of the airways by the tumour or by the oesophageal stent itself [32–34], insertion of a stent in the airways ("double stenting") is a valuable option. Close collaboration between gastroenterologists and pulmonologists is necessary, and in some centres airway stents are inserted prior to, or simultaneous with, oesophageal stents. In selected patients, an important improvement in quality of life and even survival can be obtained [32–34].

## Iatrogenic rupture of the trachea

Iatrogenic tracheal rupture is a rare complication of tracheal intubation, mechanical ventilation, resuscitation or percutaneous dilatational tracheostomy [35–37]. The tracheal tear is almost always localised in the membranous part, parallel to the longitudinal axis of the trachea.

It may be localised in the cervical of thoracic part of the trachea, and extend into one of the main bronchi. Risk factors for the development of iatrogenic rupture include: female sex; a thin posterior membrane; poor, general condition; and diabetes [38]. The use of metal guide-wires during insertion of an endotracheal tube and insertion of double-lumen tubes also increase the risk for tracheal rupture.

Diagnosis should be suspected in cases of subcutaneous emphysema in the soft tissues of the neck, pneumomediastinum and pneumothorax, difficulties in ventilator management, and in cases of dyspnoea or haemoptysis occurring after detubation [5, 36–38]. Chest radiographs or a computed tomography scan of the thorax, show subcutaneous emphysema, pneumomediastinum and pneumothorax. Diagnosis is confirmed by bronchoscopy. The diagnosis may be delayed or missed, which is associated with a significant mortality rate [36–38].

In small tears, or in patients with a high operative risk, an attempt for conservative treatment (antibiotics, parenteral nutrition, supportive measures, adequate ventilator management, pleural drainage) may be undertaken. Conservative treatment also is a valuable option in patients who no longer need positive pressure ventilation [39, 40].

Spontaneous cicatrisation occurs generally within 8–10 days. In the case of inoperable patients who still need mechanical ventilation, the endotracheal tube should be inserted with its cuff distal from the tear [40]. In cases of very distal tears involving the carinal region, a large tracheostomy can be created through which two endotracheal tubes can be inserted which are placed in both of the main bronchi [41]. In all other cases, early primary surgical repair is indicated [5, 40].

## Traumatic tracheobronchial rupture

Lesions of the tracheobronchial tree are rare complications of trauma (~0.2–5%). Approximately 70% of all bronchial or tracheal lesions are caused by penetrating trauma, whereas in 30%, blunt trauma leads to bronchial rupture [42]. Rupture is thought to occur in blunt trauma after the sudden deceleration of the tracheobronchial tree, or because of the sudden decrease in anteroposterior diameter of the thorax with a consecutive widening and distraction of the carina followed by disruption. The sudden onset and rise of thoracic pressures with occlusion of the glottis may result in an airway blow out at the point of the carina. It is known that >80% of injuries occur within 2 cm of the carina (fig. 7), and most are in young patients with elastic chest walls [43]. Depending on whether the peribronchial tissues remain intact, two clinical presentations have been documented. If the tear ruptures into the pleural cavity, a severe pneumothorax occurs which fails to resolve after chest tube insertion, often associated with subcutaneous emphysema. In these instances diagnosis in obvious and urgent surgical intervention is generally required [44]. When the peribronchial tissues remain intact, symptoms may be minimal; abnormalities on chest radiographs may be limited to a small pneumomediastinum.

If there is suspicion of post-traumatic airway injury (subcutaneous emphysema, air leak, pneumomediastinum), a bronchoscopy should be performed. Some authors recommend to perform this procedure in a fully equipped operating theatre with full anaesthesiological backup because of the risk of disrupting peribronchial tissues, in which case immediate intubation with a tube passed distally to the rupture can be performed [43].

After stabilisation of vital functions, immediate "day 1" primary surgical repair gives the best long-term results [42–45], whereas delayed repair has a less favourable outcome [46]. Whenever possible, primary bronchial suture should be performed, however, in larger tears, a lobar resection may be necessary. Pneumonectomy should be avoided whenever possible in these multiple injury patients because of a very high (75–100%) mortality rate [47].

In cases of delayed diagnosis of partial rupture, conservative therapy with endobronchial stenting seems to be an alternative treatment to surgical repair [48] others, however, advocate endobronchial stenting in complex disruptions [49].

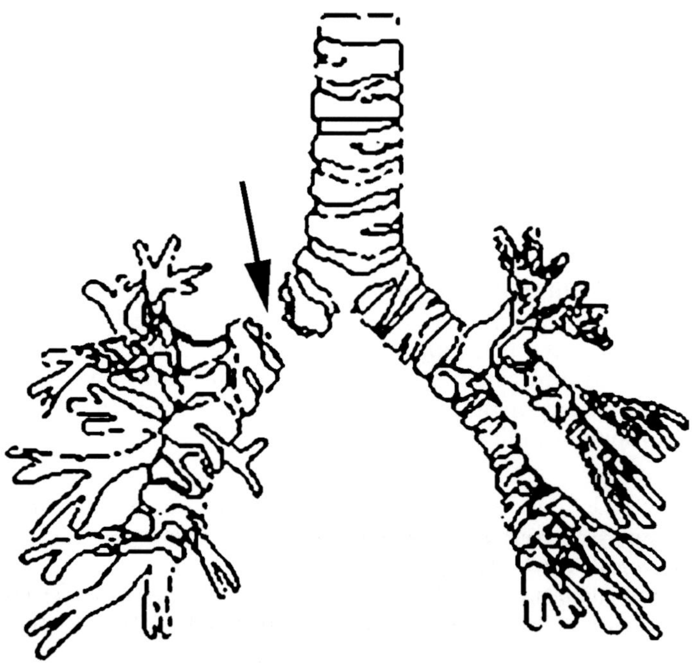

Fig. 7. – Schematic diagnosis of the tracheobronchial tree, the arrow shows a typical site of traumatic bronchial rupture.

## Conclusions

For the most benign airway injuries and sequelae, surgical repair represents the treatment of choice. For correct surgical repair, however, an experienced surgical team, an operable patient, and an operable lesion are all required. In many cases, therefore, conservative bronchoscopic treatment represents the first line of treatment. In some disorders, this treatment may even have a permanent character. Both types of treatment are, therefore, complementary.

## Summary

Surgery remains the definitive treatment for the majority of patients suffering from central airway injury of benign origin. Corrective tracheobronchial surgery, however, requires considerable surgical expertise, an operable lesion, and an operable patient. Hence this type of surgery can only rarely be performed immediately after the causative injury has occurred, and preoperative stabilisation of the patient is often necessary. Conservative, endoscopic treatment therefore is indicated for temporary treatment awaiting definitive surgical repair, and even for permanent treatment when surgery remains impossible because of patient-or lesion-related characteristics, or because of patient refusal. Conservative endoscopic treatment includes various techniques which can be applied through rigid or flexible bronchoscopy, such as mechanical and balloon dilation, Nd:YAG-laser or electrocautery resection, and airway stenting. Lesions candidate for conservative treatment include postintubation stenosis of the trachea, burn lesions of the airways, airway fistulae (bronchopleural, tracheo-oesophageal), and iatrogenic and traumatic airway rupture.
Indications, techniques and outcome of conservative endoscopic temporary or permanent treatment of these disorders are discussed. Conservative endoscopic techniques constitute a valuable treatment complement while awaiting definitive surgical repair, and can even be proposed as a permanent treatment in inoperable patients.

**Keywords:** Airway fistula, airway rupture, stenosis of trachea, interventional bronchoscopy.

***Acknowledgements.*** The authors would like to thank L. Van Gijseghem for her secretarial assistance.

## References

1. Mathisen DJ. Surgical management of tracheobronchial disease. *Clin Chest Med* 1992; 13: 151–171.
2. Courand L, Jougon JB, Velly JF. Surgical treatment of nontumoral stenoses of the upper airway. *Ann Thorac Surg* 1995; 60: 250–260.
3. Bison A, Bonnette P, Ben El Kadi N, Leroy M, Colchen A, Personne C. Tracheal sleeve resection for iatrogenic stenosis (subglottic laryngeal and tracheal). *J Thorac Cardiovasc Surg* 1992; 104: 882–887.
4. Helmy N, Platz A, Stocker R, Trentz O. Bronchus rupture in multiple injured patients with blunt chest trauma. *Eur J Trauma* 2001; 1: 31–34.

5. Brichet A, Ramon P, Marquette CH. Sténoses et complications trachéales postintubation. Réanimation [Postintubation stenosis and other tracheal complications]. *Réanimation* 2002; 11: 1–10.
6. Bolliger CT. Multimodality treatment of advanced pulmonary malignancies. *In*: Bolliger CT, Mathur PN eds. Interventional Bronchoscopy. Basel, Karger, 2000; pp. 187–198.
7. Noppen M, Meysman M, D'Haese J, Schlesser M, Vincken W. Interventional bronchoscopy: 5-year experience at the Academic Hospital of the Vrije Universiteit Brussel (AZ-VUB). *Acta Clin Belg* 1997; 52: 371–380.
8. Grillo HC, Donahue DM, Mathisen DJ, Wain JC, Wright CD. Postintubation tracheal stenosis. Treatment and results. *J Thorac Cardiovasc Surg* 1995; 109: 486–493.
9. Marquette CH, Brichet A, Verkindre C, Carlier ML, Darras J, Wurtz A. Multidisciplinary approach to management of post intubation tracheal stenoses. *Eur Respir J* 1999; 13: 888–893.
10. Baugnée P, Marquette CH, Ramon P, Darras J, Wurtz A. Traitement endoscopique des stenoses trachéales postintubation. A propos de 58 cas [Endoscopic treatment of postintubation stenosis of the trachea. A report on 58 cases]. *Rev Mal Resp* 1995; 12: 589–592.
11. Nordin U. The trachea and cuff-induced tracheal injury. *Acta Otolaryngol Suppl* 1977; 345: 1–71.
12. Grillo HC, Donahue DM. Post intubation tracheal stenosis. *Semin Thorac Cardiovasc Surg* 1996; 8: 370–380.
13. Grillo HC, Montgomery WW. Suprahyoid release for tracheal anostomosis. *Arch Otolaryngol* 1974; 99: 255–260.
14. Mehta AC, Lee FY, Cordasco EM, Kirby T, Eliachar I, De Boer G. Concentric tracheal and subglottic stenosis. Management using the Nd:YAG-laser for mucosal sparing followed by gentle dilatation. *Chest* 1993; 104: 673–677.
15. Martinez Ballarin JI, Diaz-Jiminez JP, Castro MJ, Moya JA. Silicone stents in the management of benign tracheobronchial stenoses. Tolerances and early results in 63 patients. *Chest* 1996; 109: 626–629.
16. Vergnon JM, Costes F, Polio JC. Efficacy and tolerance of a new silicone stent for the treatment of benign tracheal stenosis. *Chest* 2000; 118: 422–426.
17. Noppen M, D'Haese J, Meysman M, Monsieur I, Verhaeghe W, Vincken W. A new screw-thread tracheal endoprosthesis. *J Bronchol* 1996; 3: 22–26.
18. Deslee G, Brichet A, Lebuffe G, Copin MC, Ramon P, Marquette CH. Obstructive fibrinous tracheal pseudomembrane. A potentially fatal complication of tracheal intubation. *Am J Respir Crit Care Med* 2001; 163: 1169–1171.
19. Jones WG, Madden M, Finkelstein J, Yurt RW, Goodwin CW. Tracheostomies in burn patients. *Ann Surg* 1989; 209: 471–474.
20. Lund T, Goodwin CW, McManus WF, *et al.* Upper airway sequellae in burn patients requiring endotracheal intubation or tracheostomy. *Ann Surg* 1985; 201: 374–382.
21. Colice GL, Munster AM, Haponik EF. Tracheal stenosis complication cutaneous burns: an underestimated problem. *Am Rev Respir Dis* 1986; 134: 1315–1318.
22. Eliachar I, Moscona R, Joachims HZ, Kirschowitz B, Shilo R. The management of laryngotracheal stenosis in burned patients. *Plast Reconstr Surg* 1981; 68: 11–16.
23. Noppen M, Bertrand P, Vanrenterghem D, Vincken W. Tracheocoele as a late sequel of tracheal burn injury. *J Bronchol* 2000; 7: 152–155.
24. Gaissert HA, Lofgren RH, Grillo HC. Upper airway compromise after inhalation injury. *Ann Surg* 1993; 218: 672–678.
25. Gaissert HA, Grillo HC, Mathisen DJ, Wain JC. Temporary and permanent restoration of airway continuity with the tracheal T-tube. *J Thorac Cardiovasc Surg* 1994; 107: 600–606.
26. Hoier-Madson K, Schulze S, Pederson VM, Halkier E. Management of bronchopleural following pneumonectomy. *Scand J Thor Cardiovasc Surg* 1984; 18: 263–266.
27. McManigle JE, Fletcher GL, Tenholder MF. Bronchoscopy in the management of bronchopleural fistula. *Chest* 1990; 97: 1235–1238.

28. Hollaus PH, Lax F, Janakiev D, *et al.* Endoscopic treatment of postoperative bronchopleural fistula: experience with 45 cases. *Ann Thorac Surg* 1998; 66: 923–927.
29. Hollaus PH, Lax F, El-Nashef BB, Hauck HH, Lucciarini P, Pridun NS. Natural history of bronchopleural fistula after pneumonectomy: a review of 96 cases. *Ann Thorac Surg* 1997; 63: 1391–1396.
30. Rush VW, Capps JS, Tyler ML, Pierson DL. The performance of four pleural drainage systems in an animal model of bronchopleural fistula. *Chest* 1988; 4: 859–863.
31. Baumann MH, Sahn SA. Medical management and therapy of bronchopleural fistulas in the mechanically ventilated patient. *Chest* 1990; 97: 721–728.
32. Colt HG, Meric B, Dumon JF. Double stents for carcinoma of the esophagus invading the tracheo-bronchial tree. *Gastrointest Endosc* 1992; 38: 485–489.
33. Freitag L, Tekolf E, Steveling H, Donovan TJ, Stamatis G. Management of malignant esophagotracheal fistulas with airway stenting and double stenting. *Chest* 1996; 110: 1155–1160.
34. Noppen M, Reynaert H, D'Haese J, Vincken W. Tracheal penetration of an esophageal self-expandable Cook Z Granturco metal stent. *J Bronchol* 1999; 6: 95–97.
35. Noppen M. Percutaneous dilational tracheostomy. *In*: Bolliger CT, Mathur PN, eds. Interventional bronchoscopy. Basel, Karger, 2000; pp. 215–226.
36. Nestorowicz A, Furmanik F, Siwicki M, Kotlinska E. Tracheal rupture caused by a double-lumen endotracheal tube. *Anaesthesiol Intens Ther* 2001; 1: 21–23.
37. Devitt JH, Boulanger RH. Lower airway injuries and anesthesia. *Can J Anaesth* 1996; 43: 148–159.
38. Kaloud H, Smolle-Juettner FM, Prause G, List WF. Iatrogenic ruptures of the tracheobronchial tree. *Chest* 1997; 112: 774–778.
39. Molins L, Buitrago LJ, Vidal G. Tracheal lacerations after intubation. *Chest* 1998; 114: 179–184.
40. Ross HM, Grant FJ, Wilson RS, Burt ME. Non operative management of tracheal lacerations during endotracheal intubation. *Ann Thorac Surg* 1997; 36: 240–242.
41. Marquette CH, Bocquillon N, Roumilhac D, Nevière R, Mathie D, Ramon P. Conservative treatment of tracheal rupture. *J Thorac Cardiovasc Surg* 1999; 117: 399–341.
42. Helmy N, Platz A, Stocker R, Trentz O. Bronchus rupture in multiple injured patients with blunt chest trauma. *Eur J Trauma* 2002; 28: 31–34.
43. Stewart BT, Meridew CG, Krishnan M. Posttraumatic rupture of the right main broncus: a rare clinical entity? *JR Coll Surg Edinb* 1999; 44: 132–133.
44. Roxburg JC. Rupture of the tracheobronchial tree. *Thorax* 1987; 42: 681–688.
45. Jones WS, Mavroudis C, Richardson DJ. Management of tracheobronchial disruption resulting from blunt trauma. *Surgery* 1984; 95: 319–323.
46. Taskinen SO, Salo JA, Halttunen PE, Sovijarvi AR. Tracheobronchial rupture due tot blunt chest trauma: a follow-up study. *Ann Thorac Surg* 1989; 48: 846–849.
47. Bowling R, Mavroudis C, Richardson JD, Flint LM, Howe WR, Gray LA. Emergency pneumonectomy for penetrating and blunt trauama. *Am Surg* 1985; 51: 136–139.
48. Sim EKW, Liam BL, Lee KH, Chan WX. Treatment of delayed partial rupture with expandable metallic stents. *Singapore Med J* 1999; 40: 428–429.
49. Huh J, Milliken JC, Chen JC. Management of tracheobronchial injuries following blunt and penetrating trauma. *Am Surg* 1997; 63: 896–899.